Human Cytogenetic Cancer Markers

Contemporary Biomedicine

Human Cytogenetic Cancer Markers

Edited by

Sandra R. Wolman, MD

*Uniformed Services University of the Health Sciences,
Bethesda, MD*

and

Stewart Sell, MD

Albany Medical College, Albany, NY

Humana Press 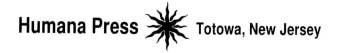 Totowa, New Jersey

© 1997 Humana Press Inc.
999 Riverview Drive, Suite 208
Totowa, New Jersey 07512

This publication is printed on acid-free paper. ♾
ANSI Z39.48-1984 (American National Standards Institute) Permanence of Paper for Printed Library Materials.

Cover illustration: Fig. 2 from Chapter 3, "*In Situ* Hybridization and Comparative Genomic Hybridization," by Anton H. N. Hopman, Christina E. M. Voorter, Ernst J. M. Speel, and Frans C. S. Ramaekers

Cover design by Patricia F. Cleary.

For additional copies, pricing for bulk purchases, and/or information about other Humana titles, contact Humana at the above address or at any of the following numbers: Tel.: 201-256-1699; Fax: 201-256-8341; E-mail: humana@mindspring.com or visit our Web site: http://lbin.com/humana.html

Printed in the United States of America. 10 9 8 7 6 5 4 3 2 1
Library of Congress Cataloging in Publication Data

Human cytogenetic cancer markers / edited by Sandra R. Wolman and Stewart Sell.
     p. cm. — (Contemporary biomedicine)
    Includes index.
    ISBN 0-89603-357-0 (alk. paper)
    1. Tumor markers. 2. Cancer—Genetic aspects. I. Wolman, Sandra R.
    II. Sell, Stewart, 1935– . III. Series.
    [DNLM: 1. Neoplasms—diagnosis. 2. Neoplasms—genetics. 3. Tumor Markers, Biological—genetics. QZ 241 H91805 1997]
    RC270.3.T84H86 1997
    616.99'4075—dc21
    DNLM/DLC
    for Library of Congress   97-7392
                                           CIP

Preface

The series on Cancer Markers published by Humana Press illustrates the expanding base of knowledge of the different types of markers and their applications to the study of cancer. In an earlier volume in this series, the development of different eras of investigation of cancer markers was described. The first era was the time of earliest recognition that tumor cell products, such as myeloma proteins, hormones, and isozymes, could be used to detect and monitor tumor growth. After some delay, the second era, beginning in the early 1960s, was notable for the discovery of developmental antigens, alphafetoprotein (AFP) and carcinoembryonic antigen (CEA), that were re-expressed in many tumors, and that were detectable by conventional antisera. The first two books in the series, published in 1980 and 1982, covered the rapid accumulation of information on these topics and included early studies on prostate-specific antigen (PSA) and other organ-specific antigens. The second book included contributions by several authors that introduced the subject of monoclonal antibodies, a new and precise approach to the identification of cancer markers. The third era, then, was characterized by the expanding uses of monoclonal antibodies to detect carbohydrates, mucins, and cytoplasmic proteins, as well as cell surface markers in different forms of cancer. These topics and many other applications of cancer markers were presented in the next three books in the series.

The current perception of the fundamental role of genetic changes in basic and clinical aspects of the study of cancer has led to the conclusion that the fourth era of cancer marker study will concentrate on nuclear events. Alterations detectable as quantitative or qualitative differences in DNA and its packaging into chromosomes may be useful in cancer diagnosis and prognosis, and also reflect the heritable, progressive, and mutable nature of the disease. Thus, *Human Cytogenetic Cancer Markers* focuses on the chromosomal era, which began with the discovery of the Philadelphia chromosome by Nowell and Hungerford in 1960, and its chapters represent the coming of age of cytogenetic markers of human cancer.

We have assembled an outstanding group of contributing authors, whose work spans from basic research to clinical diagnostic applications, and from current theory to newly developing technology. The first part of the book is devoted to a section on Perspectives. Its chapters on DNA cytometry, molecular cytogenetics, and molecular genetics provide an introductory framework for the, organ- and site-specific chapters that follow. The need for integration of these disciplines with conventional cytogenetics is apparent throughout, although, as in many emerging fields, the available data do not always appear directly correlated, and may even appear inherently inconsistent. The site-specific chapters present striking differences in the degrees of data collected, integration of information from different technologies, and clinical utilities with respect to individual tumor types.

With the exception of the leukemias and lymphomas, there have been few attempts as yet to correlate the chromosomal aberrations in cancers with expression of other types of cancer markers, and with careful histological discriminations. We hope this volume will stimulate further work in these areas.

Sandra R. Wolman
Stewart Sell

Contents

Contributors

GEORGIA BARDI • *Department of Clinical Genetics, University Hospital, Lund, Sweden; Department of Genetics, Papanikolaou Research Institute, Saint Savas Hospital, Athens, Greece*

DAPHNE W. BELL • *Department of Medical Oncology, Fox Chase Cancer Center, Philadelphia, PA*

JULIA A. BRIDGE • *Departments of Pathology, Pediatrics, and Orthopedics, University of Nebraska Medical Center, Omaha, NE*

ARTHUR R. BROTHMAN • *Departments of Pediatrics and Human Genetics, University Medical Center, Salt Lake City, UT*

LINDA A. CANNIZZARO • *Department of Pathology, Albert Einstein College of Medicine, Bronx, NY*

CEES J. CORNELISSE • *Department of Pathology, University of Leiden, The Netherlands*

NORMAN L. EBERHARDT • *Departments of Medicine and Biochemistry/Molecular Biology, Mayo Clinic, Rochester, MN*

JONATHAN A. FLETCHER • *Department of Pathology, Brigham and Women's Hospital, Boston, MA*

STEFAN K. G. GREBE • *Department of Medicine, Mayo Clinic, Rochester, MN*

CONSTANCE A. GRIFFIN • *Departments of Pathology and Oncology, Johns Hopkins University, Baltimore, MD*

SVERRE HEIM • *Department of Clinical Genetics, University Hospital, Lund, Sweden; Department of Genetics, The Norwegian Radium Hospital and Institute for Cancer Research, Oslo, Norway*

LORI HOFFNER • *Department of Pathology, Magee Womens Hospital, Pittsburgh, PA*

ANTON H. N. HOPMAN • *Department of Molecular Cell Biology and Genetics, University of Limburg, Maastricht, The Netherlands*

ROBERT B. JENKINS • *Departments of Laboratory Medicine and Pathology and Biochemistry/Molecular Biology, Mayo Clinic, Rochester, MN*

SAKARI KNUUTILA • *Department of Medical Genetics, University of Helsinki, Finland*

MIN LEE • *Department of Pathology, Henry Ford Hospital, Detroit, MI*

FELIX MITELMAN • *Department of Clinical Genetics, University Hospital, Lund, Sweden*

S. DAVID NATHANSON • *Department of Surgery, Henry Ford Hospital, Detroit, MI*

TIMOTHY J. O'LEARY • *Department of Cellular Pathology, Armed Forces Institute of Pathology, Washington, DC*

NIKOS PANDIS • *Department of Clinical Genetics, University Hospital, Lund, Sweden; Department of Genetics, Papanikolaou Research Institute, Saint Savas Hospital, Athens, Greece*

FRANS C. S. RAMAEKERS • *Department of Molecular Cell Biology and Genetics, University of Limburg, Maastricht, The Netherlands*

ADRIENNE C. SCHECK • *Department of Neurology Research, Barrow Neurological Institute, Phoenix, AZ*

STEWART SELL • *Department of Pathology, Albany Medical College, Albany, NY*

T. VINCENT SHANKEY • *Departments of Urology and Pathology, Loyola University Medical Center, Maywood, IL*

JOAN RANKIN SHAPIRO • *Department of Neurology Research, Barrow Neurological Institute, Phoenix, AZ*

MARILYN L. SLOVAK • *Department of Pathology, City of Hope National Medical Center, Duarte, CA*

ERNST J. M. SPEEL • *Department of Molecular Cell Biology and Genetics, University of Limburg, Maastricht, The Netherlands*

URVASHI SURTI • *Department of Pathology, Magee Womens Hospital, Pittsburgh, PA*

JOSEPH R. TESTA • *Department of Medical Oncology, Fox Chase Cancer Center, Philadelphia, PA*

CHRISTINA E. M. VOORTER • *Department of Molecular Cell Biology and Genetics, University of Limburg, Maastricht, The Netherlands*

BRIANA J. WILLIAMS • *Department of Urology, Louisiana State University, Shreveport, LA*

ERIC WOLMAN • *Department of Operations Research and Engineering, George Mason University, Fairfax, VA*

SANDRA R. WOLMAN • *Department of Pathology, Uniformed Services University of the Health Sciences, Bethesda, MD*

MARIA J. WORSHAM • *Department of Pathology, Henry Ford Hospital, Detroit, MI*

List of Color Plates

Color plates appear as an insert following p. 212.

Plate 1 (Fig. 1 from Chapter 3). Chromosome detection from a bladder tumor.

Plate 2 (Fig. 1 from Chapter 5). Cytospin preparation for bone marrow aspirate of a patient with myelodysplastic syndrome.

Plate 3 (Fig. 2 from Chapter 5). Alkaline phosphatase antialkaline phosphatase (APAAP) staining followed by *in situ* hybridization.

Plate 4 (Fig. 3 from Chapter 5). Fluorescence (fluorescein isothiocyanate) immunostaining with glycophorin A monoclonal antibody (erythroid cells).

Plate 5 (Fig. 4 from Chapter 5). Alkaline phosphatase antialkaline phosphatase immunostaining with CD61 megakaryocytic antibody.

Plate 6 (Fig. 1 from Chapter 6). Detection of numerical chromosomal aberrations in breast tumors by FISH.

Plate 7 (Fig. 4 from Chapter 16). Dual color FISH of a dermatofibrosarcoma protuberans metaphase cell with digoxigenin-labeled chromosome 17 paint and biotin-labeled chromosome 22 paint.

Plate 8 (Fig. 14 from Chapter 16). FISH analysis of t(12;16) from a myxoid liposarcoma using the 100C4 YAC.

Chapter 1

An Introduction to Cancer Markers and Cytogenetics

Sandra R. Wolman, Stewart Sell, and Eric Wolman

Introduction

The goal of this series of books on cancer markers is to summarize and illustrate the state of the art in the use of markers for diagnosis, prognosis, and monitoring the effect of therapy on malignant tumors *(1–5)*. The purpose of this volume in the series is to present the current status of chromosomal markers of cancer, not only for their potential and realized clinical utility in diagnosis, prognosis, and disease monitoring, but also for their contributions to understanding mechanisms of tumor development and progression. These mechanisms have been identified largely by localization of relevant oncogenes and tumor suppressor genes, and by recognition of new gene constructs (and their protein products and cellular functions) that result from translocation in the course of carcinogenesis.

At present, the practical clinical diagnosis and prognosis of cancer depend on the recognition of gross and microscopic features of the individual lesion. Grossly, the size and degree of tissue infiltration combined with the presence or absence of metastasis is used to predict the clinical outcome. Microscopically malignant features reflect the "less-differentiated" state of cancer cells and tissues as compared to well-differentiated normal tissues and cells. However, there are

From: *Human Cytogenetic Cancer Markers*   Edited by S. R. Wolman and S. Sell
Humana Press Inc., Totowa, NJ

many examples in which the diagnosis and prognosis of cancer are determined, at least in part, by serologic, molecular, or chromosomal changes in the tumor. The first two types of markers, serologic and molecular, have been the subjects of previous books in this series on cancer markers; and relationships between chromosomal and molecular genetic events are a recurring theme in this volume.

The first serologic marker, Bence-Jones protein, was identified in patients with multiple myeloma (mollities ossium) in 1846, but the applications of serologic marker analysis had little impact on clinical patient management until after the discoveries of α-fetoprotein (AFP) by Garri Abelev in 1963, and carcinoembryonic antigen (CEA) by Gold and Freeman in 1965. With the notable exception of prostate-specific antigens (PSA), most serologic markers have been disappointing as diagnostic and prognostic tools. On the other hand, many have important roles in determining the response to therapy. If the serum level of a marker (e.g., CEA, AFP, PSA, ectopic hormone, Bence-Jones protein, or cancer carbohydrate and mucin markers detected by monoclonal antibodies) is elevated in a given patient, then a falling serum level indicates a positive response to therapy. However, if the serum level fails to fall to normal and then rises, residual tumor or metastasis is likely. Occasionally, elevations of these serologic markers are also found in benign conditions, and the levels may overlap those found with malignant lesions. Nevertheless, high and sustained levels of AFP in individuals at high risk for hepatocellular carcinoma are essentially diagnostic for the presence of tumor. Similarly, very high and sustained levels of different serologic markers strongly indicate other malignant diseases. Thus, serologic and other markers are of considerable value when interpreted within the context of other clinical and pathologic findings.

Over the past decade, molecular markers have promised far more precise and specific definition of tumors and their behavior, but that promise has not yet been realized. The definitive diagnosis of cancer still depends mainly on histologic criteria. In microscopic examination of thin slices of tissues, early pathologists noted the resemblance between cancerous tissue and embryonic tissues. They used terms such as "poorly differentiated," "undifferentiated," and "well-differentiated" to describe the appearance of a tumor in embryonic terms. More recently, it has been recognized that cancerous tissues often contain detectable mutations and altered expression of genes that control cell-cycle activation or progression. This raised the possibility that measurement of these mutations or changes might be used to make the diagnosis or determine the prognosis of individual cancers. Unfortunately, although general relationships have been identified, many molecular biologic changes do not correlate closely enough with specific behavior patterns of a malignant tumor to provide "stand-alone" clinical guidelines for individual patient care. They complement, rather than replace, the standard parameters used to describe a tumor. Therefore, the diagnoses of most forms of cancer for the foreseeable future will remain linked with the classic histologic features of the tumors, although markers will modify and increase discrimination of the diagnosis. Similarly, markers will contribute to prognosis, although the location, size, histologic type and grade, and presence or absence of metastatic lesions will remain important components of that determination. Such factors as ploidy, mitotic frequency, immunohistochemical markers for proliferating cells (Ki67, PCNA), angiogenesis, and vascular invasion all correlate with prognosis; their predictive power modifies, but is not independent of, that based on histologic criteria. The same is true for serum markers (e.g., CEA, CA-15-3, CA-249), mucin cancer antigens, and tissue polypeptide antigen; and it is equally true for expression of oncogenes (e.g., *bcl*-2, p53, c-*erb*B-2, c-*myc*, and nm23), and for markers of invasion or metastasis (e.g., cathepsin D, laminin receptors, plasminogen activator, angiogenesis factors, and expression of cell adhesion molecules). Expression of all these markers correlates with degree of malignancy, and their determination adds in varying degrees to prediction of tumor behavior when histologic type and grade are known; but we do not yet have foolproof "magic markers."

This volume addresses the status of chromosomal markers. Some chromosomal markers are causally related to individual tumors and have achieved primary diagnostic "stand-alone" status, such as the t(9;22)* of chronic myelogenous leukemia and the

---

*Cytogenetic terminology is based on ISCN nomenclature. [ISCN 1985 International System for Human Cytogenetic Nomenclature (1985) March of Dimes Birth Defects Foundation and Cytogenetics and Cell Genetics S. Karger, Basel, Switzerland. (Guidelines for Cancer Cytogenetics ed. Mitelman F. Supplement 1991 and 1995)]

t(15;17) of acute promyelocytic leukemia. Others, such as the t(X;18) of synovial sarcoma, are highly discriminatory in differential diagnosis. For many forms of human cancer, however, unique and tumor-specific chromosomal patterns have not yet been discerned, largely because of the extent and complexity of chromosomal change in many solid tumors. When the critical biologic events in each tumor can be chromosomally localized, molecularly identified, and appropriately correlated with clinical findings, it is likely that markers will play a much greater role in medical management. **Because we believe that cancers are genetic diseases, genetic markers should eventually provide the most accurate means to signify their diagnosis and prognosis.** Detection may be based on classical cytogenetic means, but in solid tumors molecular cytogenetic techniques that do not depend on metaphase analysis will probably be of greater utility for finding such markers as loss of heterozygosity (LOH) of certain genes, gene amplifications, or fusion constructs such as the *BCR/ABL* translocation.

The first association between genetic and chromosomal aberrations and malignancy was made by Boveri *(6)*, who originated the theory of a somatic mutational basis for cancer. Muller *(7)* then showed that chromosome damage was one of the immediate biological results of exposure to ionizing radiation. Shortly thereafter, animal studies indicated that a later consequence of radiation exposure was tumor formation *(8)*. In the 1940s and 1950s, several investigators reported chromosome aberrations in experimental tumor models such as mouse ascites tumors. Later the atomic bomb explosions resulted, among other grim sequelae, in ample evidence of dose-related induction of tumors in humans by radiation *(9)*. Effects similar to those of radiation on chromosomes (breakage, rearrangements) could be induced by a variety of chemicals that were also implicated in tumor induction. These observations eventually led to the conviction that agents capable of inducing chromosome damage were potentially tumorigenic and, therefore, that chromosome aberrations could have an etiologic role in tumor formation.

The new age of chromosomal changes in human cancer began in 1960 with the discovery of the Philadelphia chromosome by Nowell and Hungerford *(10)*, shortly after simple modifications of technique permitted accurate recognition that the normal diploid human pattern contained 46 chromosomes. In 1970, Caspersson's application of fluorescing dyes to stain chromosomes revealed longitudinal patterns of "bands" that other investigators soon found could be elicited by many other methods. Only 3 yr later, Rowley *(11)* used chromosomal banding to demonstrate that the Philadelphia chromosome was not, as originally thought, a deletion, but a translocation between two chromosomes without apparent loss. Since that time there has been an explosion of effort directed at identification of tumor-specific chromosome alterations. Indeed, the utility of chromosomal specificity in the diagnosis, subclassification, and monitoring of human leukemias is widely recognized, and has become a component of standard practice in many institutions. More recently, with the approaches described in the chapters of this book, analysis of chromosomal aberrations has been extended to all types of tumors. Of equal interest to the diagnosis and prognosis of specific cancers by chromosomal aberrations, is the promise that germ-line chromosomal aberrations or mutations may be used to predict accurately the likelihood that a given individual will develop cancer of a particular type. This predictive capacity would allow specific preventive measures to be taken. For example, frequent retinal examinations in an infant carrier of a mutated retinoblastoma (*RB*) gene may permit early detection and laser surgery of tumors with ultimate preservation of the eye. Similarly, through detection of families with heritable high risk of breast cancer (carriers of *BRCA1*, *BRCA2*, and possibly *ATM*), hormonal cancer-suppressive treatment or prophylactic mastectomy might be offered under certain circumstances.

The enormous potential of chromosomal analysis for detection of carcinogenic exposures, for contributing to understanding of mechanisms of tumor initiation and progression, for diagnostic purposes, and ultimately, for influencing the control of cancer, has led to massive research efforts. The number of papers published on chromosomal markers grew from 200 in 1974 to 600 in 1994 (increasing at about 5.6%/yr). Although application of nonchromosomal markers appears to have attracted more general attention during this period, the rate of increase in published papers during the same time frame is similar. With the rapid accumulation of new data derived from technologic advances (particularly those described in Chapters 3 and 4 of this book), and the applications to different types of cancer (in the following chapters), there have been substantial increases in both the quantity and quality of information on chromosomal markers in cancer over the past 5 yr. Even more important is the recognition that these markers have great potential application for mechanistic understanding of initiating events and therefore for cancer prevention than is true for nonchromosomal markers. Perhaps a better sense of the growth of tumor chromosome studies is reflected in the expansion of Mitelman's *Catalog of Chromosome Aberrations in Cancer* from 3144 entries in the first edition to 22,076 in the most recent fifth edition (*see* Fig. 1). In that interval (1983–1994), the percentage of entries devoted to solid tumors more than doubled. It should also be noted that tumors with normal diploid karyotypes, those with only the t(9;22) of chronic myelogenous leukemia, and those with karyotypes obtained after prolonged culture growth in vitro have been excluded from this data base.

Three introductory chapters in this volume present the basic methods of cytometry, molecular cytogenetics, and molecular genetics that are critical for understanding chromosomal changes in specific tissues and their tumors. These chapters contain perspectives on the range of genetic analyses and techniques that may be or have been applied to the study of human tumors. Each explicitly examines the relative advantages and disadvantages of the available methods in relation to conventional cytogenetic techniques. Each set of methods also has capabilities and weaknesses associated with its ability to perceive or measure different properties of the population of cells under study. Examples are presented in later chapters wherein utilization of two or more of these approaches permits construction of a more complete picture of the types of genetic aberrations in a human tumor than is obtainable with a single mode of analysis. Thus, used in combination, these approaches allow recognition of the relative specificity of certain types of aberration, as well as identification and categorization of individual tumors and classes of lesions.

The three approaches span several levels of resolution, extending from evaluation of large populations of tumor cells (flow cytometry and image analysis), through studies of individual cells often within an organized cellular or tissue context (molecular cytogenetics), to identification of molecular alterations that may

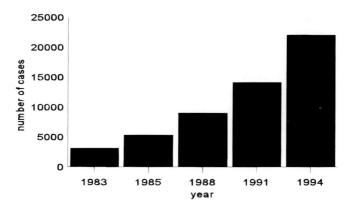

Fig. 1. Entries in *Catalog of Chromosomal Aberrations in Cancer*, by Felix Mitelman.

involve single base changes in very small numbers of cells. Each chapter delineates the technical capabilities and constraints of a set of methods that enables a class of genetic analyses and defines the level (whole tumor, individual cell, intracellular compartment) from which information is derived.

The discussion of cytometric approaches emphasizes the particular importance of these methods in solid tumor analysis, the historical context, and the extensive correlates with clinical prognosis. It presents the advantages that cytometric analysis is based on relatively large samples of the tumor population reflecting the entire cell cycle, and that it is informative of interphase cells and of cell turnover. A perspective on comparative test performance and interpretation provides an important background for review of the types of information derived from flow as opposed to image analysis, as well as presenting some reasons for discrepancies between cytogenetic and cytometric results. For interpreting cytogenetic data from cell culture, it is important to ask whether or not (and then why not) it corresponds to the DNA index (ploidy level) of the original tumor tissue, as seems generally true for lung and often untrue for prostate.

The newest approach, molecular cytogenetics, has both improved our understanding and illustrated some glaring lacks in the data obtained by classical cytogenetics. The nature of these analyses and their comparative strengths and weaknesses are an essential backdrop to our current understanding and perspective on genetic alterations in human tumors. It has become so important in a very short period of time that every chapter presents data illustrating the confirmatory and sometimes confounding, but always complementary, data from fluorescence *in situ* hybridization (FISH), *in situ* hybridization (ISH), and comparative genomic hybridization (CGH) (*see* Chapter 3). In general, the numerical karyotypic alterations observed in cultured tumor cells have been supported by FISH data on tissue sections or disaggregated cells from the primary lesions. In contrast, CGH data are notable for revealing losses and amplifications that were not prominent in classical cytogenetic or FISH analyses. For example, molecularly determined amplification of *ERBB2* has sometimes not corresponded to the more distal 17q location of amplification by CGH (*see* Chapter 6); the prevalence of amplification of the androgen receptor in prostate cancer, not recognized by other techniques, was demonstrated by CGH (*see* Chapter 10); and previously unrecognized sites of amplification have been identified in breast and lung cancers and other tumors.

The introduction to molecular genetics offers an exposition of relationships with molecular pathology. It focuses explicitly on translocation analysis rather than molecular detection of deletion or amplification because of the direct comparability with cytogenetic analysis, and because this is generally perceived to have been the most fruitful area of investigation in terms of understanding basic mechanisms of tumorigenesis. The disruption of normal gene products and functions, and the construction and altered function of new protein transcripts, explain much of the consequent acquisition of tumor-related altered growth properties by the translocation-bearing cells. One attractive feature of this chapter is that it draws clear distinctions between those tests that are technically feasible, but not contributory to clinical management, and the far fewer instances where the derived information is clinically meaningful for diagnosis, prognosis, or treatment decisions. The power of molecular assays to define with precision the nature of genetic alterations in cancer, and thus to permit mechanistic interpretations and applications to therapy, shows as yet only a hint of its enormous potential. The balanced discussion and comparisons of methods clearly illustrate that molecular assays must be developed and interpreted in the context of classical histologic and cytogenetic information.

The remaining contributions (with a single exception that describes new technology) are organ oriented, principally in relation to solid tumors. Information regarding the conventional cytogenetics of leukemias and lymphomas has been reviewed extensively elsewhere, largely because of the ready availability of representative metaphase cells directly from blood, marrow, and disaggregated lymphoid tissues. Such studies are sufficiently well known not to warrant extensive coverage in this volume. Instead we have focused on a newer approach (Morphology, Antibody, Chromosomes ([MAC]—*see* Chapter 5) that yields potential insights into chromosomal relationships to cell differentiation in the leukemic disorders, with much of the translocation cytogenetics of leukemias and lymphomas included in discussion of molecular detection methods.

Representation of the different solid tissue systems is intended to be extensive but not comprehensive, and the tissues reviewed illustrate widely varying levels and sources of data. The data available on the soft tissue sarcomas (STSs) reflect the relative ease with which these cells of mesodermal origin adapt to short-term growth in tissue culture, possibly because the basic conditions of cell culture were originally developed to support the growth of fibroblasts. STSs are the only solid tumors for which disease-specific translocations, analogous to those typical of some leukemias, have been identified. In contrast, tumors of epithelial origin have been difficult to adapt to growth in culture, and much less is known with respect to tissue- or disease-stage-specificity of the accompanying cytogenetic alterations. Often, suitable phenotypic markers are lacking that would enable definitive identification of the cells that do survive and grow in culture. Thus, the degree to which the cultured cells represent the original, often heterogeneous tumors is poorly understood. This contributes to the discrepancies among modes of analysis noted above. In the absence of extensive data derived from primary cultures, complementary methods, such as cytometry and *in situ* hybridization, become essential to flesh out the picture for many solid tumors.

The highly specific, balanced reciprocal translocations that characterize many leukemias and some soft tissue sarcomas are relatively uncommon in many solid tumors. Thus, the early (initiating) events that contribute to mechanisms of tumorigenesis in the former groups cannot be applicable to the initial biologic mechanisms responsible for the bulk of solid tumors. Some have suggested that genomic instability and simple trisomies are an alternative pathway.

It is a source of some uneasiness, although an underlying premise of this volume, that chromosome aberrations are considered among the most reliable of cancer-specific markers. The basis for discomfort is that, for most cell types, there is no correlation with the expression or lack of expression of other cancer-specific markers that will validate, in turn, the significance of the cytogenetic markers. Yet, immunophenotyping in a different context (e.g., vimentin, keratin) is appropriate for solid tumors, and other "second marker" applications are feasible. Although combined application of immunocytochemistry with cytogenetics is still infrequent in most solid tumor studies, examples appear in several chapters (e.g., individual types of STS in Chapter 16). A notable exception is the system described in Chapter 5 that focuses on the correlation of cell morphology, immunophenotype, and cytogenetics in the most accessible of tumor cell populations, the leukemias.

What is desired is the classification on a genetic basis of an otherwise amorphous grouping of tumors. In some tissues, this hope appears realizable. For example, the findings of diploidy and mismatch DNA repair (RER+) in a subset of colon cancers (*see* Chapter 7) offer the prediction of a relatively benign course for the individual patient. In other tissues, the existing data are perplexing and their clinical utility dubious. Observations of extensive or clonal aberrations without clinical significance in some benign neoplasms highlight the problem of a possibly meaningless genetic classification. Despite the cytogenetic distinction between chromophobe adenoma and oncocytoma, individual tumors sometimes show a hybrid of histologic features of both lesions. Even when cytogenetic specificity leads to better molecular understanding of the disease (as it does in papillary thyroid cancer, where chromosomal and molecular alteration of chromosome 10 led to localization of the RET oncogene to 10q11), we must still ask whether it is useful clinically: Papillary cancer is readily identifiable as a pathologic entity and there is a continuum between the benign and malignant forms of proliferation that is not resolved by the availability of more precise genetic markers.

The interpretation of the identification of diploid cells among tumor-derived metaphase preparations remains controversial, but in colorectal and some other malignancies (e.g., *see* Chapters 7 and 13), and in the leukemias, their presence is associated with longer patient survival, indicating biological significance. Is it possible that there may be more than one clone of proliferating cells in the primary tumor (*see* Chapters 6 and 12)? There is general agreement that apparently diploid tumor cells may have submicroscopic genetic lesions. However, the dearth of appropriate phenotypic markers has clouded resolution of this and other issues. Similar controversy over the relevance of trisomy 7 has largely been resolved with the advent of FISH studies, which have permitted definitive localization of the aberration within epithelial tumor cells in rectal polyps, renal tumors, glial tumors, follicular adenomas of the thyroid, and others. Similarly, loss of the second sex chromosome, sometimes interpreted as either an artifact of culture or a phenomenon of aging, has been verified as tumor-specific by application of FISH to tissue sections. A possible explanation for the high frequency of trisomy 7 in epithelial tumors has been suggested by the recent localization of a candidate gene to 7q31.1 (*see* Chapter 7). In fact, a few recurrent observations extend to many unrelated tumor groups and may reflect on effects of aberrations on tumor behavior, the most common among these being trisomy 7 and loss of sex chromosomes. The frequent losses from 3p, 9p, and 17p are readily associated with some known tumor-suppressor genes and are likely to lead to identification of others. Isochromosome formation, probably resulting from rearrangements at or near centromeric heterochromatin, is also relatively common.

Heterogeneity within individual tumors is widely recognized as a potential source of discrepant results. In a single microscopic region differences in nutrients, oxygenation, pH, waste disposal, and local and temporal alterations in blood flow can act as selective influences. We expect tumors and their chromosomal markers to evolve with time, and, therefore, advanced and more accessible tumors with pleural or peritoneal spread may show many changes not found in the primary lesion and possibly more representative of late-stage malignancies in general than of the particular tissue of origin. We also know that many forms of adjuvant therapy, including radiation and chemotherapeutic agents, have clastogenic and other damaging effects on chromosomes. For the latter reasons, some of our authors have restricted their remarks to cytogenetic studies on primary lesions from individuals who received no therapy other than surgery.

Many of the discussions (e.g., renal, STSs) are of particular interest to pathologists. These center on the realized or potential value of cytogenetics in refining histologic discrimination and the consequent clinical distinctions (benign vs malignant, differences in prognosis). For example, the progression of aberrations from benign to malignant lesions of papillary renal tumors contributes to understanding of tumor origins and evolution. In these tumors the increasing complexity of apparently random cytogenetic aberrations also appears to mirror the relative malignancy of the individual lesion. Furthermore, the focus in the chapter on renal and bladder tumors on diagnostic and prognostic correlates suggests a "paradigm for the potential uses of cytogenetics in other types of solid tumors" because the nonrandom chromosomal aberrations appear uniquely associated with specific histologic subtypes.

Integration of conventional cytogenetics with FISH and molecular biological data is a major theme of most of the organ-oriented chapters. However, with the exception of colorectal and lung cancers and melanomas, there are relatively few instances where those data are placed in the context of more inclusive although less specific cytometric information. The clinical importance of, and considerable focus of research support for, breast cancer have led to a plethora of genetic studies at all levels of analysis for these tumors. The studies have yielded complex and confusing data, possibly reflecting a group of cancers that have not been resolved into clinically meaningful subgroups. Similarly, although some overall differences are reported between squamous cancers and adenocarcinomas of lung, the overwhelming karyotypic complexity of lung cancers, with as many as 70 structural and numerical changes in a single tumor, makes it difficult to sift relevant from random changes. The preponderance of extensive and complex chromosome changes, even in newly diagnosed primary tumors, may well reflect the highly malignant character of most lung cancers. Those cases in which cell cultures yield simple trisomies may be attributable to contamination with stromal or tumor-adjacent cells, but it is notable that these appear to originate from very well-differentiated neoplasms. Studies of bladder tumors have made considerable progress in localizing tumor suppressor genes based on approaches that integrate cytogenetics, LOH, and CGH. Results in many tumor systems provide a reminder that losses identified by molecular LOH studies are in many cases the result of visible chromosomal deletion.

In conclusion, one broad generalization that can be made from studies of the different tumor systems is that increasing quantity and complexity of chromosome aberrations within a single tumor type is usually indicative of poorer prognosis than for otherwise similar tumors with fewer cytogenetic changes. This conclusion may suggest an important clinical application for CGH as a prognosticator, which needs to be confirmed by statistically significant clinical data. In prostate cancer, the presence of any clonal chromosome change appears associated with worse prognosis. It is also clear that the types of brain tumors more often characterized by diploid metaphases are the less aggressive tumors. Quantitative differences in genetic deviation among cells within a given lesion also may distinguish between benign and malignant forms of proliferation, for example, in thyroid disease.

Appropriately, emphasis is placed throughout this book on the requirement for accurate pathologic assessment of tumor type and grade in attempting to determine the significance of chromosomal aberrations. Conflicting schemes for pathologic classification exist for many solid tumors, contributing greatly to the difficulties of assignment of cytogenetic specificity. Without clear consensus on histology, the basis for determination of chromosome specificity is flawed or absent. Perhaps one reason for the discriminant value of cytogenetics in STSs is the general acceptance of standards for histopathologic classification. On the other hand, some cytogenetic observations may alter histologic definitions; e.g., one STS, the malignant fibrous histiocytoma (MFH), is a controversial classification to some pathologists, although the cytogenetic and clinical data support recognition of at least one form of MFH as a distinct clinical entity.

For many of the common solid tumors of epithelial origin, obtaining a successful and informative karyotypic harvest from direct tumor preparation or short-term tissue culture is still infrequent. Nevertheless, classical cytogenetics continues to provide direction that, in conjunction with the newer cytogenetic approaches of FISH and CGH, and within the context of cytometric information and the greater precision of molecular assays, will contribute to unraveling the genetic basis for individual cancers. In contrast, in pituitary and other endocrine tumors where markers to distinguish benign from malignant lesions are badly needed, the cytogenetic abnormalities do not appear to correlate well with histology or to be predictive of clinical behavior. Future studies, perhaps using techniques not now available, should build upon existing data to increase our understanding of the genetic control of tumor growth and behavior, and to provide the tools for better diagnostic and prognostic markers of cancer.

References

1. Sell S (ed.): Cancer Markers: Diagnostic and Developmental Significance. Clifton, NJ: Humana, 1980.
2. Sell S, Wahren B (eds.): Human Cancer Markers. Clifton, NJ: Humana, 1982.
3. Sell S Reisfeld R (eds.): Monoclonal Antibodies in Cancer. Clifton, NJ: Humana, 1985.
4. Sell S (ed.): Serological Cancer Markers. Totowa, NJ: Humana, 1992.
5. Garrett CT and Sell S (eds.): Cellular Cancer Markers. Totowa, NJ: Humana, 1995.
6. Boveri T: Auf Fragender Entstehung maligner Tumoren, Fisher, Jena (English translation: Boveri, M: The Origin of Malignant Tumors, Baltimore, MD: Williams and Wilkins, 1929.)
7. Muller HJ: Measurement of gene mutation rate in Drosophila, its high variability, and its dependence upon temperature. Genetics 13:279–357, 1928.
8. Furth J, Furth OB: Neoplastic diseases produced in mice by general irradiation with x-rays. Am J Cancer 28:54–65, 1936.
9. National Research Council, Advisory Committee on the Biological Effects of Ionizing Radiations. The Effects on Populations of Exposure to Low Levels of Ionizing Radiation. Washington, DC: National Academy of Sciences, chapter V, pp. 135–471, 1980.
10. Nowell PC, Hungerford DA: A minute chromosome in human chronic granulocytic leukemia. Science 132:1497, 1960.
11. Rowley JD: A new consistent chromosomal abnormality in chronic myelogenous leukemia identified by quinacrine fluorescence and Giemsa staining. Nature 243:290–293, 1973.
12. Mitelman F: Catalog of Chromosome Aberrations in Cancer, 1st, 2nd, and 3rd editions, New York: Liss, 1983, 1985, 1988; 4th and 5th editions, New York, Wiley-Liss, 1991, 1994.

Part I

Perspectives

*Relation of Other Genetic
Measures to Cytogenetics*

Chapter 2

Assessment of Genetic Changes in Human Cancers Using Flow and Image Cytometry

T. Vincent Shankey and Cees J. Cornelisse

Introduction

Genetic changes are a hallmark of all cancers. As first shown by Nowell and Hungerford *(1)*, analysis of chromosome structure, even at the relatively low resolution available from unbanded metaphase spreads, provided evidence for association of a chromosomal structural change (Ph[1]) with a particular hematopoietic malignancy (chronic myelogenous leukemia [CML]). The subsequent increase in resolution available from chromosome banding techniques *(2,3)* coupled with the use of in vitro blockage of cells in the G_2M phase of the cell cycle to provide metaphase chromosomes, established the use of karyotyping in the study of genetic changes in human tumors, and allowed identification of specific chromosomes involved in malignancies. Karyotyping studies thus established the characteristic translocation, t(9;22), seen in CML as the first genetic marker (Ph[1]) associated with a human cancer *(4)*.

Much of our current understanding of the specific genetic changes in human cancers developed from cytogenetic studies. Most of these early studies focused on leukemias and lymphomas, in part

From: *Human Cytogenetic Cancer Markers* Edited by S. R. Wolman and S. Sell
Humana Press Inc., Totowa, NJ

because of the ease of obtaining and isolating tumor cells in high purity, and in part because of the relatively high proliferating fraction of these tumors, making it possible to obtain significant numbers of mitotic cells after short-term culture in vitro with mitotic blocking agents. These studies (many performed by Janet Rowley and colleagues) identified reciprocal translocations between pairs of chromosomes in many hematopoietic malignancies, such as the t(9;22) in CML, t(8;21) or t(3;21) in acute myelogenous leukemia (AML), t(15;17) in acute promyelocytic leukemia (APL), t(14;19) in B-lymphocyte malignancies, and t(8;14) in Burkitt's lymphoma. These observations were important in developing concepts for the genetic basis of cancers, and for the later understanding that specific genes play unique roles in the development of specific types of cancers. The increasing sophistication of techniques in molecular genetics at this same time, which permitted identification of specific genes (such as C-*MYC*) involved in human cancers, led some researchers to conclude that further information from karyotyping studies would be unlikely to provide significant new insights into genetic mechanisms of tumorigenesis and genetic evolution. However, many molecular genetic studies (particularly in hematopoietic malignancies) have relied on the fundamental information regarding gross chromosomal changes established by karyotyping as a starting point to target searches for specific genes involved in these cancers.

During this same period of increasing understanding of genetic changes in hematopoietic tumors, much less progress was made in elucidating genetic changes in solid tumors using karyotyping techniques. Cytogenetic analysis of solid tumors is limited by the difficulties in isolating tumor cells, in maintaining cell viability even during short-term tissue culture, and in obtaining metaphase events in sufficient numbers from cells truly representative of the tumor cell population. Frequently, cells that survive isolation from solid tumors and proliferate in vitro are either normal fibroblasts, or are cells from high grade (undifferentiated) tumors. As illustrated in the Clinical Utility of DNA Content Measurements by Flow Cytometry section, it is in the analysis of solid tumors that flow and image cytometry have provided important insights into genetic changes and, for some types of human tumors, have also provided important prognostic information.

It should be noted that prior to the development of karyotyping techniques, and even preceding the experimental work that established the relationship of DNA and the expression of inherited traits, Torbjorn Caspersson *(5)* reported the results of his extensive studies involving quantitative microspectrophotometric evaluation of human cancers. From these pioneering studies using quantitative image cytometry, Caspersson concluded that tumor cells contain increased amounts of nucleic acids as compared with normal cells, and that nucleic acids must convey genetic information. These studies preceded the studies of Avery et al. *(6)* on the so-called transforming factor (DNA), and the current era of cytogenetics (and molecular genetics) by over 30 yr. In addition, Caspersson established the utility of single cell quantitative measurements (cytometry) in elucidating the biological basis for human cancers, and in providing clinically useful information. It is likely that in the future, the combination of molecular genetic techniques with cytometric analysis for the simultaneous measurement of multiple genetic (and phenotypic) markers at the single cell level will have a significant impact on our understanding of genetic changes in human tumors.

As described in the sections on DNA Ploidy and Image Analysis Measurements of DNA Content, measurements of genetic changes in cancers using flow or image cytometry are based on a determination of the total amount of DNA in each cell. The major limitations of these types of measurements, compared to cytogenetic approaches are the lower resolution and lower sensitivity of cytometric measurements. However, measurement of DNA content of individual cells using flow or image cytometry offers a number of advantages over cytogenetic analysis. These include the ability to analyze significantly larger numbers of cells that are not subjected to potentially selective conditions of in vitro culture with mitotic blocking agents. In addition, cytometric techniques analyze interphase cells, can sample all cells isolated from the tumor, and can provide the additional prognostic information available from tumor S-phase measurements.

Flow Cytometric Measurement of DNA Content

Flow cytometry involves the measurement of one or more characteristics (light scatter, fluorescence, or absorbance) performed on single cells (or nuclei) in suspension as they pass through an illumination and detection point. Most modern instruments utilize laser illumination, which provides high photon densities that can be focused at a small, fixed point in space. An additional advantage is that lasers provide only a single wavelength of illumination, eliminating the need for filters to remove unwanted or interfering wavelengths from the illuminating light. With the recent development of low-cost, air-cooled lasers, and high efficiency light-collecting optics, newer laser-based instruments offer significant advantages over older flow cytometers using mercury-arc lamp light sources. For further technical details regarding flow cytometry instrumentation, the reader is referred to an excellent text by Howard Shapiro *(7)* that covers instrumentation, as well as other aspects of flow cytometry.

Fundamental Concepts

The fundamental concept for DNA content measurements using flow cytometry is that DNA binding dyes, such as propidium iodide (PI) or 4′,6-diamidino-2-phenylindole (DAPI) are nonfluorescent or weakly fluorescent in free solution, and greatly increase fluorescence yield when bound to DNA. Dye bound to DNA fluoresces at a wavelength higher than the wavelength used to excite the dye-DNA complex (Stokes shift), and for some dye-DNA complexes, the shift can be considerable (>130 nm). As explained in the Multiparameter Measurements by Flow Cytometry section, this characteristic allows simultaneous analysis of two (or more) dyes for a single cell, such as PI bound to DNA and fluorescein isothiocyanate (FITC) bound to antibodies, even with illumination by a single wavelength (488 nm). PI, which is commonly used for DNA flow cytometry, can be excited by either UV (354 nm) or blue (488 nm) light, producing DNA-dye fluorescence that peaks at 610–615 nm following excitation at either wavelength.

DNA-dye binding is through noncovalent interactions, and it is important that the appropriate ratio of dye to DNA be maintained for cytometric measurement of DNA content. This is because the fluorescence signal obtained from each cell must be proportional to the amount of DNA present. Too low a dye-to-DNA ratio (undersaturation) produces a fluorescence signal that underestimates the total amount of DNA per cell. Many DNA-binding dyes can quench the fluorescence signal at high ratios of dye to DNA *(8)*. Under conditions of oversaturation, the fluorescence signal would also underestimate the total amount of DNA per cell. It is thus important that an appropriate ratio of dye to DNA be maintained for all measurements used to determine the amount of DNA per cell using fluorescence measurements. For additional technical details regarding sample staining for DNA flow cytometry, the reader is referred to ref. *9*. Other important factors which can affect the fluorescent signal include cell fixation procedures *(9)* and nuclear chromatin configuration *(10)*. Different dyes have different sensitivities to chromatin-DNA structure, and dyes such as 7-aminoactinomycin D (7-AAD), whose binding is highly sensitive to chromatin-DNA configuration, can produce different fluorescence intensities for cells with the same total amount of DNA, but at different stages of differentiation.

Flow cytometric measurement of DNA content requires that single cells or nuclei are isolated from the tumor. For hematopoietic malignancies, tumor cells are readily obtained from whole blood, lymph nodes, or from bone marrow aspirates using simple preparation steps (mechanical dissociation of lymph nodes). Whereas physical enrichment steps are sometimes used to isolate the malignant cell population (to enrich lymphocytes and remove platelets and red blood cells), some isolation techniques can cause loss of specific types of cells (i.e., loss of large granular lymphocytes during isobuoyant density centrifugation), and should be avoided. The use of whole-cell preparations (rather than nuclei) has the advantage that cell surface markers are preserved; therefore, phenotyping can be used in conjunction with DNA content analysis of the malignant cell population. With the use of the appropriate combinations of cell surface markers to identify both normal and malignant cells, it is possible to detect small increases or decreases in DNA content (near-diploid, DNA-aneuploid malignancies). For hematopoietic malignancies, this is an important technical detail for flow cytometric measurements, as many leukemias and lymphomas demonstrate relatively small changes in the total DNA content as compared to appropriate DNA-diploid control cells. For further information regarding the techniques of cell isolation and multiparameter flow cytometric analysis of hematopoietic malignancies, the reader is referred to an excellent reference by Braylan *(11)*.

The isolation of single cells from unfixed, solid tumors, which is necessary for flow cytometric measurement of DNA content, is generally accomplished using either mechanical disruption or enzymatic digestion of tumor tissue, or a combination of these techniques. Tumors that lack strong intracellular connections and are not tightly attached to basement membranes generally give a high yield of intact tumor cells following mechanical scrapping or chopping of tumor-containing tissue. Tumors that have tightly interconnected cells (squamous cell cancers) or cells tightly attached to basement membranes generally require enzymatic treatment (proteases, trypsin, or pepsin, sometimes used in conjunction with collagenases). In a comparison of the use of mechanical versus enzymatic treatments, Smeets and coworkers *(12)* demonstrated that mechanical dissociation more frequently resulted in the isolation of DNA-aneuploid and karyotypically abnormal tumor cells from transitional cell bladder tumors. In contrast, mechanical disruption of squamous cell head and neck tumors resulted in less frequent isolation of DNA-aneuploid tumors, as compared to enzymatic digestion *(13)*. In general, enzymatic digestion may add little to the dissociation of many glandular epithelial tumors (adenocarcinomas), whereas prostate cancers and tumors with squamous differentiation require this approach. Mixtures of collagenases and proteases have been reported to increase the yield of tumor cells in some studies, likely because of the disruption of connective tissues by collagenase. Some investigators have used DNase in conjunction with mechanical or enzymatic techniques, to prevent aggregation of isolated cells by DNA strands released from disrupted cells. It must be appreciated that variations in the structure of tumors can result in two- to fivefold differences in cell yield for different tumors of the same cell type *(14)*. Unfortunately, there are no clearcut or standardized techniques for the isolation of representative tumor cells from all types of tumors. For reviews covering techniques and strategies for the isolation of tumor cells from solid tumors, the reader is referred to references by Pallavacini and coworkers *(15)* and by Visscher and Crissman *(16)*.

Flow cytometric analysis of nuclei isolated from paraffin-embedded tumor tissue was originally reported by Hedley and coworkers *(17)*. The technique has allowed many flow and image cytometry studies to be performed using archival tumor material.

The technique utilizes thick sections (50–90 μ), which are dewaxed, rehydrated, and digested with pepsin (or proteinase) to release single nuclei. As indicated, flow cytometric analysis of nuclei isolated in this manner provides a measurement of the DNA content (DNA-ploidy and S-phase) of all nuclei isolated. Although direct comparisons of the results of flow or image analysis studies of these nuclei with karyotypic analysis are not possible, numerous reports have compared the results of flow cytometric analysis with fluorescence *in situ* hybridization (FISH) (*see* Chapter 3). These types of studies have demonstrated that DNA-diploid tumors frequently contain gains or losses of chromosomes, as determined using centromere-specific probes *(18,19)*. In addition, DNA aneuploid tumors by flow cytometry frequently have heterogeneous copy numbers for one or more chromosomes, providing evidence for genetic heterogeneity in a significant portion of some types of tumors.

DNA Ploidy

Under conditions where the amount of fluorescence is directly proportional to the amount of DNA present in each cell or nucleus, flow cytometric analysis provides a direct measurement of gains or losses in the total amount of DNA in tumors. Representative results of the analysis of a human tumor with an abnormal amount of DNA is shown in Fig. 1. The tumor population analyzed has a DNA content 1.8-times greater than cells with a diploid DNA content (the first peak in the DNA histogram). By convention *(20)*, the results of DNA ploidy measurements by flow cytometry are expressed as DNA index (DI), or the mean channel of the tumor G_0/G_1 peak divided by the DNA diploid G_0/G_1 mean peak channel. The DNA aneuploid tumor shown in Fig. 1 would thus have a DNA index of 1.8. Similarly, DNA diploid tumors would have a DI of 1.0. It is apparent that this tumor has a gain in total DNA content but, unlike the results of karyotyping analysis, no information is provided by flow cytometry regarding gains (or losses) of specific chromosomes, or portions of chromosomes, or changes in DNA sequences on specific chromosomes.

It is important to make a distinction between the results of cytogenetic and flow or image cytometric measurements. Although terminology used to describe the results of flow cytometry is not

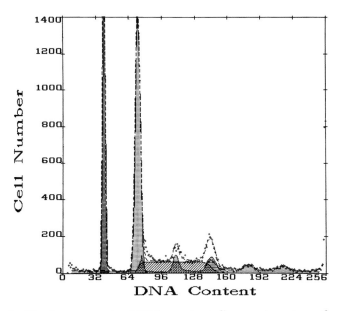

Fig. 1. Single parameter DNA content flow cytometry of a human tumor, demonstrating the presence of a DNA aneuploid population. The first peak (left side of histogram, at channel 40) represents the DNA diploid cells present in the cell mixture isolated from the tumor, whereas the second peak represents the tumor G_0/G_1 population (tumor cells either not in cell cycle, or in the preDNA synthesis portion of the cell cycle). The third major peak in the histogram (at channel 144) represents tumor cells in the G_2 (post-DNA synthesis) and M (mitosis) phases of the cell cycle. Cells between the tumor G_0/G_1 peak and the G_2/M peak are S-phase cells, or tumor cells synthesizing DNA. The tumor has a DNA content 1.8-times that of the DNA diploid cell reference. The tumor has a relatively high S-phase (22%). Important aspects of quality control for DNA content measurements by flow cytometry that are shown here include the low coefficient of variation (CV) for the DNA diploid cells (2.7%), the low percentage of events in the histogram that represent background debris (events shown in shadow to the left of the DNA diploid peak and to the right of the DNA aneuploid G_2/M peak), and aggregates of any two or more nuclei (small peaks at channels 110, 180, and 200). Collectively, these background events are referred to as the percent background aggregates and debris, or % B.A.D.

universally applied, a convention for nomenclature for all DNA cytometry was recommended in 1984 *(20)*. These guidelines recommended that the use of cytogenetic terminology (hypodiploidy, peritetraploidy, etc.) should not be employed for cytometry studies where there was no direct measurement of changes in the number or composition of individual chromosomes. Rather, the guidelines recommended the use of the terms DNA diploid and DNA aneuploid to denote a tumor with or without the same DNA ploidy with appropriate DNA diploid control populations. As indicated previously, the guidelines recommended the use of DI as a measurement of the degree of deviation of the tumor from diploid DNA content.

A critical aspect of DNA ploidy measurements is the use of an appropriate standard for diploid DNA content values. Since most tumors contain normal and reactive (DNA diploid) cells as well as tumor, the isolation of cells or nuclei from tumor samples also provides a DNA diploid cell population in most cases, which can serve as an internal diploid control. As recommended by the DNA consensus guidelines *(21)*, the best DNA-diploid standard is the normal counterpart of the neoplastic cells. The use of cells added to the tumor sample (e.g., normal lymphocytes, chicken, or trout erythrocytes) as a DNA-content standard should be avoided. These added cells can be useful in determining which peak is the DNA-diploid population in samples of fresh tumor material, provided one aliquot of the tumor sample is analyzed without added cells (to prevent the confounding impact of aggregates of these added cells on identifying which peak represents the DNA-diploid population). Variations in dye-DNA binding by different diploid or reference cell populations can produce ambiguity in the correct diploid DNA content. For nuclei isolated from paraffin-embedded tissues, the absence of a known DNA-diploid reference population makes it advisable to assume that the first peak on the histogram represents the DNA-diploid population *(21)*.

S-Phase

Additional information obtained from flow cytometric analysis, also shown in Fig. 1, includes a measurement of tumor S-phase, or the proportion of tumor cells in the DNA synthesis phase of the cell cycle. For the tumor shown in Fig. 1, the S-phase was 22%, a relatively high value for most solid tumors. As indicated in the section on Clinical Utility of DNA Content Measurement by Flow Cytometry, this information has been shown to have prognostic value in a number of human tumors. Flow cytometric analysis of DNA ploidy has been relatively easy to reproduce in interlaboratory comparisons *(22)*, but S-phase measurements frequently vary considerably for measurements performed by different laboratories using identical samples *(23)*. This lack of reproducibility of S-phase values is because of different techniques used to stain and analyze samples, and because of the lack of uniform agreement on standards for S-phase measurements. For these reasons, it is not now possible to compare the results of S-phase analyses directly between laboratories. Each laboratory performing S-phase analysis on clinical specimens must establish its own values for low, intermediate, and high S-phase, and for the associated risks for progression, response to therapy or survival for each group as analyzed by that laboratory. S-phase values that place a patient with a particular type of tumor at low or intermediate risk in one laboratory might represent an S-phase of intermediate or high risk based on values from another laboratory. For further descriptions of these technical points on S-phase analysis, the reader is referred to the reference by Rabinovitch *(9)*.

Clinical Utility of DNA Content Measurements by Flow Cytometry

Cytometric analysis has been performed on human tumors for over 30 yr and has demonstrated that genetic changes (as determined by DNA ploidy) occur in many human tumors. For studies of hematopoietic malignancies, the measured tumor DNA ploidy is frequently similar to that of appropriate diploid DNA-control cells. These findings are consistent with the results of cytogenetic studies indicating a high frequency of balanced translocations that would not change the DNA ploidy compared with appropriate DNA-diploid controls. For hematopoietic malignancies with balanced translocations, karyotyping analysis can provide significantly more information regarding the presence or absence of genetic abnormalities than can flow cytometric DNA ploidy measurements. A consensus conference on the clinical utility of DNA content measurements of leukemias and lymphomas *(24)* concluded that, overall, DNA ploidy determinations are of limited value in predicting treatment response. Although there is some value of DNA ploidy measurements in non-Hodgkins lymphomas, it is likely that S-phase measurements are of more clinical value in lymphomas *(11)*.

For solid malignancies, the appearance of DNA aneuploidy generally correlates with tumor grade and stage, with superficial, low-grade tumors predominantly DNA-diploid, and invasive or high-grade tumors predominantly DNA-aneuploid. These results suggest that gross genetic abnormalities (as detected by cytometric measurements) are less frequently seen in low-grade or stage-solid tumors, and that during tumor evolution additional chromosomes (or parts of chromosomes) are added to (or lost from) the neoplastic cell genome. DNA ploidy (and to a larger extent, tumor S-phase) has demonstrated clinical utility in predicting disease course or response to therapy in some (but not all) types of solid tumors *(25)*. For example, in transitional cell cancers (TCC) of the bladder, the majority of low-grade, superficial tumors are DNA-diploid, whereas most high-grade, superficial tumors are DNA-aneuploid. Since progression of these tumors is predicted well by grade, DNA ploidy does not add significant prognostic information *(26)*. However, the disease course for intermediate grade, superficial TCC is variable, and for these tumors, DNA ploidy provides an independent predictor of outcome *(26)*. An additional use of DNA ploidy for TCC is in the detection of exfoliated tumor cells from bladder washing samples *(26)*. In bladder washings, DNA-aneuploid tumors can be detected with high sensitivity, although the presence of only DNA-diploid cells in the sample does not rule out the possible presence of a DNA-diploid tumor. On the other hand, in colon cancers, the clinical utility of DNA ploidy measurements, although probably limited to Duke's stage B and C disease, and S-phase measurements are likely to provide markers of equal or greater significance than those provided by grade and stage *(27)*. Breast cancers have been perhaps the most studied clinical samples using flow cytometry. The predictive value of DNA ploidy measurements by flow cytometry remain somewhat controversial, but it is most likely that DNA ploidy is less useful than grade and stage in predicting outcome *(28)*. Although studies on the predictive value of S-phase in breast cancers have been limited, S-phase is likely to provide a clinically useful predictor of outcome *(28)*. For prostate cancers, DNA ploidy measurements probably offer an independent measurement of progression and survival, particularly in more advanced disease (stage T3–4, N0/+, M0/+), and are likely to provide a predictor of response to antiandrogen therapy *(29)*.

Multiparameter Measurements by Flow Cytometry

Current flow cytometry instrumentation has the ability to measure simultaneously three or four different fluorochromes bound to a single cell. In addition to DNA content analysis using a single laser (commonly the 488 nm line from a argon laser), it is possible to measure DNA with propidium iodide, plus a second antigen using FITC-conjugated antibodies, and a third antigen using phycroerythrin (PE)-conjugated antibodies. The major advantage of using one or more antibody probes is that they provide markers for the identification of the normal counterpart of the neoplastic cell population, such as the use of antibodies to cytokeratins *(30)*, or the identification of diploid lymphocytes, monocytes, or granulocytes that have infiltrated the tumor, using anti-CD 45 antibodies *(31)*. With these types of markers, the internal DNA-diploid cell population can be readily identified, making the identification of near-diploid, DNA-aneuploid tumor populations unambiguous.

Using two different antibodies with different fluorochromes, it is possible to identify the presence or absence of cytoplasmic proteins that may have additional prognostic significance, in conjunction with the use of lineage-specific markers, such as intermediate filament proteins. An example of such an application is shown in Fig. 2, demonstrating the simultaneous analysis of DNA content, cytokeratins, and p53 protein expression. For these experiments, a mixture of normal human lymphocytes (DNA-diploid, cytokeratin negative, p53 negative) and cells from the T24 bladder tumor cell line (DNA-aneuploid, cytokeratin, and p53 positive) were stained with PI, PE-labeled anticytokeratin (pan-cytokeratin) antibodies, and FITC-labeled anti-p53 (clone DO7) antibodies. As shown in Fig. 2, only the DNA-aneuploid cell population (T24 cells) is positive for both cytokeratin and p53 (the cell line contains a mutant p53 gene and constitutively expresses the p53 protein), whereas the DNA-diploid lymphocytes are negative for both protein markers. The analysis shown here was

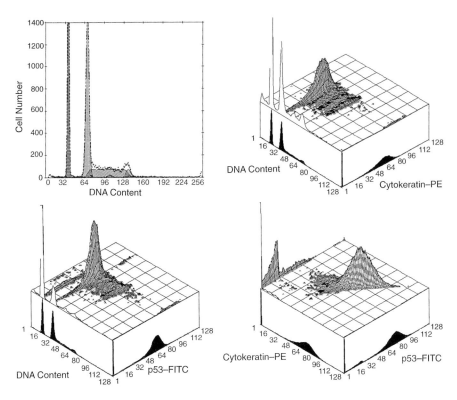

Fig. 2. Multiparameter flow cytometric analysis of a mixture of human lymphocytes (DNA diploid, cytokeratin negative and p53 negative) and T24 bladder tumor cell line (DNA aneuploid, cytokeratin and p53 positive). Cell mixture was stained with directly conjugated antibodies to cytokeratins (Phycoerythrin) and to p53 (FITC), and the DNA was stained using propidium iodide. Top Left: DNA content measurement of cell mixture. Top right: Two parameter analysis of DNA (PI content) plus cytokeratin, demonstrating cytokeratin only in the DNA aneuploid (T24) cells. Bottom left: Two parameter analysis of DNA plus p53, demonstrating that only DNA aneuploid cells express p53. Bottom right: Two parameter analysis of cytokeratin vs p53 expression demonstrating that cytokeratin positive cells express p53. Note that <2% of cells are Ck⁻ and p53⁺, or Ck⁺ and p53⁻ (an indication of the quality of the antibody staining proceedure used).

performed on a single laser, bench-top instrument (Coulter Epics XL, Miami, FL), using directly fluorochrome-conjugated antibodies. The use of direct antibody-fluorochrome conjugates significantly reduces the technical complexity of these types of experiments, and greatly shortens the amount of time necessary for sample preperation. With the increasing appearance of high-quality, directly conjugated antibodies to intracellular markers of potential clinical value (cell cycle proteins, markers for apoptosis), such multiparameter analyses are likely to become increasingly common.

One other area of potential application for flow cytometry is in the determination of the amount of a specific receptor protein on tumor cells. Examples include quantification of the levels of estrogen or progesterone receptors in breast cancer cells, epidermal growth factor (EGF) receptors in bladder cancer, and tumor growth factor (TGFβ) receptors in prostate cancer. Although flow cytometric techniques have the capacity to provide quantitative measurements, aside from DNA content measurements, quantitative measurements are rarely performed. Such receptor quantification measurements may represent the ultimate application of flow cytometry in diagnostic pathology, and could serve as an important adjunct to routine immunohistochemical staining for applications where the quantity of the receptor may define specific risk groups, or those individuals most likely to respond to new therapies aimed at the specific receptors on tumor cells.

Image Analysis Measurements of DNA Content

As indicated previously, the earliest studies of DNA content in human tumors were performed by Caspersson *(see* ref. *5)* using image analysis techniques. These studies were performed using absorbance measurements of individual cells illuminated with UV (350 nm) light. At this wavelength, nucleic acids (DNA and RNA) absorb light with relatively high efficiency. The technical difficulties in these types of measurements were significant, and included the needs to develop special objective lenses that would not absorb UV light, to develop light sources with sufficient light output in the UV range, and to develop techniques to mask individual cells for measurement.

Fundamental Concepts

Starting in the 1950s, image analysis techniques for single cell DNA content measurements were developed using chemical modification of DNA to produce residues capable of absorption after illumination with visible light. The best known, the Feulgen stain, uses acid hydrolysis of DNA, followed by a Schiffs reaction to facilitate the blue-colored DNA stain. Although fluorescence-based image analysis is possible using the same dyes commonly used for flow cytometry (PI, DAPI, etc.), quantitative measurements require that fluorescence is collected over a constant and highly reproducible time period. The need for time-gated fluorescence signal acquisition is not necessary for flow cytometric measurements because the cells pass through the laser and detection point at a highly regulated rate. For image analysis measurements, relatively small changes in illumination and fluorescence detection times significantly change the signal obtained from each cell.

Image analysis is performed by calculating the amount of absorbance (or fluorescence) for each nucleus in the field under study. Generally, a threshold is first set to allow the software to distinguish the absorbance signal from the background (slide and cytoplasm) from that of the nuclei. The software then must define the boundaries of each nucleus (segmentation), and measure the absorbance signal from each nucleus. Image analysis systems can use either a charge-coupled device (CCD) or video cameras to collect the absorbance signal. Digital images are collected on a grid of individual detectors, called pixels, with most current cameras used for image analysis dividing the entire field into a 512×512 pixel array. After segmentation to define which pixels contain signals from inside a nucleus, the absorbance signal (optical density) from each included pixel is summed to give the integrated optical density, or the sum of absorbance values from each pixel. The optical density value stored in each pixel is generally on a linear scale with an optical density value from 0–255. As indicated earlier for flow cytometric measurements of DNA content (*see* Fundamental Concepts), the absorbance obtained must be proportional to the total amount of DNA present in each nucleus.

Image analysis of DNA content has been performed using single whole-cell or nuclear preparations on glass slides, tissue touch preparations, and tissue sections. Cell isolation techniques have the same impact on image analysis measurements as discussed for flow cytometric techniques. The advantage of image analysis is that cell (or nuclear) morphology can sometimes be used to identify tumor or appropriate DNA-diploid control cells (lymphocytes, fibroblasts). This is generally useful for intermediate and high-grade tumors where distinct cell or nuclear features permit easy identification of tumor cells. For low-grade tumors, morphologic criteria alone are frequently insufficient to identify isolated tumor cells or nuclei. In such cases, multiparameter image analysis (using multiple fluorescent or absorption dye-labeled antibodies) could greatly enhance image analysis measures, assuming that multiparameter staining and analysis techniques will be developed for routine image cytometry applications. However, given the relative ease of multiparameter flow cytometry analysis, image analytical approaches are less likely to contribute a significant impact to the analysis of those single cell or nuclear samples where morphology alone is insufficient to identify tumor cells.

The application of image cytometry techniques to the analysis of tissue touch preparations and tissue sections represents a potentially important use of this technology. Here, the cues used for histopathological evaluation of tumors are potentially available, allowing the analysis to focus on tumor cells, or areas of premalignant cells. However, several practical limitations exist for DNA-content analysis using tissues. From a practical point, the Feulgen stain results in a cellular and nuclear morphology quite different from that of routine hematoxylin and eosin (H&E) stains. Personnel performing image analysis of tissues must become familiar with the morphological appearance of Feulgen-stained tissues, which provide distinctively different cues from those presented by textbook H&E-stained histological criteria. An additional limitation for tissue sections is the problem with sliced and overlapping nuclei. Thin sections (2–4-µ thick) contain a significant percentage of sliced nuclei, and these contain different percentages of the original amount of DNA present in the intact nucleus. Thicker sections (10–15 µ) contain fewer sliced nuclei, but include a higher percentage of nuclei that overlap, making segmentation of these events as independent nuclei difficult. Although currently available image analysis instruments have software algorithms capable of eliminating a percent of sliced or overlapping nuclei from DNA-content measurements, they all perform this function at the expense of eliminating a significant percent of the nuclei present from the measurement.

DNA Content Measurements

As early as the 1950s, adsorption microphotometric techniques were used for DNA-content measurements of Feulgen-stained slides from imprints or tissue sections from solid tumors *(32)*. Prior to the development of digital image analysis techniques and relatively inexpensive, powerful computers roughly a decade ago, DNA cytometry using slides was a laborious and time-consuming procedure that could not compete with the speed, elegance, and resolution provided by flow cytometry. Current commercially available image analysis systems need much less user interaction and provide DNA profiles with significantly improved resolution, because of improvements in both the hardware used for imaging systems, and in the Feulgen staining techniques used to measure DNA content.

Representative results of an image cytometry analysis of a tissue section from a prostate carcinoma are shown in Fig. 3. As is typical for such studies, this analysis was restricted to areas of prostate cancer and as shown, both DNA-diploid and DNA-aneuploid nuclei are observed, with the majority of events measured as DNA-aneuploid. Although the peak of the aneuploid population appears to have a 4C DNA content, it is difficult to assign precise values of DNA index from image analysis studies. Slicing of nuclei reduces the amount of DNA measured in a significant percentage of nuclei in 5–6-μ thick tissue sections, as used here, and the amount of DNA lost is related to the section thickness and the volume of the tumor nuclei. The first peak in this histogram (2C peak) represents DNA-diploid tumor nuclei. These generally have a significantly lower volume than DNA-aneuploid prostate cancer nuclei, and are less subject to artificial loss of DNA content caused by nuclear slicing.

Concordance of image analysis with the results of flow cytometric DNA ploidy is generally good in the few comparative studies that have used large numbers of specimens *(33,34)*. One potential exemption to this is in the use of tissue sections for DNA content

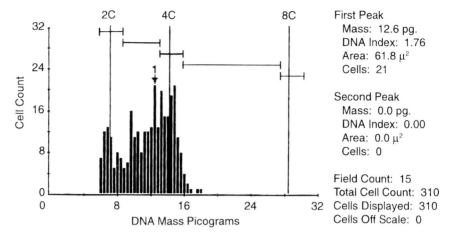

Fig. 3. DNA content image analysis of Feulgen-stained tissue section (5–6-μ thick) from prostate carcinoma specimen, demonmstrating the presence of DNA ploidy heterogeneity in this prostate tumor. The majority of the tumor nuclei analyzed were DNA aneuploid (here measured as 4C), though the sample contained a significant number of DNA diploid tumor nuclei (only nuclei from tumor containing areas included in this histogram). The diploid DNA content is established by measuring nuclei from an area of BPH (benign prostatic hypertrophy) in the same tissue section (results not shown).

analysis by image cytometry. As shown in Fig. 4, comparison of the results of image analysis of tissue sections (5–6-μ thick) with DNA content by flow cytometry of nuclei isolated from adjacent sections from the same prostate cancer frequently demonstrates a significantly lower DNA content for the image analysis sample. This is likely the result of a significant percent of large volume tumor nuclei being sliced during the preperation of the tissue section. A number of technical aspects unique to image analysis measurements of DNA content using absorption methods generate errors not found in flow cytometric measurements (glare correction, pixel limits, binning errors). Both flow and image cytometric measurements of DNA ploidy are affected by differences in measured DNA content based on chromatin compactness (between normal and tumor cells, or between normal, diploid cells at different stages of differentiation).

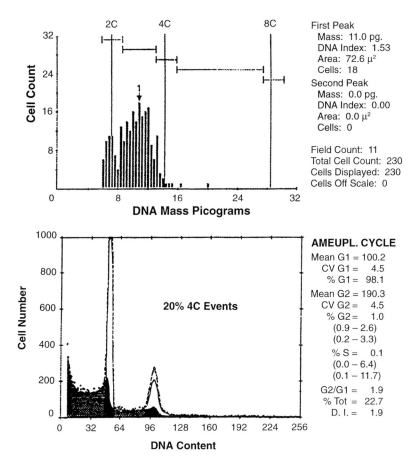

Fig. 4. Comparison of the results of image (top) and flow cytometric (bottom) analysis of the same human prostate cancer specimen. For image analysis, a 5–6-µ thick tissue section was Feulgen stained and only tumor nuclei were included in the DNA content measurement. For flow cytometric analysis, adjacent 50-µ thick sections from the same tissue block were digested using the Hedley technique (ref. *17*) and nuclei analyzed after PI staining of the DNA. As shown here, the flow cytometric analysis shows the presence of DNA tetraploid (4C) tumor nuclei, whereas the results of image analysis shows a DNA aneuploid tumor population with significantly less DNA per nucleus. The lower DNA content measured by image analysis (tissue sections) is likely because of loss of DNA content in the majority of tumor nuclei caused by slicing artifacts.

Recently published guidelines for the standardization of DNA image cytometry *(35)* should improve the reproducibility of image cytometric measurements of DNA ploidy.

Some investigators have suggested that S-phase estimates are possible from image cytometry measurements; these are unlikely to be accurate. In images derived from tissue sections, an unknown number of sliced G_2/M events and overlapping G_0/G_1 nuclei will be measured as events in the S-phase of DNA content. In measurements of isolated cells or nuclei where sliced and overlapping nuclei are less likely to present a problem, the statistical variability that results from counting small numbers of S-phase events makes the accuracy of S-phase determinations unacceptably low. Although it is possible to count 1000 S-phase events to make the count reproducible *(36)*, the amount of time involved using manual image processing techniques makes this unacceptable in a clinical setting.

One alternative that permits tumor proliferation by image analysis is to stain the sample with an antibody that marks only proliferating cells, and to use image analytical techniques to measure the percent of positively stained tumor nuclei. Antibodies to proliferation-associated antigens such as proliferating cell nuclear antigen (PCNA) and Ki-67 have been extensively used in image analysis determinations of tumor proliferation. Limitations of this approach include the need to stain two different samples, one for DNA content, the other for the proliferation antigen (unless fluorescence staining and analysis techniques are used), and the difficulty in obtaining a proliferation marker that is found exclusively in cycling cells. For example, whereas PCNA is a part of the DNA synthesis complex (replicons), it is also involved in nonreplicative DNA repair, and can be expressed in irradiation damaged cells that are not proliferating. For an excellent review of image analysis techniques on tumor samples, including DNA content and proliferation markers, the reader is referred to Weinberg *(37)*.

Image cytometry and flow cytometry should be considered as complementary rather than as competing techniques for measuring DNA content. Visual or automated selection of cells meeting specific morphological criteria is a strong point of image analysis. An additional asset is the feasibility of measuring very small cell or tissue samples. Flow cytometry, on the other hand, provides greater accuracy, better statistics, higher resolution, the potential to sort selected populations for subsequent analysis, and the capability of simultaneous measurement with several different probes.

Strengths and Weaknesses of Cytogenetics and DNA Ploidy

Cytometric measurements of genetic changes using flow cytometry involve staining a preparation of single cells or isolated nuclei with a dye that qualitatively binds to the DNA in each nucleus. Unlike cytogenetic analysis where 20–40 cells are routinely analyzed, cytometric analyses can measure hundreds (image analysis) or tens of thousands (flow cytometry) of cells. One of the most important advantages of cytometric DNA content analysis is that it does not rely on metaphase cells, and all cells that are isolated from the tumor are analyzed. In addition, cells in all phases of the cell cycle are included in flow or image analysis. Cytogenetic analysis relies on extensive periods of time to culture, blocking of cells in metaphase, and the preparation, banding, and analysis of metaphase spreads (including locating, photographing, and carefully analyzing individual chromosomes). In contrast, cytometric techniques are technically simple and require minimal time. Flow (and possibly image) cytometry also offers the potential for quantifying multiple markers simultaneously for each cell. With the development of appropriate antibodies for the measurement of cell cycle and apoptosis pathway-related proteins, flow cytometric analysis of tumors will likely be able to pinpoint some genetic mutations (p53, cyclins) that could have clinical significance for predicting disease course or response to therapy.

Personnel involved in cytogenetic studies must be carefully trained in cell culture and photographic techniques, and must be able to scan numerous microscope slides patiently, to identify abnormal chromosomes, and to cut and paste images of individual chromosomes to assemble a karyogram. The automated or semi-automated karyotyping instruments that are available are expensive, and are restricted by the fundamental limitations of karyotyping. On the other hand, flow cytometry instrumentation is complex, even more expensive, and requires training to operate and maintain the instrument. In addition, the use of antibodies for multiparameter measurements significantly increases both the cost and the complexity of the measurements.

DNA ploidy measurements, based on cytometric techniques can provide an assessment of genetic changes that occur in human cancers. Using appropriate standards and controls, it is possible to detect changes in the total amount of DNA in individual tumor cells, as compared to the DNA content found in normal DNA-diploid cells. However, flow or image cytometry can only detect gains or losses to the total amount of DNA per cell. Even highly sensitive flow cytometers are limited to the detection of a change (gain or loss) of roughly 5% in total DNA per cell. This corresponds to the gain or loss of at least one large (such as an A group) chromosome. The actual sensitivity depends upon the individual chromosome and the specific dye used. The signal obtained by flow cytometry for dye-DNA complexes is dependent on the dye used (some dyes are AT- or CG-specific) as well as the chromosome that is changed (some regions and chromosomes are more AT- or CG-rich than others).

Comparisons of DNA content measurements made between flow cytometry and cytogenetic analysis have been reported for a number of different types of tumors. Overall, these have shown that DNA-content values measured by flow cytometry are generally 10–30% higher than that predicted by chromosome counts for the same tumors, and that the differences are generally more pronounced for tumors with a triploid (or greater) chromosome number. Typical results comparing DNA ploidy measurements using flow cytometry (DNA index) with karyotyping analysis of the same tumor material are shown in Fig. 5 (reproduced from ref. *38*). Bladder cancers have been perhaps the best studied using a comparison of the two techniques. In some cases, the differences between flow cytometry and karyotypic analysis have been attributed to an increase in the proportion of large to small chromosomes, or the presence of large abnormal marker chromosomes *(39)*. In other cases, the differences have been attributed to an increase in DNA-binding dye uptake by tumor-specific chromosomes in flow cytometry studies. Different dyes have different affinities for AT or GC basepairs, and addition of AT-rich regions can increase or decrease the total fluorescence per nucleus, depending on the DNA-binding

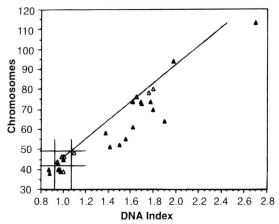

Fig. 5. Comparison of chromosome counts and DNA indices obtained by flow cytometry for 29 cell populations from 25 human breast tumors; low-grade tumors (△), high-grade tumors (▲). The limits of the flow cytometer-defined DNA-diploid range have been drawn on the diagram (lower left). Relevance of DNA ploidy as a measure of genetic deviation: A comparison of flow cytometry and cytogenetics in 25 cases of human breast cancer. Adapted from ref. *38*.

dye used. Small differences in DNA ploidy and specific aneusomies (particularly in DNA-diploid tumors that, by flow cytometry, have small increases or decreases in modal chromosome number) are likely a result of the lower sensitivity of flow cytometry. Studies in human breast cancers have demonstrated DNA-diploid tumors by flow cytometry that have 35–40 chromosomes by karyotyping *(38)*. These decreases in chromosome number are likely below the resolution of the flow cytometer used in the study.

Conclusions

An important advantage of DNA ploidy measurements is that they provide information on predominating mechanisms of karyotype evolution and the degree of inter- and intratumor heterogeneity for large numbers of solid tumors of different histogenetic origin. Such information is difficult or impossible to obtain on a similar scale using cytogenetic analysis, because of the inherent limitations discussed in this chapter. By pooling DNA indices for individual tumors of a given type, population histograms are obtained whose shape indicates the frequency distribution of ploidy variations for that tumor. For example, in breast, bladder, and testicular cancers, this distribution is bimodal, with clustering around near-diploid and DI ~ 1.5 *(40–42)*. Apparently, endoreduplication is a common event in karyotype evolution in these cancers, which is supported by flow cytometric *(41)* and by cytogenetic data *(43)*.

The degree of regional ploidy heterogeneity has long been underestimated in both cytometric and cytogenetic studies, because of limited sampling. With more extensive sampling, many primary breast *(44,45)* and prostate *(46)* cancers appear to contain multiple stemlines of differing ploidy and DNA index. This extensive regional heterogeneity may be a complicating factor in the clinical use of ploidy data and may explain why in breast cancers, DNA ploidy is not a strong prognostic factor *(28)*. Overall, a high concordance has been found between the DNA index of stemlines in primary tumors and their metastases, indicating that clonal evolution is limited once local-regional and distant metastases have been established. Thus, ploidy analysis of primary tumors and their metastases can yield information on clonal divergence, the stability of subclones, and their metastatic capacity. Although the stability of DNA indices after metastasis may help to discriminate multiple primary tumors from metastatic disease, as has been explored for ovarian carcinomas, molecular-genetic analysis using microsatellite markers provides a more powerful analytical technique *(47,48)*.

Finally, flow sorting of tumor cells on the basis of DNA ploidy can yield highly enriched tumor cell populations for molecular genetic analysis. This approach offers a direct method to study the question of clonal divergence at the DNA ploidy level as well as at the karyotypic level, and provides a basis for association for these changes with concomitant changes at the molecular-genetic level *(49)*.

References

1. Nowell P, Hungerford DA: A minute chromosome in human granulocytic leukemia. Science 132:1497–1499, 1960.
2. Caspersson T, Farber S, Folley G, et al.: Chemical differentiation along metaphase chromosomes. Exp Cell Res 49:219–222, 1968.

3. Latt SA, Brodie S, Munroe S: Optical studies of complexes of quinacrine with DNA and chromatin: implications for the fluorescence of cytological chromosome preperations. Chromosoma 49:17–28, 1974.

4. Rowley JD: A new consistent chromosomal abnormality in chronic myelogenous leukemia identified by quinacrine fluorescence. Nature 243:290–294, 1973.

5. Caspersson T: Uber den chemischen Aufbau der Strukturen des Zellkernes. Skand Arch Physiol 73(Suppl. 8):1–151, 1936.

6. Avery OT, MacLeod CM, McCarty MJ: Studies on the chemical nature of the substance inducing transformation of pneumococcal types: Induction of transformation by a desoxyribonucleic acid fraction isolated from Pneumococcus Type III. Exp Med 79:137–159, 1944.

7. Shapiro H: Practical Flow Cytometry, 3rd ed. New York: J Wiley, 1995.

8. Latt SA, Wohlleb JC: Optical studies of the interaction of 33258 Hoechst with DNA, chromatin, and metaphase chromosomes. Chromosoma 52: 297–316, 1975.

9. Rabinovitch PS: DNA ploidy and cell cycle analysis. In: Bauer KD, Duque RE, Shankey TV, (eds.), Clinical Flow Cytometry: Principles and Application. Baltimore; MD: Williams & Wilkins, pp. 117–142, 1993.

10. Darzynkiewicz Z, Traganos F, Kapuscinski J, Staiano-Coico L, Melamed MR: Accessibility of DNA in situ to various fluorochromes: relationship to chromatin changes during erythroid differentiation of Friend leukemia cells. Cytometry 5:355–363, 1984.

11. Braylan R: Lymphomas. In: Bauer KD, Duque RE, Shankey TV (eds.), Clinical Flow Cytometry: Principles and Application, Baltimore; MD: Williams & Wilkins, pp. 203–234, 1993.

12. Smeets AWGB, Pauwels RPE, Beck HLM, Feitz WFJ, Geraedts JPM, Debruyne FMJ, Laarakkers L, Vooijs GP, Ramaekers FCS: Comparison of tissue disaggregation techniques of transitional cell bladder carcinomas for flow cytometry and chromosomal analysis. Cytometry 8:14–19, 1987.

13. Ensley JF, Maciorowski Z, Pietraskiewicz H, Hassan H, Kish J, Al-Sarraf M, Jacobs J, Weaver A, Atkinson D, Crissman J: Solid tumor preperation for clinical application of flow cytometry. Cytometry 8:479–487, 1987.

14. Costa A, Silvestrini R, Del Bino G, Motta R: Implications of disaggregation procedures on biological representation of human solid tumors. Cell Tissue Kinet 20:171–180, 1987.

15. Pallavicini M, Taylor IW, Vindelov LL. Preperation of cell/nuclei suspensions from solid tumors for flow cytometry. In: Melamed MR, Lindmo T, Mendelsohn WL (eds.), Flow Cytometry and Sorting, 2nd ed. New York: Wiley-Liss; pp. 187–194, 1990.

16. Visscher D, Crissman JD: Dissociation of intact cells from tumors and normal tissues. In: Darzynkiewicz Z, Robinson JP, Crissman HA (eds.), Flow Cytometry. San Diego; Academic, pp. 1–12, 1994.

17. Hedley DW, Freidlander ML, Taylor IW, Musgrove L: Method for analysis of cellular DNA content of paraffin-embedded pathological material using flow cytometry. J Histochem Cytochem 31:1333–1335, 1983.

18. Hopman AH, Poddighe PJ, Smeets AW, Moesker O, Beck JL, Vooijs GP, Ramaekers FC: Detection of numerical chromosome aberrations in bladder cancer by in situ hybridization. Am J Pathol 135:1105–1117, 1989.
19. Hopman AH, Moeskar O, Smeets AW, Pauwels RP, Vooijs GP, Ramaekers FC: Numerical chromosome 1, 7, 9, and 11 aberrationss in bladder cancer detected by in situ hybridization. Cancer Res 51:644:651, 1991.
20. Hiddeman W, Schumann J, Amdreeff M, Barlogie B, Herman CJ, Leif RC, Mayall BH, Murphy RF, Sandberg AA: Convention on nomenclature for DNA cytometry. Cytometry 5:445–446, 1984.
21. Shankey TV, Rabinovitch PS, Bagwell B, Bauer KD, Duque RE, Hedley DW, Mayall BH, Wheeless L: Guidelines for the implementation of clinical DNA cytometry. Cytometry 14:472–477, 1994.
22. Coon JS, Deitch AD, de Vere White RW, Koss LG, Melamed MR, Reeder JE, Weinstein RS, Wersto RP, Wheeless LL: Interinstitutional variability in DNA flow cytometric analysis of tumors. The National Cancer Institute's Flow Cytometry Network Experience. Cancer 61:126–130, 1988.
23. Silvestrini R, the SICCAB Group for Quality Control of Cell Kinetic Determinations. Quality control for evaluation of the S-phase fraction by flow cytometry: a multicentric study. Comm Clin Cytometry 18:11–16, 1994.
24. Duque RE, Andreeff M, Braylan RC, Diamond LW, Peiper SC: Consensus review of the clinical utility of DNA flow cytometry in neoplastic hematopathology. Cytometry 14:492–496, 1993.
25. Wheeless LL, Hedley DW, Shankey TV. DNA cytometry consensus conference. Cytometry 14:471–500, 1993.
26. Wheeless LL, Badalamant RA, deVere White R, Fradet Y, Tribukait B: Consensus review of the clinical utility of DNA cytometry in bladder cancer. Cytometry 14:478–481, 1993
27. Bauer KD, Bagwell B, Giaretti W, Melamed M, Zarboe RJ, Witzig TE, Rabinovitch PS: Consensus review of the clinical utility of DNA cytometry in colorectal cancer. Cytometry 14:486–491, 1993.
28. Hedley DW, Clark GM, Cornelisse CJ, Killander D, Kute T, Merkel D. Consensus review of the clinical utility of DNA cytometry in carcinoma of the breast. Cytometry 14:482–485, 1993.
29. Shankey TV, Kallioniemi O-P, Koslowski JM, Lieber ML, Mayall B, Miller G, Smith GJ: Consensus review of the clinical utility of DNA content cytometry in prostate cancer. Cytometry 14:497–500, 1993.
30. Shankey TV: Antibodies to intermediate filament proteins as probes for multiparameter flow cytometry. In: Darzynkiewicz Z, Robinson JP, Crissman HA (eds.), Flow Cytometry, Part B. San Diego, CA: Academic, pp. 209–229, 1994.
31. Zarbo RH, Visscher DW, Crissman JD: Two-color multiparametric method for flow cytometric DNA analysis of carcinomas using staining for cytokeratin and leukocyte-common antigen. Anal Quant Cytol Histol 11:391–402, 1989.

32. Leuchtenberger C, Leuchtenberger R, Davis AM: A microspectrophotometric study of the deoxyribonucleic acid (DNA) content in cells of normal and malignant tissue. Am J Pathol 30:65–85, 1954.

33. Bertino B, Knape WA, Pytlinska M, Strauss K, Hammou JC: A comparative study of DNA content as measured by flow cytometry and image analysis in 1864 specimens. Anal Cell Pathol 6:377–394, 1994.

34. Uyterlinde AM, Baak JP, Schipper NW, Peterse H, Matze E, Meijer CJ: Further evaluation of the prognostic value of morphometric and flow cytometric parameters in breast-cancer patients with long follow-up. Int J Cancer 45:1–7, 1990.

35. Böcking A, Giroud F, Reith A: Consensus report of the ESACP task force on standardization of diagnostic DNA image cytometry. Anal Cell Pathol 8:67–74, 1995.

36. Rabinovitch PS: DNA content histogram and cell-cycle analysis. In: Darzynkiewicz Z, Robinson JP, Crissman HA (eds.), Flow Cytometry, Part A 2nd ed. San Diego, CA: Academic, pp. 263–296, 1994.

37. Weinberg DS: Relative applicability of image analysis and flow cytometry in clinical medicine. In: Bauer KD, Duque RE, Shankey TV (eds.), Clinical Flow Cytometry: Principles and Application. Baltimore; MD: Williams & Wilkins, pp. 359–371, 1993.

38. Remvikos Y, Gerbault-Seurreau M, Vielh P, Zafrani B, Margdelenat H, Dutrillaux B: Relevance of DNA ploidy as a measure of genetic deviation: A comparison of flow cytometry and cytogenetics in 25 cases of human breast cancer. Cytometry 9:612–618, 1988.

39. Tribukait B, Granberg-Öhman I, Wijkström H: Flow cytometric and cytogenetic studies in human tumors: a comparison and discussion of the differences in modal values obtained by the two methods. Cytometry 7:194–199, 1986.

40. Hedley D: Breast cancer. In: Bauer KD, Duque RE, Shankey TV (eds.), Clinical Flow Cytometry: Principles and Application. Baltimore; MD: Williams & Wilkins, pp. 247–261, 1993.

41. Shackney SE, Berg G, Simon SR, Cohen J, Amina S, Pommersheim W, Yakulis R, Wang S, Uhl M, Smith CA, Pollice AA, Hartsock RJ: Origins and clinical implications of aneuploidy in early bladder cancer. Comm Clin Cytometry 22:307–316, 1995.

42. Oosterhuis JW, Castedo Sergio MMJ, Jong Bd, Corneliosse CJ, Dam A, Sleiffer Dth, Schraffordt Koops H: Ploidy of primary germ cell tumors of the testis. Lab Invest 60:14–21, 1989.

43. Dutrillaux B, Gerbeault-Seureau M, Remvikos Y, Zafrani B, Prieur M: Breast cancer genetic evolution. I. Data from cytogenetics and DNA content. Breast Cancer Res Treatment 19:245–255, 1991.

44. Beerman H, Smit VTHBM, Kluin PM, Bosning BA, Hermans J, Cornelisse CJ: Flow cytometric analysis of DNA stemline heterogeneity in prmary and metastatic breast cancer. Cytometry 12:145–157, 1991.

45. Bosning BA, Beerman H, Kuipers-Dijkshoorn N. Fleuren GJ, Cornilesse CJ: High levels of DNA index heterogeneity in advanced breast carcinomas. Cancer 71:382–391, 1993.

46. Shankey TV, Jin J-K, Doughlerty S, Flanigan RC, Graham S, Pyle JM: DNA ploidy and proliferation heterogeneity in human prostate cancers. Cytometry 21:30–39, 1995.

47. Smit VTHBM, Fleuren GJ, Van Houwelingen JC, Zegveld ST, Kuipers-Dijkshoorn NJ, Cornelisse CJ: Flow cytometric analysis of synchronously occurring multiple malignant tumors of the female genital tract. Cancer 66:1843–1849, 1990.

48. Abeln ECA, Kuipers-Dijkshoorn NJ, Berns EMJJ, Henzen-Longmans SC, Fleuren GJ, Cornelisse CJ: Molecular genetic evidence for unifocal origin of advanced epithelial ovarian cancer and for minor clonal divergence. Brit J Cancer 72:1330–1336, 1995.

49. Abeln ECA, Corver WE, Kuipers-Dijkshoorn NJ, Fleuren GJ, Cornelisse CJ: Molecular genetic analysis of flow sorted ovarian tumor cells: improved detection of loss of heterozygosity. Br J Cancer 70:225–256, 1994.

Chapter 3

In Situ Hybridization and Comparative Genomic Hybridization

Anton H. N. Hopman, Christina E. M. Voorter, Ernst J. M. Speel, and Frans C. S. Ramaekers

Introduction

Quantitative and structural aberrations in the genomic content of malignancies or premalignant lesions are in many cases correlated with the prognosis of the disease. Since such genetic changes are central to the initiation and progression of neoplasms, techniques have been developed for their detection and characterization.

Cytogenetic, flow cytometric, and molecular genetic studies have provided convincing evidence that development and progression of human malignancies involves multiple genetic changes. In this respect, karyotyping of tumors allows the determination of numerical and/or structural chromosomal defects. Chromosome banding techniques play an important role, mainly in the detection of genetic aberrations of hematological malignancies. Although karyotyping is routinely applicable in leukemia, karyotyping of solid tumors is often very cumbersome; selection of a fast growing subpopulation could give unreliable information about the total tumor population. Moreover, paraffin-embedded material from patients with known clinical outcome is as yet not available for such

From: *Human Cytogenetic Cancer Markers*   Edited by S. R. Wolman and S. Sell
Humana Press Inc., Totowa, NJ

cytogenetic analyses. Molecular genetic techniques such as Southern blot, restriction fragment length polymorphism (RFLP) analyses, polymerase chain reaction (PCR)-based microsatellite analysis, or single-stranded conformation polymorphism (SSCP) analysis provide information about changes in the number of copies of DNA sequences, loss of heterozygosity, or even mutations in the gene. Because of the integral nature of these approaches, such studies are limited to description of the characteristics of tumors as a whole, without further information about the heterogeneity of cells within the tumor.

The fluorescence *in situ* hybridization (FISH or ISH) technique using chromosome-specific probes allows a targeted detection of genetic aberrations in metaphase chromosomes and in the interphase nucleus, in the latter case referred to as "interphase cytogenetics." The developments in probe-labeling techniques, the generation of different types of probes, and the technical improvements for processing of biological material, have now reached a point that the FISH technique can be considered as a significant adjunct to more established methods for detection and characterization of genetic aberrations in cancer. The FISH methods have not only been applied to several types of malignancies, but have also been applied successfully to a variety of cell and tissue preparations, such as single cells isolated from solid cancers collected as paraffin-embedded material or as frozen tissue blocks. The FISH technique offers the possibility to correlate genomic changes with cellular phenotypes on a single cell basis. A correlation with histological features, with proliferative index, or with protein markers has become feasible because of new protocols for application of FISH to tissue sections or FISH in combination with immunocytochemical approaches.

Recently, comparative genomic *in situ* hybridization (CGH) has been developed based on ISH using isolated tumor DNA as a probe; it is possible to generate a copy number karyotype from a solid tumor by comparing the DNA of the tumor with that of normal cells. In contrast with the targeted analysis of FISH, neither intact tumor cells nor the preparation of high-quality metaphase spreads from tumor cells is required. Furthermore, CGH enables a complete mapping of genetic imbalances of the total tumor genome and is not restricted to the region of a specific FISH probe or RFLP probe.

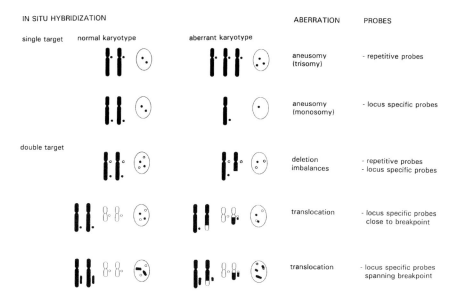

Fig. 1. Schematic illustration of FISH on metaphase chromosomes and interphase nuclei.

DNA Probes and Probe Modification

Probes

For the detection of numerical and structural chromosome aberrations in metaphase preparations and interphase nuclei several different types of probes are available (*1–8*) (*see* Fig. 1).

Probes Recognizing Highly Repetitive Sequences

DNA probes recognizing tandemly repeated DNA sequences (referred to as repetitive probes, repeat sequence probes, or satellite probes), mostly present in the centromeric and telomeric regions, are now applicable in daily practice. The sequences targeted by these probes are typically alpha satellite or satellite III sequences that are usually repeated several hundred- to several thousand-fold (*9*). This results in DNA targets up to several thousand kilobase pairs localized in the compact centromeric and telomeric regions of the individual chromosomes. Such repetitive probes have been developed for most of the human chromosomes and many are now

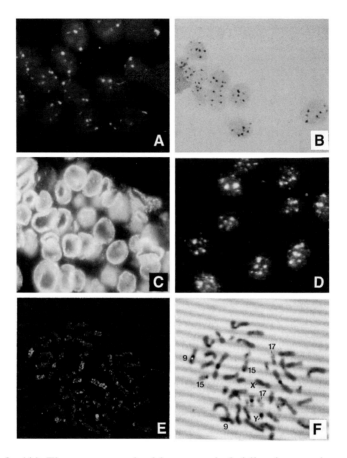

Fig. 2. (**A**) Fluorescence double-target hybridization on interphase nuclei isolated from a bladder tumor showing trisomy for chromosome 1 (Biotin-labeled) and disomy for chromosome 18 (Digoxigenin-labeled). Centromeric repeat probes were detected in TRITC- and FITC-labeled secondary antibodies, respectively. (**B**) Brightfield detection of triple-target ISH in T24 cells. DNA probes used were centromeric repeat probes for (sub)centromeric regions of chromosomes 1 (biotin-labeled), 7 (digoxigenin-labeled), and 17 (fluorescein-labeled). Detection of the chromosomes 1, 7, and 17 in brown (peroxidase-DAB), red (alkaline phosphatase-Fast Red), and green (peroxidase-TMB), respectively. (**C**) Combined immunocytochemistry for lamin and FISH with a centromeric repeat probe for chromosome 7 (FITC-labeled). Lamin was used to mark the nuclear contour and detected with alkaline phosphatase labeled antibodies and developed with Fast Red (red fluorescence).

commercially available. The FISH signal intensity of these probes is high and the hybridization signal is tightly localized within metaphase and interphase nuclei. Since the number of signals is constant during the cell cycle, these probes can be scored rapidly and accurately *(1–8,10–13) (see* Fig. 2A,B).

Chromosome Painting Probes

Another type of DNA probe comprises many different elements distributed densely and more or less continuously over the chromosome so that the probe specifically stains almost the complete chromosome or human chromosome fragment *(14,15).* These so-called whole chromosome probes or chromosome painting probes, are based on chromosome purification by fluorescence-activated sorting and subsequent cloning into a vector. Different cloning systems have been developed. Painting probes are now commercially available for several human chromosomes. ISH with these probes stains entire chromosomes in metaphase and in interphase nuclei. In the interphase nucleus the FISH domain size is much larger than for the repeat sequence probes. Domain overlap and/or fragmentation hampers chromosome counting in tumors with a complex karyotype.

Locus-Specific Probes

These probes are useful for analysis of small DNA sequences. They target to unique sequences ranging in size from about 2 kb to a few hundred. Different cloning systems e.g., cosmid, phage, or plasmid vectors and yeast artificial chromosomes (YAC), have been used *(1,3,4,6,8).* For chromosome painting probes as well as

---

Fig. 2. *(continued)* **(D)** Nuclear proliferation marker Ki67-Ag stained with alkaline phosphatase-Fast Red (red fluorescence) and chromosome 7 (FITC-labeled). **(E,F)** Comparative genomic hybridization. Metaphase spread of normal human lymphocytes hybridized with DNA from a bladder tumor detected by FITC (tumor DNA) and TRITC (control DNA). (E) False color image of FITC to TRITC fluorescence ratio of the metaphase spread. Chromosomal regions over-represented in the tumor genome are displayed in green, whereas under-represented regions are shown in red. (F) Digital inverted image of the DAPI-counterstained chromosomes to allow chromosomal identification. (*See* color insert following p. 212.)

specific locus probes, suppression of hybridization signals from ubiquitous repeated sequences, such as the Alu and Kpn1 elements, is necessary. This can be achieved by using either total human DNA or Cot1 DNA in a reannealing procedure, and is, therefore, also referred to as chromosome *in situ* suppression (CISS) hybridization. In interphase cytogenetics a high hybridization efficiency is obtained with probes of 30 kb (unique sequences) or larger for analysis of the copy number and structural integrity of several genes (e.g., tumor suppressor genes, oncogenes). In some cases overlapping probes (contig probes) are used to span a large target on the chromosome to generate a larger signal. Several probes e.g., for the detection of translocations (e.g., *bcr/abl*), or oncogenes (N-*MYC*, HER-2/*neu*), are available. Additional probes will be available in the near future as a result of the human genome project.

Probe Modification

Probes can be radioactively or non-isotopically labeled. Non-isotopic ISH has the advantage of good topological resolution, no environmental hazards, short procedure times, and relatively easy labeling. Several methods for non-isotopic detection are described (*16–19*). They are based on the introduction of a reporter molecule into the DNA probe that can then be detected (immuno)cytochemically after hybridization to its specific target. In the last decade about 20 different hapten- and fluorochrome-labeling procedures have been developed. These haptens or fluorochromes are incorporated in the probe by nick translation, random priming, or during PCR, using hapten- or fluorochrome-labeled triphosphates. Currently, three of them, the biotin, digoxigenin, and fluorochrome labeling, are the most frequently used hapten modifications.

Processing of Biological Material

Standard tissue fixatives, such as methanol/acetic acid (3/1) used for karyotyping analysis, 70% ethanol for flow cytometric analyses, methanol/acetone for cytological analysis, and 4% formaldehyde in phosphate-buffered saline (PBS) for histopathological analyses, are fully compatible with the ISH procedure (*1,6,16,20*). Depending on the amount of cytoplasm or crosslinking of nuclear proteins, a proteolytic pretreatment is needed to permeabilize the cell for macromolecular reagents such as DNA probes and antibodies, and to allow ISH of the probe.

Single cell suspensions can be easily prepared by mechanical or enzymatic disaggregation of fresh solid tumors. Also direct imprints of the fresh tumor may be used *(21)*. Nuclear suspensions can be prepared by enzymatic disaggregation of thick frozen or fixed tissue samples and cytological preparations (e.g., effusions, fine needle aspiration biopsies). A standard digestion schedule of 100 µg pepsin/mL in 0.01N HCl for 20 min could be used for several tumor types, including bladder cancer, renal cell cancer, leukemia, and several different ethanol-fixed tumor cell lines. Cell or nuclear suspensions can be cytocentrifuged on a slide for FISH. Protocols for efficient interphase cytogenetics of solid tumors on single cells have been developed and are based on methanol/acetic acid fixation or enzymatic pretreatments.

Sections can be made from paraffin-embedded tissue material as well as frozen tissue. A limited number of studies have dealt with the application of ISH for the study of chromosomal aberrations in tissue sections (e.g., *20,22–25)*. Frozen sections can be mildly fixed in methanol/acetone or more strongly in formaldehyde in PBS. Proteolytic digestion should be modified so as not to overdigest the cells resulting in a complete loss of morphology. As opposed to frozen tissue samples, tuning of proteolytic pretreatment for routinely processed paraffin-embedded tissue sections is more difficult. The proteolytic pretreatment step has to be optimized for each paraffin block. This can be done by exposure to a series of digestion time periods. The success rate of ISH, in general, is mainly dictated by the accessibility of the target DNA. Proteolytic enzymes such as pepsin and proteinase K are generally and efficiently used to permeabilize the tissue section to allow penetration of modified probes and antibodies. Additional steps to improve this ISH reaction have been suggested. These include:

1. Deparaffinization in warm xylol;
2. Freezing and thawing of the cells;
3. Prolonged digestion time;
4. Increased denaturation temperatures; and
5. Different treatment steps prior to the enzymatic digestion.

However, no data concerning reproducibility on large series of paraffin-embedded tumor blocks are available. To improve the efficiency of the ISH procedure using pepsin in 0.2N HCl for permeabilization of the section, we included a DNA-nucleohistone denaturation or dissociation step by heating the section in hot 1M sodium thiocyanate (80°C) *(25)*. Pretreatment of the sections in this way greatly improved the effect of the proteolytic digestion step, resulting in reproducible and efficient ISH results. A standard digestion time for a 4–6-μm thick section is 30 min at 37°C in 4 mg pepsin/mL 0.2M HCl and a denaturation time of 8 min at 80°C.

Hybridization and Immunocytochemical Detection

Modified probes are hybridized under standard conditions for the different types of probes. Hybridization mixtures contain formamide, salt, carrier DNA or RNA, and dextran sulfate. Protocols have been developed to denature target DNA and probe DNA simultaneously or separately. After hybridization, in most cases overnight, washing procedures are used to remove specifically bound probe. After these washings, the hybridized probes are detected cytochemically.

In most cases the haptens are detected by standard affinity cytochemical techniques as indicated in Table 1 *(17–19)*. In the case of biotin, the reporter molecule can be detected with labeled (strept)avidin molecules or monoclonal antibiotin followed by incubation with labeled secondary antibodies. Labels can be fluorochromes, like fluorescein (FITC), rhodamine (TRITC) or aminomethyl-coumarin-acetic acid (AMCA), or enzymes such as peroxidase and alkaline phosphatase (*see* Table 2). With fluorochrome-labeled DNA probes, no immunological detection is needed, although a cytochemical amplification step to obtain a higher signal intensity using antifluorochrome antibodies and secondary antibodies is possible. The choice of detection system will depend on the area of application of the ISH and choice of microscope (*see* Tables 1 and 2). When enzymatic detection (visualization by brightfield microscopy) is used, the preparation will be permanent. Moreover, detection and evaluation are not influenced by autofluorescence of the specimen, and different substrates can

Table 1
Detection of Labeled Probes[a]

Label	Immunochemical detection/affinity detection system		
	Primary layer	Secondary layer	Tertiary layer
Biotin	Avidin[b]		
	Avidin[b]	Biotinylated-anti-avidin	Avidin[b]
	Mouse-antibiotin[b]	Rabbit-anti-mouse[b]	
		Biotinylated-anti-mouse	Avidin[b]
Dig	Mouse-anti-dig[b]	Anti-mouse[b]	
		Biotinylated-anti-mouse	Avidin[b]
		Dig-labeled-anti-mouse	Anti-dig[b]
	Rabbit-anti-dig[b]	Anti-rabbit[b]	
FITC	Rabbit-anti-FITC	Anti-rabbit[b]	
	Mouse-anti-FITC	Anti-mouse[b]	

[a]Dig, digoxigenin; FITC, fluorescein.
[b]Proteins are conjugated with a fluorochrome or enzyme.

result in different colors of precipitated products. With fluorescent detection (visualization by fluorescence microscope), a higher detection intensity is obtained (detection limit up to a few kilobases) and the localization is better. In the latter case, simultaneous detection of several DNA targets in one and the same cell, chromosome spread, or tissue section, is possible with probes carrying different haptens, and which are then visualized with different distinguishable affinity systems *(26–32)*. The resolution between two different ISH signals using different fluorochromes, e.g., fluorescein (FITC, yellow-green) in combination with rhodamine (TRITC or Texas Red, red) or coumarin (AMCA, blue) is excellent. For example, in chronic myelogenous leukemia (CML) the reciprocal translocation responsible is characterized by the fusion of the *BCR* gene on chromosome 22 and the *ABL* oncogene on chromosome 9. By red labeling at the *bcr* locus and yellow-green labeling at the *abl* locus, the so-called Philadelphia chromosome is visualized in the interphase nucleus by a colocalization of red and yellow-green *(3,26) (see* Fig. 1). Similar approaches have been used to analyze other translocations. Multitarget FISH with multiple-color

Table 2
Nonradioactive ISH Detection Systems[a]

Enzymes	Substrate[b]	Detection[b]
Fluorochromes	FITC	Green, yellow (FM)
	AMCA	Blue (FM)
	TRITC; CY3	Red (FM)
	TexRed	Red (FM)
	CY5	Infrared (FM)
Peroxidase	H_2O_2/DAB	Brown color (BFM)
	H_2O_2/chloronaphthol	Purple color (BFM)
	H_2O_2/TMB	Green color (BFM)
Alkaline	BCIP/NBT	Blue color (BFM)
phospatase	Naphthol-p/Fast red	Red color (BFM)
		Red fluorescence (FM)
	Naphthol-p/New Fuchsin	Red color (BFM)
		Red fluorescence (FM)

[a]Double enzymatic detection based on peroxidase and alkaline phosphatase. Multiple fluorescence detection based on combinations of green, red, and blue fluorescence or mixed ratios of fluorochromes.

[b]Abbreviations: BCIP, bromo-chloro-indolyl phosphate; BFM, bright field microscopy; DAB, diaminobenzidine; FM, fluorescence microscopy; NBT, nitro blue tetrazolium; TMB, tetramethylbenzidine.

probes now enables the detection of 2–12 different probes in a single cell based on combinations of the three fluorescent colors mentioned *(27–32)*. Multiple-target FISH can be used to demonstrate numerical as well as structural chromosome aberrations and to interrelate such genetic changes.

For brightfield microscopical evaluation, detection of probes is performed by using different enzymes and color-producing substrates *(see* Table 2). Double enzymatic detection is mostly based on peroxidase and alkaline phosphatase *(28,33)*, whereas a triple enzymatic detection can be performed by combining, for example, two peroxidase and one alkaline phosphatase reaction *(34)* *(see* Fig. 2B).

Recently, a very sensitive detection system, based on haptenized substrates for peroxidase, has been developed *(35)*. Biotinylated tyramine (BT) as a substrate enables the accumulation of a large number of biotin molecules that subsequently can be cyto-chemically detected. The first results already demonstrate that the ISH detection limit of DNA and RNA sequences for fluorescence and bright field microscopy can be further increased *(36,37)*. Also, fluorochrome-labeled tyramines have been synthesized enabling a direct fluorescent enzymatic deposit reaction. It is to be expected that this amplification system in paraffin-embedded tissue sections will enable a detection sensitivity that is comparable with hybridizations in methanol/acetic acid fixed fresh material *(36)*.

Evaluation and Interpretation of ISH Signals

Fluorescent ISH signals are evaluated by counting spots in from a few hundred up to several thousands of interphase nuclei *(11,20,38–40)*. The following criteria can be applied for a proper evaluation with minimal inter- and intra-observer variation:

1. Overlapping nuclei are not counted;
2. Only nuclei in which the ISH signals have more or less the same homogeneous fluorescence intensity are evaluated, unless indications of a partial deletion or polymorphism exist;
3. Minor hybridization signals, which can be recognized by a lower intensity and spot size, are not counted; and
4. Fluorescent spots or patches of fluorescence in nuclei are included when the signals are completely separated.

In case of centromeric repeat probes, several sources can lead to an improper evaluation of the chromosome copy number *(20)*. The percentage of cells without ISH signal differs from experiment to experiment and percentages up to 10% artificial "nullisomy" are not uncommon. The percentage of nuclei with one ISH signal in diploid cells ranges from 5–20%, again depending on the efficiency of the ISH procedure, the chromosome, and the type of tissue. There is always a certain percentage of nuclei that show one ISH signal as a result of colocalization of ISH signals. One should realize that in a mixed normal cell and tumor cell population the number of interphase nuclei to be analyzed for a valid evaluation of a monosomy or trisomy will depend on the frequency of tumor cells in the total cell population *(38)*.

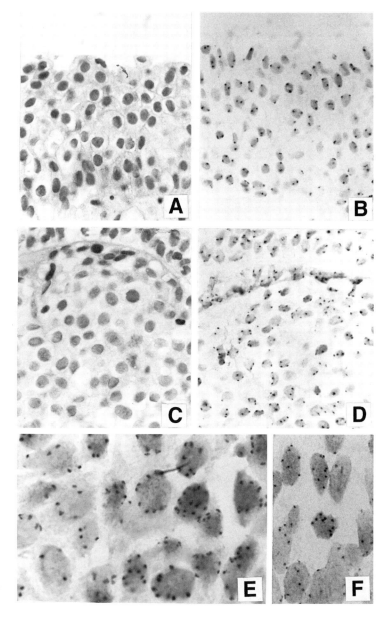

Fig. 3. Hybridization results on 4–6-µm thick tissue sections of paraffin-embedded bladder tumors using a (sub)centromeric repeat probe for chromosome 1 developed with peroxidase-DAB. (**A,B**) Normal urothelial cells, with disomy for chromosome 1. As a result of nuclear truncation, nuclei with no, one, and two signals are seen.

Not only the frequency, but also the percentage, of false positive cells is important. The percentage of false-positive cells is strongly dependent on the nature of pretreatment of the biological material. Some typical pitfalls that may occur during the interpretation of chromosome aneuploidy using ISH can be summarized as follows *(20)*:

1. Pairing of chromosomes results in one ISH signal that could be interpretated as a monosomy *(41)*;
2. Translocations of short arm sequences from chromosome 15 onto other D-group chromosomes occur frequently. ISH studies with a chromosome 15 repetitive probe will then show three ISH signals in the interphase nuclei suggesting a trisomy for chromosome 15 *(42)*; and
3. chromosomal polymorphisms in chromosomes 1 and 9 result in heterogeneity of ISH signal intensities with chromosome-specific satellite DNA sequences.

The unique advantages of ISH on tumor tissue sections (*see* Fig. 3) as compared to ISH on isolated tumor cells can be summarized as follows *(23–25,43,44)*:

1. Local tumor cell areas with chromosome aberrations can be recognized in the sections and be correlated with histologic appearance;
2. No selection of cells occurs as a result of the isolation procedure;
3. Heterogeneity, as well as tetraploidization within the tumor, can be recognized;
4. It allows retrospective analysis using archival material (also after isolation of cells).

In principle the same criteria can be followed for the evaluation of ISH signals in paraffin sections or frozen sections as are used for single cell suspensions *(20,25)*. However, for sections the percentage

---

Fig. 3. (*continued*) **(C,D)** Nest of "von Brunn" in the bladder consisting of inbudded surface epithelium, with cells aberrant for chromosome 1. Overlying epithelium showed a normal copy number for chromosome 1. Counterstained with Mayers hematoxylin (A,C). **(E,F)** Transitional cell carcinoma marked by nuclear variability and hyperchromasia. In this case the nuclei contain extra homologs of chromosome 1, up to 20 copies/nucleus. (F) Hybridization on mitotic figure illustrating the high chromosome copy number.

of cells with no or one signal for normal ploidy will be higher (about 25%) as compared to the single cell suspension (about 5%). In paraffin and frozen sections the results have to be evaluated more qualitatively (selection of tumor area, normal tissue, stromal cells), since no simple correction factors for truncation of nuclei are available. Recent statistical approaches to analyze monosomies and trisomies have been published that attempt to deal with the quantitative evaluation of tissue section hybridizations *(43,45)*. Others have calculated the ratio between spot numbers as detected in the normal (lymphocyte cells) and tumor cells *(44)*. We compared the number of ISH signals as detected in ethanol fixed, single-cell suspensions of a large series of bladder tumors to the ISH results obtained in paraffin sections of the same tumors. By hybridization of serial sections (in one experiment using the same section thickness and the same proteolytic pretreatment) or double-target hybridizations using different chromosomal probes, the imbalance between chromosome copy numbers can be determined. In cell-dense areas, overlap of nuclei complicates the evaluation of signals per individual nucleus, since the morphology is partly disrupted during the hybridization. In these cases a lamin immunocytochemical staining of the nuclear contour facilitates evaluation of the ISH signals *(46)* (Fig. 2C). Hybridization of thick tissue sections and evaluation of ISH signals by confocal microscopy is another approach, albeit rather complicated for routine application *(47)*. An alternative approach for valid detection of the true chromosome copy number in paraffin, as well as frozen sections, is the isolation of nuclei from thick tissue sections. Truncation of nuclei will be reduced as compared to the thin sections used for direct hybridization on sections *(48,49,22)*.

Multiparameter Analysis

The FISH technique offers the opportunity to correlate genomic changes with cellular phenotypes on a single cell basis *(50–54)*. The application of alkaline phosphatase (APase)-Fast Red reaction for the immunocytochemical (ICC) detection of proteins before the ISH step has been reported recently. This detection method produces a strongly red fluorescent reaction product with a virtually permanent character that is stable during pretreatments (enzymatic) for ISH and during the total ISH procedure. The accurate detection of these parameters in the same cell makes this procedure extremely suitable for detection of tumor cell heterogeneity, rare event detection, and in cases where only a few cells can be obtained for analysis (e.g., in aspirate cytology or in biopsy material). Furthermore, in cases where extensive proteolytic digestion for FISH is needed (i.e., in paraffin sections), ICC based on APase-Fast Red can be advantageous. By this approach cellular markers such as neural cell adhesion molecules, cytokeratin filaments, lamin, or the Ki67 antigen have been combined with ISH using centromere-specific DNA probes (*see* Fig. 2D).

Comparative Genomic Hybridization Methods

Recently, the technique of comparative genomic ISH has been developed *(55)* and pioneered by different groups *(55–59)*. With this technique, based on the biochemical isolation of the tumor DNA, it is possible to generate a copy number karyotype from a solid tumor by comparing its DNA with that of normal cells. In contrast with the targeted analysis of FISH, no intact tumor cells are needed nor is the preparation of high quality metaphase spreads from tumor cells required. Furthermore, CGH enables a total mapping of genetic imbalances in the whole tumor genome and is not restricted to the FISH probe regions only. The principle of the CGH procedure is outlined schematically in Fig. 4. Genomic test DNA (tumor DNA), isolated from a tumor specimen, is labeled with a hapten (e.g., biotin), whereas genomic control DNA, isolated from normal lymphocytes, is labeled with another hapten (digoxigenin). An equimolar mixture of these differently labeled genomic DNA probes is used for CISS on normal metaphase spreads. The hybridized test (tumor) and control DNA sequences are detected by different fluorochromes (e.g., FITC, TRITC). Since test and control DNA sequences compete for the same target chromosomes (sequences), the relative copy number of homologous sequences is directly reflected by the ratio of the FITC/TRITC fluorescence intensities. The fluorescence signal intensities are measured by quantative microscopy by means of (cooled) CCD cameras and ratios are calculated by software *(see 55,57,60)*. After determination of thresholds, the balanced copy numbers and relative loss or gain of sequences can be detected. Karyotyping is done on the basis

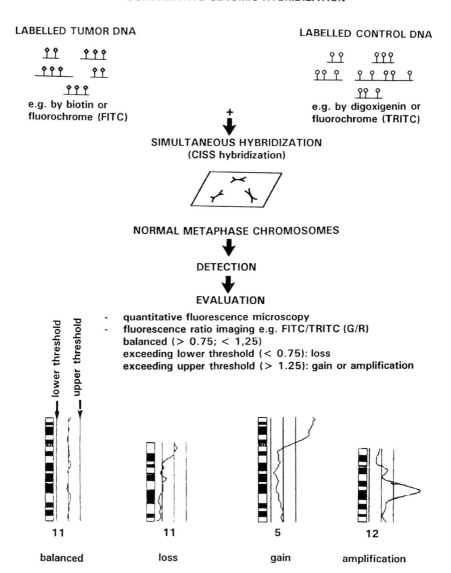

Fig. 4. Schematic illustration of CGH.

of DAPI staining of the chromosomes (*see* Figs. 2E and F). Amplifications and deletions of 1–10 Mb are detectable, and this sensitivity will be further increased by optimization of the method in the next few years. For certain amplifications even smaller regions (~100 kb) can be detected when such an amplicon is present in excess (20 times or more). In this respect double minutes (DM) or homogeneous staining regions (HSR) present in the tumor were shown to be the amplified sequences as analyzed by targeted analyses after CGH. Imbalances of chromosomes or chromosome arms can also be detected with CGH. As compared with the other techniques available to date for evaluation of genetic aberrations of solid tumors, CGH has several major advantages:

1. A complete copy number karyotype can be obtained with this technique, truly representing the isolated tumor DNA. As compared with (targeted) FISH, the specificity is not limited to the analysis of a specific target gene or chromosomal region, but covers the whole genome.
2. Since the technique is based on biochemical isolation of DNA, the amount of available tumor material is no longer limiting, because that DNA can be increased by standard PCR technology. However, the DNA must be amplified by e.g., degenerated oligonucleotide primer (DOP)-PCR, which is a general DNA amplification method.
3. Single cells, frozen tissue blocks or sections, as well as paraffin-embedded tumor tissue samples can be used.

This approach also has its limitations and problems. Balanced chromosome rearrangements and information about the composition of marker chromosomes cannot be detected. Furthermore, since only the ratio between fluorescence intensities is measured, no information about ploidy is obtained. Additional targeted analyses to determine the chromosome ploidy can be made. To enable a CGH analysis, at least 50% of the tumor source should consist of tumor cells, because mixing with DNA from normal cells will effectively mask chromosomal gains and losses. To enrich the fraction of tumor cells from a biopsy, flow cytometric sorting on the basis of DNA content and/or specific immunocytochemical markers can be performed. DNA from these sorted cells can then be isolated and amplified by DOP-PCR. Isolation of different parts of a tumor by microdissection or immunosorting also enables the study of tumor heterogeneity.

Technical Aspects

Although the protocol for CGH is very similar to FISH protocols, a considerable amount of time and energy is needed to establish

CGH even in laboratories experienced in molecular cytogenetics. Success seems to be dependent on a summation of numerous steps in the protocol that have been extensively reviewed *(56–58,60–64)*. These steps include:

1. Specimen preparation: This is one of the most critical parameters for successful CGH. Pretreatment of the metaphase chromosomes by proteolytic digestion can improve the accessibility of the probes. However, such treatment may also result in a higher granularity of the signal generated by the genomic DNA, hampering the CGH analysis. Furthermore, an overdigestion of the chromosomes will hamper karyotyping after CGH as a result of a poor banding quality (DAPI reverse banding).

2. Probe labeling: DNA probes (control and test DNA) can be labeled either directly (FITC-dXTP and TRITC-dXTP) or indirectly (Digoxigenin-dXTP and Biotin-dXTP). Although directly labeled probes generate smooth fluorescence along the chromosomes, which is preferred for the analysis, indirect detection procedures are also appropriate. Labeling is performed by nick translation. The length of the probe molecules after labeling is a very critical factor for good quality comparative genomic hybridizations. It is important to adjust not only for the length of the fragments, but also to achieve similar lengths for test and control DNA. Tuning of DNase 1 for nicking during the polymerase reaction is critical to achieve this. Fragment length should vary between 0.5–2 kb (in comparison the length for targeted analysis is 100–200 nucleotides).

   Probe isolation: CGH analysis requires about 1 µg of labeled DNA for hybridization. Thus far CGH has been applied to analyze genetic alterations in tumor tissue. However, since the amount of tumor is often too small to yield DNA sufficient for CGH, amplification of the DNA by universal PCR can be applied. The possibility of performing CGH from very few cells by combining it with DOP-PCR *(65)* has been demonstrated. The lowest number of cells to yield DNA needed for amplification in CGH reactions is estimated in the range of 5–10. Whether or not one to two cells can be used for this type of analysis is still to be determined.

3. Suppression: The large amounts of probe DNA provide high frequencies of labeled interspersed repetitive sequences to be suppressed. Suppression of these sequences must be as complete as possible to enable proper fluorescence intensity measurements. An excess of unlabeled Cot1 DNA is used and/or the annealing

time (after probe denaturation) is prolonged. Typical concentrations of Cot1 DNA are 40–70 µg/1 µg test DNA and control DNA. The intensity of hybridization signals in CGH experiments is improved by extension of the hybridization time from overnight to 2 or 3 d.

4. Equipment: CGH analysis by quantitative measurements put high demands on the equipment necessary for evaluation *(60)*. This includes the microscope, the camera system, and the computer software. The relevant instrumentation parameters specific for CGH are described in detail elsewhere. These parameters include hardware requirements: microscope optics, filters, CCD camera, image analysis hardware, and software requirements: image acquisition, image quality assessment, quantitation of fluorescence and ratio profiles. The guidelines are discussed and agreed to by research groups that have developed, pioneered, and used CGH image analyis. These efforts have resulted in commercially available systems as supplied (e.g., by Applied Imaging, Vysis, Meta Systems, Oncor, etc.).

Applications

The CGH technique has been utilized to detect chromosomal regions gained or lost in a variety of tumor specimens, derived cell lines, and archived specimens. These include breast, bladder, gliomas, liposarcomas, colon cancer, head and neck carcinomas, lung carcinomas, or leukemia *(66–73)*. Microdissection combined with universal DNA amplification will enable the analysis of small tumor areas or samples from which only limited numbers of cells can be obtained. At present a few hundred cells are necessary for a routine CGH analysis. However, the lowest limit of cells needed for CGH has still to be determined. To validate the impact of detected genetic data by CGH and complementarity of different methods, CGH results are to be compared with data obtained by RFLP analysis and targeted FISH.

Acknowledgment

This work was supported by the Netherlands Organization for Scientific Research NWO, 900-534-102 and Dutch Cancer Society IKL 88-7, 92-7.

References

1. T, Cremer T: Chromosome analysis by non-isotopic in situ hybridization. In: Human Cytogenetics: A Practical Approach. Oxford, UK: IRL Press, pp. 157–192, 1992.
2. Trask B: Fluorescence in situ hybridization: applications in cytogenetics and gene mapping. Trends Genet 7:149–154, 1991.
3. Tkachuk DC, Pinkel D, Kuo W-L, Weier H-U, Gray J: Clinical applications of fluorescence in situ hybridization. Genet Anal Technol Appl 8:67–74, 1991.
4. Bentz M, Döhner H, Cabot G, Lichter P: Fluorescence in situ hybridization in leukemias: "the FISH are spawning." Leukemia 8:1447–1452, 1994.
5. Poddighe PJ, Ramaekers, FCS, Hopman AHN: Interphase cytogenetics of tumors. J Pathol 166:215–224, 1992.
6. Joos S, Fink TM, Rätsch A, Lichter P: Mapping and chromosome analysis: the potential of fluorescence in situ hybridization. J Biotechnol 35:135–153, 1994.
7. Hopman AHN, Voorter CEM, Ramaekers FCS: Detection of genomic changes in cancer by in situ hybridization. Mol Biol Rep 19:31–44, 1994.
8. Lichter P, Boyle AL, Cremer C, Ward DC: Analysis of genes and chromosomes by non-isotopic in situ hybridization. Genet Anal Technol Appl 8:24–35, 1991.
9. Willard FW, Waye JS: Hierarchical order in chromosome-specific human alpha satellite DNA. Trends Genet 3:192–198, 1987.
10. van Dekken H, Pizzolo JG, Reuter VE, Melamed MR: Cytogenetic analysis of human solid tumors by in situ hybridization with a set of 12 chromosome-specific DNA probes. Cytogenet Cell Genet 54:103–107, 1990.
11. Devilee P, Thierry RF, Kievits T, Kolluri R, Hopman AHN, Willard HF, Pearson PL, Cornelisse CJ: Detection of chromosome aneuploidy in interphase nuclei from human primary breast tumors using chromosome-specific repetitive DNA probes. Cancer Res 48:5825–5830, 1988.
12. Poddighe PJ, Moesker O, Smeets D, Awwad BH, Ramaekers FCS, Hopman AHN: Interphase cytogenetics of hematological cancer: comparison of classical karyotyping and in situ hybridization using a panel of eleven chromosome specific probes. Cancer Res 51:1959–1967, 1991.
13. Cremer T, Landegent J, Bruckner A, Scholl HP, Schardin M, Hager HD, Devilee P, Pearson P, van der Ploeg M: Detection of chromosome aberrations in the human interphase nucleus by visualization of specific target DNAs with radioactive and non-radioactive in situ hybridization techniques diagnosis of trisomy 18 with probe L1.84. Hum Genet 74:346–352, 1986.
14. Cremer T, Lichter P, Borden J, Ward DC, Manuelidis L: Detection of chromosome aberrations in metaphase and interphase tumor cells by in situ hybridization using chromosome-specific library probes. Hum Genet 80:235–246, 1988.
15. Pinkel D, Landegent J, Collins C, Fuscoe J, Segraves R, Lucas J. Gray J: Fluorescence in situ hybridization with human chromosome-specific libraries: detection of trisomy 21 and translocations of chromosome 4. Proc Natl Acad Sci USA 85:9138–9142, 1988.

16. Raap AK, Hopman AHN, van der Ploeg M: Hapten labeling of nucleic acid probe for DNA in situ hybridization. In: Bullock GR, Petrusz P (eds.), Techniques in Immunocytochemistry. Cambridge, UK: Cambridge University Press, pp. 167–198.

17. Raap AK, Wiegant J, Lichter P: Multiple fluorescence in situ hybridization for molecular cytogenetics. In: Techniques and Methods in Molecular Biology: Non-Radioactive Labeling and Detection of Biomolecules. Berlin, Germany: Springer Verlag, pp. 343–354, 1992.

18. Speel EJM, Ramaekers FCS, Hopman AHN: Cytochemical detection systems for in situ hybridization, and the combination with immunocytochemistry. "Who is still afraid of Red, Green and Blue?" Histochem J 27: 833–858, 1995.

19. Hopman AHN, Speel EJM, Voorter CEM, Ramaekers FCS: Non-isotopic methods in molecular biology. A practical approach. In: Levy ER, Herrington CS (eds.), IRL, Probe Labelling Methods. Oxford, UK: Oxford University Press, pp. 1–21, 1995.

20. Hopman AHN, Poddighe P, Moesker O, Ramaekers FCS: Interphase cytogenetics: an approach to the detection of genetic aberrations in tumours. In: McGee JOD, Herrington CS (eds.), Diagnostic Molecular Pathology: A Practical Approach. Oxford, UK: IRL Press, pp. 142–167, 1992.

21. Waldman FM, Carroll PR, Kerschmann R, Cohen MB, Field FG, Mayall BH: Centromeric copy number of chromosome 7 is strongly correlated with tumor grade and labeling index in human bladder cancer. Cancer Res 14:3807–3813, 1991.

22. Hyytinen E, Visakorpi T, Kallioniemi A, Kallioniemi O-P, Isola JJ: Improved technique for analysis of formalin-fixed, paraffin-embedded tumors by fluorescence in situ hybridization. Cytometry 16:93–99, 1994.

23. van Dekken H, Bosman FT, Teijgeman R, Vissers GJ, Tersteeg TA, Kerstens HM, Vooijs GR, Verhofstad AA: Identification of numerical chromosome aberrations in archival tumours by in situ hybridization to routine paraffin sections evaluation of 23 phaeochromocytomas. J Pathol 171:161–171, 1992.

24. Emmerich P, Jauch A, Hofmann M-C, Cremer T, Walt H: Interphase cytogenetics in paraffin embedded sections from human testicular germ cell tumor xenografts and in corresponding cultured cells. Lab Invest 61: 235–242, 1989.

25. Hopman AHN, van Hooren E, van de Kaa CA, Vooijs GP, Ramaekers FCS: Detection of numerical chromosome aberrations using in situ hybridization in paraffin sections of routinely processed bladder cancers. Mod Pathol 4:503–513, 1991.

26. Arnoldus EPJ, Wiegant J, Noordermeer IA, Wessels JW, Beverstock CC, Grosveld GC, van der Ploeg M, Raap AK: Detection of the Philadelphia chromosome in interphase nuclei. Cytogenet Cell Genet 54:108–111, 1990.

27. Dauwerse JG, Wiegant J, Raap AK, Breuning MH, van Ommen GJB: Multiple colors by fluorescence in situ hybridization using ratio-labelled DNA probes create a molecular karyotype. Hum Mol Genet 1:593–598, 1992.

28. Hopman AHN, Wiegant J, Raap AK, Landegent J.E, van der Ploeg M, van Duijn P: Bi-color detection of two target DNAs by non-radioactive in situ hybridization. Histochemistry 85:1–4, 1986.

29. Nederlof PM, Robinson D, Abuknesha R, Wiegant J, Hopman, AHN, Tanke HJ, Raap AK: Three-color-fluorescence in situ hybridization for the simultaneous detection of multiple nucleic acid sequences. Cytometry 10:20–28, 1989.

30. Nederlof PM, van der Flier S, Wiegant J, Raap AK, Tanke HJ, Ploem JS, van der Ploeg M: Multiple fluorescence in situ hybridization. Cytometry 11:126–131, 1990.

31. Ried T, Baldini A, Rand TC, Ward DC: Simultaneous visualization of seven different DNA probes by in situ hybridization using combinatorial fluorescence and digital imaging microscopy. Proc Natl Acad Sci USA 89:1388–1392, 1992.

32. Wiegant J, Weismeijer CC, Hoovers JMN, Schuuring E, d'Azzo A, Vrolijk J, Tanke HJ, Raap AK: Multiple and sensitive fluorescence in situ hybridization with rhodamine-, fluorescein-, and coumarin-labeled DNAs. Cytogenet Cell Genet 63:73–76, 1993.

33. Kerstens HMJ, Poddighe PJ, Hanselaar AGJM: Double-target in situ hybridization in brightfield microscopy. J Histochem Cytochem 42:1071–1077, 1994.

34. Speel EJM, Jansen MPHM, Ramaekers FCS, Hopman AHN: A novel triple-color detection procedure for brightfield microscopy, combining in situ hybridization with immunocytochemistry. J Histochem Cytochem 42:1299–1307, 1994.

35. Bobrow MN, Shaughnessy KJ, Litt GJ: Catalyzed reported deposition, a novel method of signal amplification. J Immunol Methods 137:103–112, 1991.

36. Kerstens HJM, Poddighe PJ, Hanselaar AGJM: A novel in situ hybridization signal amplification method, based on the deposition of biotinylated tyramine. J Histochem Cytochem 43:347–352, 1995.

37. Raap AK, Van de Corput MPC, Vervenne RAW, Van Gijlswijk RPM, Tanke HJ, Wiegant J: Ultra-sensitive FISH using peroxidase-mediated deposition of biotin- or fluorochrome tyramide. Hum Mol Genet 4:529–534, 1995.

38. Kibbelaar RE, Kok F, Dreef EJ, Kleiverda JK, Cornelisse CJ, Raap AK, Kluin PhM: Statistical methods in interphase cytogenetics: an experimental approach. Cytometry 14:716–724, 1993.

39. Hopman AHN, Ramaekers FCS, Raap AK, Beck JLM, Devilee P, Van der Ploeg M, Vooijs GP: In situ hybridization as a tool to study numerical chromosome aberrations in solid bladder tumors. Histochemistry 89:307–316, 1988.

40. Anastasi J, Le Beau MM, Vardiman JW, Westbrook CA: Detection of numerical chromosomal abnormalities in neoplastic hematopoietic cells using in situ hybridization with a chromosome specific probe. Am J Pathol 136:131–139, 1990.

41. Arnoldus EPJ, Noordermeer IA, Peters ACB, Voormolen JHC, Bots GTAM, Raap AK, van der Ploeg M: Interphase cytogenetics of brain tumors. Genes, Chrom Cancer 3:101–107, 1991.

42. Smeets DFCM, Merkx GFM, Hopman AHN: Frequent occurence of translocations of the short arm of chromosome 15 to other D-group chromosomes. Hum Genet 87:45–48, 1991.

43. van Dekken H, Kerstens HM, Tersteeg TA, Verhofstad AA, Vooijs GP: Histological preservation after in situ hybridization to archival solid tumor sections allows discrimination of cells bearing numerical chromosome changes. J Pathol 168:317–324, 1992.

44. Dhingra K, Sneige N, Pandita TK, Johnston DA, Lee JS, Emami E, Hortobagyi GN, Hittelman WN: Quantitative analysis of chromosome in situ hybridization signal in paraffin-embedded tissue sections. Cytometry 16:100–112, 1994.

45. Pahlplatz MMM, De Wilde PCM, Poddighe P, Van Dekken H, Vooijs GP, Hanselaar AGJM: A model for evaluation of in situ hybridization spot count distributions in tissue sections. Cytometry 20:193–202, 1995.

46. Herbergs J, Speel EJM, Ramaekers FCS, de Bruïne AP, Arends J-W, Hopman AHN: Combination of lamin immunocytochemistry and in situ hybridization for the analysis of chromosome copy numbers in tumor cell areas with high nuclear density. Cytometry 23:1–7, 1996.

47. Thompson CT, LeBoit PE, Nederlof PM, Gray JW: Thick-section fluorescence in situ hybridization on formalin-fixed, paraffin-embedded archival tissue provides a histogenetic profile. Am J Pathol 144:237–243, 1994.

48. Arnoldus EPJ, Dreef EJ, Noordermeer IA, Verheggen MM, Thierry RP, Peters AC, Cornelisse CJ, van der Ploeg M, Raap AK: Feasibility of in situ hybridization with chromosome specific DNA probes on paraffin embedded tissue. J Clin Pathol 44:900–904, 1991.

49. van Lijnschoten G, Albrechts J, Vallinga M, Hopman AHN, Arends JW, Geraedts JPM: Fluorescence in situ hybridization on paraffin-embedded abortion material as a means of retrospective chromosome analysis. Hum Genet 94:518–522, 1994.

50. Speel EJM, Herbergs J, Ramaekers FCS, Hopman AHN: Combined immunocytochemistry and fluorescence in situ hybridization for simultaneous tricolor detection of cell cycle, genomic, and phenotypic parameters of tumor cells. J Histochem Cytochem 42:961–966, 1994.

51. Weber-Matthiesen K, Deerberg J, Müller-Hermelink A, Schlegelberger B, Grote W: Rapid immunophenotypic characterization of chromosomally aberrant cells by the new fiction method. Cytogenet Cell Genet 63:123–125, 1993.

52. van den Berg H, Vossen JM, Langlois van den Bergh R, Bayer J, van Tol MJ: Detection of Y chromosome by in situ hybridization in combination with membrane antigens by two-color immunofluorescence. Lab Invest 64:623–628, 1991.

53. Herbergs J, de Bruïne AP, Marx PTJ, Vallinga MIA, Stockbrügger RW, Ramaekers FCS, Hopman AHN: Chromosome aberrations in adenomas of the colon. Proof of trisomy in tumor cells by combined interphase cytogenetics and immunocytochemistry. Int J Cancer 57:781–785, 1994.

54. Strehl S, Ambros PF: Fluorescence in situ hybridization combined with immunohistochemistry for highly sensitive detection of chromosome 1 aberrations in neuroblastoma. Cytogenet Cell Genet 63:24–31, 1993.
55. Kallioniemi A, Kallioniemi O-P, Sudar D, Rutovitz D, Gray JW, Waldman F, Pinkel D: Comparative genomic hybridization for molecular cytogenetic analysis of solid tumors. Science 258:818–821, 1992.
56. Kallioniemi O-P, Kallioniemi A, Sudar D, Rutovitz D, Gray JW, Waldman F, Pinkel D: Comparative genomic hybridization: a rapid new method for detecting and mapping DNA amplification in tumors. Cancer Biol 4:41–46, 1993.
57. Manoir du S, Speicher MR, Joos S, Schröck E, Popp S, Döhner H, Kovacs G, Robert-Nicoud M, Lichter P, Cremer T: Detection of complete and partial chromosome gains and losses by comparative genomic in situ hybridization. Hum Genet 90:590–610, 1993.
58. Speicher MR, du Manoir S, Schröck E, Holtgreve-Grez H, Schoell B, Lengauer CH, Cremer T, Ried T: Molecular cytogenetic analysis of formalin-fixed, paraffin-embedded solid tumors by comparative genomic hybridization after universal DNA-amplification. Hum Mol Genet 2:1907–1914, 1993.
59. Joos S, Scherthan H, Speicher MR, Schleger J, Cremer T, Lichter P: Detection of amplified DNA sequences by reverse chromosome painting using genomic tumor DNA as probe. Hum Genet 90:584–589, 1993.
60. Comparative genomic hybridization. Special section. Cytometry 19:1–42, 1995.
61. Kallioniemi O-P, Kallioniemi A, Piper J, Isola J, Waldman F, Gray G, Pinkel D: Optimizing genomic hybridization for analysis of DNA sequence copy number changes in solid tumors. Genes Chrom Cancer 1:231–243, 1994.
62. Houldsworth J, Chaganti RSK: Comparative genomic hybridization: an overview. Am J Pathol 145:1253–1260, 1994.
63. Isola J, DeVries S, Chu L, Ghazvini S, Waldman F: Analysis of changes in DNA sequences copy number by comparative genomic hybridization in archival paraffin-embedded tumor samples. Am J Pathol 145:1301–1308, 1994.
64. Lichter P, Bentz M, Joos S: Detection of chromosomal aberrations by means of molecular cytogentics: painting of chromosomes and chromosomal subregions and comparative genomic hybridization. Methods Enzymol 254:343–359, 1995.
65. Telenius H, Pelmear AH, Tunnacliffe A, Carter NP, Behmel A, Ferguson-Smith MA, Nordenskjöld M, Pfragner R, Ponder BAJP: Cytogenetic analysis by chromosome painting using DOP-PCR amplified flow-sorted chromosomes. Genes, Chrom Cancer 4:257–263, 1992.
66. Mohamed AN, Macoska JA, Kallioniemi A, Kallioniemi O-P, Waldman F, Ratanatharathorn V, Wolman SR: Extrachromosomal gene amplification in acute myeloid leukemia; characterization by metaphase analysis, comparative genomic hybridization and semi-quantitative PCR. Genes Chrom Cancer 8:185–189, 1993.
67. Kallioniemi A, Kallionimei O-P, Piper J, Tanner M, Stokke T, Chen L, Smith HS, Pinkel D, Gray JW, Waldman FM: Detection and mapping of amplified DNA sequences in breast cancer by comparative genomic hybridization. Proc Natl Acad Sci USA 91:2156–2160, 1994.

68. Schröck E, Thiel G, Lozanova T, du Manoir S, Meffert M-C, Jauch A, Speicher MR, Nürnberg P, Vogel S, Jänisch, Donis-Keller H, Ried T, Witkowski R, Cremer T: Comparative genomic hybridization of human malignant gliomas reveals multiple amplification sites and nonrandom chromosomal gains and losses. Am J Pathol 144:1203–1218, 1994.

69. Suijkerbuijk RF, Olde Weghuis DEM, Van den Berg M, Pedeutour F, Forus A, Myklebost O, Glier C, Turc-Carel C, Geurts van Kessel A: Comparative genomic hybridization as a tool to define two distinct chromosome 12-derived amplification units in well-differentiated liposarcomas. Genes Chrom Cancer 9:292–295, 1994.

70. Ried T, Petersen I, Holtgreve-Grez H, Speicher MR, Schröck E, du Manoir S, Cremer T: Mapping of multiple DNA gaines and losses in primary small cell lung carcinomas by comparative genomic hybridization. Cancer Res 54:1801–1806, 1994.

71. Speicher MR, Howe C, Crotty P, du Manoir S, Costa J, Ward DC: Comparative genomic hybridization detects novel deletions and amplifications in head and neck squamous cell carcinomas. Cancer Res 55:1010–1013, 1995.

72. Kallioniemi A, Kallioniemi O-P, Citro G, Sauter G, DeVries S, Kerschmann R, Caroll P, Waldman F: Identification of gains and losses of DNA sequences in primary bladder cancer by comparative genomic hybridization. Genes Chrom Cancer 12:213–219, 1995.

73. Voorter C, Joos S, Bringuier P-P, Vallinga M, Poddighe P, Schalken J, du Manoir S, Ramakers FCS, Lichter P, Hopman A: Detection of chromosomal imbalances in transitional cell carcinoma of the bladder by comparative genomic hybridization. Am J Pathol 146:1341–1354, 1995.

Chapter 4

Nucleic Acid Amplification Methods for Identifying Cytogenetic Abnormalities

Timothy J. O'Leary

Introduction

The recognition that malignant neoplasms result from one or more genetic aberrations, together with the development of improved methods for identifying these abnormalities, has given rise to a new discipline, typically referred to as "molecular pathology." The role of molecular methods in routine diagnosis remains ambiguous, however, because there is a stunning array of different molecular methods for identifying "the same" abnormalities, and because the relationships among the results of "molecular" assays, traditional cytogenetics, and classical histology are incompletely defined.

In this chapter we provide an overview of gene amplification methods, and their utility in the identification of chromosomal translocations. In so doing, we ignore a wide range of molecular testing that can be performed using in vitro amplification methods, including such important applications as identification of immunoglobulin and T-cell receptor gene rearrangements, detection of gene amplifications and deletions, and localization of point mutations.

From: *Human Cytogenetic Cancer Markers*   Edited by S. R. Wolman and S. Sell
Humana Press Inc., Totowa, NJ

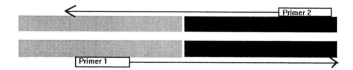

Fig. 1. PCR across a chromosomal translocations. PCR primers are designed to amplify the region at which the two chromosomes have joined.

Amplification Methods

The use of amplification methods for identifying chromosomal translocations is made possible by the fact that translocations result in the formation of new "genes" containing segments characteristic of each of the chromosomes involved in the translocation (Fig. 1). Development of a new amplification assay for identifying chromosome translocations is a four-step process:

1. The presence of a characteristic translocation is identified and localized using traditional (metaphase spread and chromosome banding) cytogenetics.
2. The translocation is more precisely localized, using DNA sequence markers that are characteristic of particular chromosomal regions.
3. DNA sequences spanning the regions of translocation are cloned using positional cloning techniques. Clones must generally be obtained from several different tumors.
4. The DNA sequences at and around the sites of translocation are determined by standard DNA sequencing methods.

Initial assay development, therefore, requires considerable effort. Only after the DNA sequences at and around the sites of translocation have been established may an amplification assay be implemented readily in other laboratories.

Amplification methods provide extremely sensitive ways by which to detect small numbers of these newly formed "genes"—as few as 1 in 10^6 cells need carry the translocation for the assays to yield a positive result. This extreme sensitivity is simultaneously the power and the pitfall of the amplification methods—although minimal numbers of "diseased" cells will yield a positive result, a positive result may also be obtained from small numbers of abnormal cells that are not and will not be associated with clinically significant disease. One of the challenges facing the laboratory worker using an amplification-based method, therefore, is determining the clinical significance of a positive result.

The amplification methods described in this chapter are typically employed with digested tissue. For this reason, chromosomal translocations identified with the amplification methods cannot, in general, be localized to cells with specific cytologic characteristics. Some localization is possible if reactions are performed on cells separated by flow cytometric methods *(1)*, or by using *in situ* polymerase chain reaction (PCR) *(2)*. The latter technique has proven technically difficult, and many labs have not been able to obtain results satisfactory for routine clinical use.

PCR

PCR was the first-identified of the gene amplification methods. PCR is a three-step process:

1. The genomic DNA is denatured by heating either purified DNA, or a cell lysate, in the presence of an overwhelming excess of specific oligonucleotide primers.
2. The genomic DNA/primer solution is rapidly cooled, allowing primers to bind to the genomic DNA. For identification of chromosomal translocations, primer sets that span the chromosomal breakpoint are used (Fig. 1).
3. The solution is again warmed, allowing a thermostable DNA polymerase (typically the DNA polymerase from *Thermus aquaticus*, or *Taq*-polymerase) to replicate the DNA sequences downstream from the primer binding sites.

This process is repeated 20–40 times. When a DNA sequence spanned by the primer pairs is present, the sequence between the primer pairs nearly doubles with every cycle. If the sequence spanned by the primer pairs is not present, then no amplification occurs.

Following amplification, the amplification products are separated by gel electrophoresis, transferred to a nylon gel by Southern blotting, and probed using a specific nucleic acid probe. If cells bearing the translocation are present, a band should be observed in the resulting autoradiogram.

The use of PCR to detect a translocation requires that the chromosome breaks associated with that translocation occur within one or more fairly small regions, so that a PCR product smaller than about 1000 bp-long (250 bp for formalin-fixed, paraffin-embedded tissue) can be formed using primers that invariably span the chromosomal break point. Somewhat wider latitude may be possible when an RNA fusion transcript is formed by the "new" gene, since sequences corresponding to introns are not present in the fusion transcript. The RNA fusion product is detected by first incubating isolated RNA in the presence of reverse transcriptase to make cDNA copies, and then by carrying out PCR using primers directed against the cDNA.

Transcription-Based Amplification (TAS)

TAS is a multicycle, two-step process *(3)*. In the first, cDNA synthesis step, a double-stranded DNA template is produced for each copy of the DNA or RNA target in the sample. This template incorporates a sequence recognized by DNA-dependent RNA polymerase. In the second step, the DNA-dependent RNA polymerase transcribes template molecules into multiple RNA copies, which may then be detected by a blotting or bead-based hybridization capture technique.

TAS results in 30–50-fold amplification per cycle; thus, four cycles may be expected to yield greater than 10^6 RNA copies. Low-temperature amplification may result in nonspecific priming and decreased specificity, however. Although TAS has been successfully used for detection of human immunodeficiency virus (HIV), it has not been employed for identification of chromosomal translocations.

Self-Sustained Sequence Replication (3SR) and Nucleic Acid-Based Sequence Amplification (NASBA)

Both 3SR *(4)* and NASBA *(5)* are modifications of TAS. RNAs H is added to the reaction mixture, so that the RNA associated with TAS RNA–DNA hybrids is digested. This allows continuous, isothermal cDNA synthesis to occur. Although 3SR and NSABA have been experimentally demonstrated, they have not as yet been incorporated into promising diagnostic tests for cytogenetic applications.

Strand-Displacement Amplification (SDA)

SDA is an isothermal amplification technique based on a four-step cycle *(6)*:

1. A primer consisting of the sequence 5′-GTTGAC-complementary sequence is hybridized to a single-stranded target DNA.
2. An exonuclease-deficient form of *Escherichia coli* DNA polymerase I extends the 3′ ends of the duplex, using dGTP, dCTP, dTTP and dATP{αS}, giving rise to a hemiphosphorothioate recognition site.
3. HincII nicks the unprotected primer strand of the hemiphosphorothioate recognition site, leaving the newly synthesized strand intact.
4. The exonuclease-deficient DNA polymerase extends the 3′ end of the nick, displacing the downstream complement of the target strand.

The nick–elongate–displace sequence of Steps 3 and 4 reiterate until the reaction is terminated by depletion of reagents or degradation of enzyme. Furthermore, strands displaced in Step 4 become templates for Step 1, giving rise to exponential amplification, which is typically maintained for approximately 1 hr. Although SDA has been utilized for detection of mycobacteria, it has not been applied to the identification of cytogenetic abnormalities. Furthermore, the sequence fidelity of the amplification reaction has yet to be established.

Q-Beta Replicase (QBR) Probe Amplification

The QBR scheme depends on modification of the QBR template, MDV-1, to incorporate sequences complementary to a target DNA. The MDV probes are incubated together with the target DNA, then excess probe is removed. Only probe that has been specifically bound to the target DNA is then available for replication by the QBR enzyme, a unique RNA polymerase that does not require primer to initiate RNA synthesis. Each MDV-1 molecule can be amplified to make billions of copies *(7)*. Although QBR techniques are useful for the identification of infectious organisms with specific mutations, the variability of chromosomal breakpoints limits applicability of the technique for cytogenetic purposes.

Ligase Amplification Reaction (LAR)

The LAR, also known as the ligase chain reaction (LCR), is in many ways similar to PCR in that it also may be thought of as a multicycle, three-step, exponential amplification system *(8,9)*. As with PCR, the first step is heat denaturation. This is followed by a second step in which oligonucleotide primers are hybridized to both strands of the denatured DNA. Unlike PCR, however, two primers are used for each of the DNA strands; these primers correspond to immediately adjacent DNA sequences. In the third step, ligation of these adjacent sequences is used to produce a new target. Following multiple cycles of amplification, the DNA product may be detected by a variety of methods, as with PCR. In a variation of this method, "gap-LCR," one may leave a gap between the two primers annealing to a single strand of DNA. The gap is "filled in" by a thermostable DNA polymerase prior to ligation.

Although LCR has proven practical for identification of many infectious agents, as well as for detection of common mutations, it is not particularly well suited to the identification of chromosomal translocations. Although these translocations occur at conserved regions, the breakpoints can occur anywhere within a few to several thousand base pairs, making synthesis of adjacent, conserved primer pairs for each DNA strand impossible.

Quality Assurance for PCR-Based Assays

The extraordinary sensitivity of PCR methods necessitates extreme care in their use. Special attention must be paid to prevention of contamination of samples or reagents by human DNA from any other source and, more especially, from previously prepared PCR products. Prudent practice requires that separate work areas for reagent preparation, sample preparation, amplification, and product analyses be maintained. Use of amplification-product inactivation methods, such as enzymatic, photochemical, or chemical inactivation methods, further reduces the risk of false-positive results, but does not mitigate the need for separate work areas or meticulous laboratory technique.

PCR tests for chromosomal translocations should incorporate several different types of controls:

1. Positive controls demonstrate the translocation for which the test is designed. Positive controls can be incorporated as sensitivity controls, which enables the pathologist/cytogeneticist to determine the fraction of cells that must bear a particular translocation that is sufficient to detect a positive result. The positive control should be qualitatively similar to the patient sample. For example, positive controls used with formalin-fixed, paraffin-embedded patient samples should also be formalin-fixed and paraffin-embedded.
2. Tissue controls are used to demonstrate that the patient specimen contains amplifiable DNA or RNA. Typically, controls for DNA amplification are highly conserved single-copy genes, such as those for β-globin or interferon-γ. Controls for RNA amplification are the RNA products of ubiquitously expressed housekeeping genes, such as actin.

   Tissue controls are useful, because failure to detect product indicates that nucleic acids in the tissue are not amplifiable, and that one should not, therefore, expect to demonstrate a chromosomal translocation even if present, by PCR. Since tissue-control genes are generally present in relatively high abundance, however, the demonstration of amplifiable DNA or RNA does not guarantee that a translocation that is present in the tissue will actually be identified, particularly if it is present in only a small fraction of cells (as would be expected for minimal residual disease, for example).
3. Negative controls are used to indicate the presence of crossover contamination. These samples, which must contain tissue that does not demonstrate the expected translocation, are scattered among the patient samples and are subjected to the same manipulations as all other samples. Demonstration of signal associated with a chromosomal abnormality indicates the possibility of sample contamination, and may indicate the need to repeat the test. "Clean" negative controls do not guarantee that patient sample contamination has not occurred, however. For this reason, patient results must always be interpreted in the light of other laboratory and clinical information.

Several useful sources of quality assurance information are available *(10–12)*.

Strengths and Limitations of Amplification Methods

PCR-based methods for cytogenetic analysis have several advantages and disadvantages when compared to traditional and fluorescent *in situ* hybridization (FISH) assays.

Relative Advantages of PCR Methods

PCR methods are extremely sensitive. Thus, they may be expected to detect abnormalities present in cells too few to be identified using traditional cytogenetic or FISH methods. PCR and RT-PCR may be performed on routinely obtained formalin-fixed, paraffin-embedded tissue. PCR primers and probes are relatively easy to design and synthesize. This allows most laboratories to "home-brew" a diagnostic assay relatively quickly. In contrast, implementation of a FISH assay requires, for most laboratories, the availability of commercial reagents. Neither cell culture nor the preparation of metaphase spreads is typically required for PCR; this may enable some laboratories not capable of cell culture to implement PCR-based assays. Finally, equipment costs are lower than those for FISH, and not significantly different from those for equipping a traditional cytogenetics laboratory. PCR methods giving turnaround times of only a few hours have been devised. Such turnaround times are also achievable with FISH assays, but cannot usually be obtained with traditional cytogenetic methods.

Relative Disadvantages of PCR Methods

The high sensitivity of PCR-based methods gives rise to the need for much space, as well as "obsessive-compulsive" laboratory technique, to prevent contamination. Cytogenetic abnormalities either not diagnostic of disease, or not useful in therapeutic decision making, may be detected. Correlation with cytologic characteristics is not generally possible. The per-assay cost for PCR is relatively high (approx $100/assay), although less than that typical of a complete cytogenetic analysis and comparable to that for FISH.

The greatest disadvantage of PCR-based assays, in comparison with traditional cytogenetics methods utilizing metaphase spreads and chromosome banding, is the inability to detect cytogenetic abnormalities other than those for which the test was designed. In aggregate, only a small percentage of known translocations can be detected by either PCR or FISH. In contrast, traditional cytogenetic methods are capable, in principle, of detecting all major cytogenetic abnormalities, including those that were not initially anticipated by the clinician or laboratorian.

Another major disadvantage of amplification methods is the need to know the sequence surrounding the translocation. Neither classical cytogenetic assays nor the use of FISH require that detailed sequence information be available. It is thus easier initially to implement a FISH assay than a PCR assay. Thus, each method—PCR, FISH and traditional cytogenetics—has relative advantages and disadvantages. Selection of the most appropriate method requires careful consideration of both the clinical situation and readily available resources.

Identification of Specific Chromosomal Abnormalities

The identification of specific chromosomal translocations is a clinically and therapeutically important aspect of disease characterization for a number of malignant neoplasms, particularly those affecting the hematopoietic and lymphatic systems. Cytogenetic characteristics may rival or exceed cytologic and histologic features in clinical importance. Typically, the cytogenetic features associated with these diseases have first been identified by classical metaphase spread/chromosome banding methods. Molecular characterization has followed, usually by many years, as increasingly detailed physical chromosome maps have facilitated positional cloning and sequence analysis. In this section, we describe a few of the more important PCR-based assays available for detection of tumor-associated cytogenetic abnormalities, together with some of their specific advantages and limitations.

Leukemias

Molecular assays have become part of the "standard of care" for diagnosing a number of leukemias. Although diagnosis of chronic myelocytic leukemia (CML) via identification of the Philadelphia chromosome *BCR/ABL* translocation is best known, molecular assays are also useful in the assessment of both acute

lymphocytic and acute myelocytic leukemias. We now briefly discuss four of the more commonly employed amplification-based
assays.

Acute Lymphoblastic Leukemia (ALL)

Whole chromosomal duplications, typically involving chromosomes X, 4, 6, 10, and 21 are frequently observed in ALL. Although
it is possible to devise "differential PCR" (DPCR) tests for gene
quantification, the detection of two-fold changes is not easily
achieved. For this reason, PCR-based methods are not currently useful for identification of chromosome duplications. Whole or partial
deletions of chromosomes 6, 9, and 12 are also frequently observed
in ALL. Although DPCR methods can detect such deletions, they
are too cumbersome for routine use.

Approximately three-fourths of all cases of ALL have an early
pre-B or pre-B phenotype. Ten to fifteen percent of these malignancies demonstrate either t(9;22)(q34;q11), t(1;19),(q23;p13), or
t(4;11) (q21;q23). The presence of any of these three translocations
is associated with a high risk of treatment failure with traditional
chemotherapy; thus, identification of the translocations is required
to select patients for more aggressive treatment protocols.

The t(9;22)(q34;q11), Philadelphia chromosome, derived from
the fusion of *BCR* (chromosome 22) and *ABL* (chromosome 9) is
found in about one-fourth of adult and one-twentieth of childhood
ALL cases. In about half the adult ALL cases showing this translocation, the *bcr* breakpoint localizes to a "major breakpoint cluster"
in exons 12–16 *(13)*. In most other adult ALL cases, the breakpoint
occurs in the first intron *(14)*. Although the chromosome breaks
occur over too wide a region to permit a direct DNA PCR, reverse
transcriptase (RT)-PCR assays are capable of detecting virtually all
t(9;22) translocations associated with adult ALL *(15)*. When insufficient metastases are present for cytogenetic analysis *(16)*, or when
bone marrow aspirates are unobtainable *(17)*, the RT-PCR assay frequently permits identification of the fusion transcript. In addition,
RT-PCR assays are useful to assess presence or absence of minimal
residual disease following clinical remission *(18)*.

The t(1;19)(q23;p13) translocation, derived from the fusion of the
E2A immunoglobulin enhancer binding protein gene (chromosome 19)

and the *PBX1* DNA binding protein gene (chromosome 1), is observed in approximately one-fourth of pediatric pre-B cell ALL patients. RT-PCR assays can demonstrate this translocation not only in virtually all cytogenetically positive cases *(19,20)*, but also in cases demonstrating normal metaphase spreads and minimal residual disease *(19,21)*; patients with translocations detected by RT-PCR have a poorer prognosis than those without *(21)*.

The t(4;11)(q21;q23) translocation results from the fusion of the *MLL* DNA binding protein gene (chromosome 11) with the *AF4* nuclear protein gene (chromosome 4); chimeric genes are found on both derived chromosomes. This translocation is seen in up to 70% of ALL cases in infants, and is associated with a poor response to conventional therapy *(22)*. RT-PCR assays based on the der(11) chromosome detect all cytogenetically abnormal cases, of in contrast with assays based on der(4), which detect only about 5 in 6 *(23,24)*; only one in 10^5 cells need demonstrate the translocation to obtain a positive RT-PCR result, which is predictive of a poor response to conventional therapy. Failure to identify an 11q23 abnormalities by RT-PCR, in contrast, portends a relatively good prognosis for infants with ALL *(22)*.

ALL cells expressing mature surface immunoglobulin (as well as Burkitt's lymphoma cells) frequently demonstrate t(8;14)(q24; q32), in which the *MYC* gene is translocated into the immunoglobulin heavy chain gene on chromosome 8. Although detailed sequence analyses are available, molecular methods are not useful in routine diagnosis of these diseases. Similarly, T-cell ALL demonstrates several characteristic translocations for which sequence information has been obtained. Nevertheless, cytogenetic and molecular analyses do not currently provide additional clinically useful information.

Chronic Myelocytic Leukemia

The Philadelphia chromosome *(25)*, resulting from t(9;22) (q34;q11) is present in more than 95% of CML cases. Whether associated with CML or ALL, this translocation results from translocation of the *ABL* protooncogene (chromosome 9) onto the *BCR* gene (chromosome 22); transcription of the chimeric gene results in an 8.5-kb product *(26)*. Although the breakpoints within both *BCR* and *ABL* are variable, RNA splicing results in precise joining of *BCR* and *ABL* exons so that the hybrid mRNA has one of two sequences that differ only in the presence or absence of bcr exon 3. As a result, detection of the fusion gene product by RT-PCR is straightforward *(15,27)*. These assays identify virtually all cases in which conventional cytogenetics demonstrates the Philadelphia chromosome, as well as those that do not. Thus, demonstration of *BCR/ABL* gene rearrangement, whether by Southern blotting or by RT-PCR, has become the "gold standard" for diagnosis of CML.

Lymphomas

Follicular Lymphoma

Follicular lymphoma is characterized by the presence of t(14;18)(q32;q21) in more than 80% of cases *(28,29)*; those patients whose tumors lack the rearrangement appear to have a more favorable prognosis than those whose tumors demonstrate t(14;18) *(30)*. The translocation juxtaposes portions of the *BCL*-2 oncogene (chromosome 18) to the immunoglobulin heavy chain locus (chromosome 14), resulting in overexpression of a *BCL*-2 product and apparent blockage of programmed cell death *(31–33)*. Chromosome 18 breaks typically occur at one of two "breakpoint clusters." Nucleic acid sequences surrounding the translocation breakpoints have been established *(34–39)*.

Direct PCR methods for detecting t(14;18) can detect as few as one cell per million normal cells *(40–42)*, enabling identification of cells bearing t(14;18) in bone marrow and peripheral blood *(43–48)*. PCR testing for t(14;18) has been used to evaluate bone marrow for autologous bone marrow transplantation in follicular lymphoma, although the observation that t(14;18) can be detected in circulating cells of follicular lymphoma patients throughout long clinical remissions *(49,50)* limits the clinical utility of detecting "minimal residual disease" using this assay.

Modiying PCR, using such techniques as primer nesting, can further improve sensitivity. High-sensitivity assays have demonstrated cells bearing t(14;18) in lymph node and tonsils with histologic follicular hyperplasia *(51,52)*, and in Hodgkin's disease *(1,53)*; t(14;18) is not observed in hyperplastic tissues when PCR methods of lower sensitivity are used *(54)*. The less sensitive PCR methods can complement histologic examination and immunocytochemical methods for differentiation of follicular hyperplasias and lymphomas.

Mantle Cell Lymphoma

Many cases of mantle zone lymphoma are associated with t(11;14)(q13;q32), in which the *BCL*-1 (cyclin D1) locus (chromosome 11) is juxtaposed with immunoglobulin heavy chain sequences (chromosome 14) *(55–58)*. Although 11q13 translocation breakpoints may appear anywhere within about a 100-kb region, most localize to a 300-bp region within the *BCL*-1 major translocation cluster *(56,58)*. This has enabled development of several direct PCR assays for the translocation *(55,58)*. These assays identify the t(11;14) in approx 40% of mantle cell lymphomas *(55,57)*, but not in other lymphomas. The clinical utility of this assay is not yet established; it may prove useful for identification of minimal residual disease in a subset of patients with mantle cell lymphoma.

Anaplastic Large Cell Lymphoma (Ki-1 lymphoma)

Fusion of the N-terminal portion of nucleophosmin (*NPM*, chromosome 5) with the kinase domain of a transmembrane protein kinase (*ALK*, chromosome 2), gives rise to a characteristic translocation (t(2;5) *(59)* associated with CD-30-positive large cell anaplastic lymphoma. The translocation is readily identified by RT-PCR *(59,60)* Although the RT-PCR assay appears to have a sensitivity of >95% by comparison with cytogenetic analysis, Lopategui et al. *(61)* demonstrated t(2;5) by RT-PCR in only 16% of CD30-positive lymphomas, in contrast with approx 60% of the cases assayed by Downing et al. *(59)*. The reason for the discrepancy is unclear.

RT-PCR assays have also demonstrated t(2;5) in large cell lymphoma *(59)*, immunoblastic lymphoma *(59)*, and Hodgkin's disease (HD)*(62)*, although it has been suggested that HD specimens exhibiting t(2;5) are not typical *(63)*. However, the RT-PCR product in these cases is of identical size and sequence. Both the clinical and biological significance of the translocation, and thus the clinical utility of the RT-PCR assay, are uncertain.

Solid Tumors of Childhood

Histologic differentiation of pediatric small round cell tumors is often quite difficult. The development of immunohistochemical and molecular techniques for identification of hematopoietic and lymphoid malignancies, together with the application of cytogenetic and molecular techniques to classify tumors such as alveolar rhabdomyosarcoma, Ewing's sarcoma/peripheral neuroepithelial tumor (PNET), and neuroblastoma has greatly improved the accuracy of diagnosis. Classical karyotyping, FISH, and RT-PCR assays generally yield identical results. Comparative analysis suggests that RT-PCR assays are more sensitive than classical cytogenetics in detecting the translocations of Ewing's sarcoma/PNET and alveolar rhabdomyosarcoma, and that the technical success rate for RT-PCR assays on frozen tissue (99%) is substantially higher than that for classical cytogenetics (39%) or FISH (75%) *(64)*.

RT-PCR assays detect cells bearing the t(11;22) in peripheral blood of nearly all patients with Ewing's sarcoma/PNET, which may sometimes enable both accurate diagnosis without biopsy and easy monitoring of residual disease *(65)*.

Solid Tumors of Adults

Cytogenetic analysis of adult solid tumors is of less clinical value than the corresponding analysis of pediatric tumors. In part, this reflects the relative paucity of information associated with the greater difficulty in culturing adult tumors; it also reflects the often greater complexity of the cytogenetic findings, and lesser ambiguity of histologic and immunohistochemical findings in adult cancers. Characteristic translocations leading to detailed molecular sequence analysis have been identified for three adult sarcomas; chromosomal translocation assays may occasionally prove clinically useful in their further characterization.

Clear Cell Sarcoma

Clear cell sarcoma of tendons and aponeuroses, also known as malignant melanoma of soft parts, is frequently characterized by t(12;22)(q13;q12); duplication or other structural abnormality of chromosome 22 is found in almost all cases lacking this translocation (which is not observed in malignant melanoma). The association of t(12;22) helps to establish clear cell sarcoma as a distinct entity *(66–71)*. RT-PCR assays have been used to characterize the molecular cytogenetic changes of myxoid liposarcoma *(72–73)*, but results regarding the clinical utility of RT-PCR methods have not been published.

Synovial Sarcoma

Synovial sarcoma exhibits a unique translocation t(X;18) (p11;q11) involving one of two homologous genes, SS1 and SS2, from the X chromosome and SYT from chromosome 18. This translocation can be detected in approx 90% of cases using either an RT-PCR or FISH assay *(74,75)*. The assay may prove to be useful in distinguishing some cases of monophasic synovial sarcoma from other tumors which may mimic it histologically.

Conclusions

Nucleic acid amplification assays, particularly PCR and RT-PCR assays, are useful for identification of an increasing number of characteristic nonrandom translocations associated with various leukemias, lymphomas, and solid tumors. Once the DNA sequence surrounding the translocation breakpoints has been sufficiently well-characterized, PCR assays may be readily implemented. PCR assays may be conducted more quickly than traditional assays, and may be often performed using tissue unsuitable for culture. Well-designed PCR assays typically demonstrate high degrees of concordance with traditional methods. Discrepant results frequently reflect the higher sensitivity of PCR methods, which make them suitable for identification of minimal residual disease.

Despite these advantages, several drawbacks are associated with the use of PCR-based tests. Unlike FISH or conventional cytogenetic tests, PCR assays generally destroy tissue architecture. As a result, the relationship between the translocation and the underlying disease process may not always be apparent. In addition, amplification assays cannot demonstrate translocations not anticipated in the assay design. By contrast, metaphase culture and chromosome banding may demonstrate unanticipated cytogenetic abnormalities that may prove clinically significant. Thus, amplification assays should be considered complementary to traditional cytogenetic assays, rather than as a technique aimed at replacing these other useful methods.

Editors' Note

The power of molecular assays to define with precision the nature of genetic alterations in cancer, and, thus, to permit mechanistic interpretation and potential approaches to therapy, is overwhelming. As the preceeding discussion has shown, these assays must be developed and interpreted in the context of classical histologic and cytogenetic information.

References

1. Reid AH, Cunningham RE, Frizzera G, O'Leary TJ: bcl-2 rearrangement in Hodgkin's disease. Results of polymerase chain reaction, flow cytometry, and sequencing on formalin-fixed, paraffin-embedded tissue. Am J Pathol 142:395–402, 1993.
2. Nuovo GJ: PCR *In Situ* Hybridization: Protocols and Applications. New York: Raven, 1992.
3. Kwoh DY, Davis GR, Whitfield KM, Chapelle HL, DiMichele LJ, Gingeras TR: Transcription based amplification system and detection of amplified human immunodeficiency virus type I with a bead-based sandwich hybridization format. Proc Natl Acad Sci USA 86:1173–1177, 1989.
4. Guatelli JC, Whitfield KM, Kwoh DY, Barringer KJ, Richman DD, Gingeras TR: Isothermal, in vitro amplification of nucleic acids by a multienzyme reaction modeled after retroviral replication. Proc Natl Acad Sci USA 87:1874–1878, 1990.
5. Compton J: Nucleic acid sequence based amplification. Nature 350:91, 92, 1991.
6. Walker GT, Little MC, Nadeau JG, Shank D: Isothermal in vitro amplification of DNA by restriction enzyme/DNA polymerase system. Proc Natl Acad Sci USA 89:392–396, 1992.
7. Lizardi PM, Guerra CE, Lomeli H, Tussie-Luna I, Kramer FR: Exponential amplification of recombinant-RNA hybridization probes. Bio/Technology 6:1197–1202, 1988.
8. Wu DY, Wallace RB: The ligase amplification reaction (LAR): amplification of specific DNA sequences using sequential rounds of template-dependent ligation. Genomics 4:560–569, 1989.
9. Barany F: The ligase chain reaction in a PCR world. PCR Methods Appls 1:5–16, 1991.
10. O'Leary TJ, Brindza L, Kant JA, Kaul K, Sperry L, Stetler-Stevenson MA: Immunoglobulin and T-Cell Receptor Gene Rearrangement Assays: Proposed Guideline. National Committee on Clinical Laboratory Standards Document MM2-P (Vol. 14. No. 13). Lancaster, PA: National Committee on Clinical Laboratory Standards, 1994.

11. Spadoro JP, Dragon E: Quality control of the polymerase chain reaction. In: Farkas DH, (ed.), Molecular Biology and Pathology: a Guidebook for Quality Control. San Diego, CA: Academic, 1993.

12. Enns RK, Bromley SE, Day SP, Inderlied CB, Madej RM, Nolte FS, Nutter C, Persing DH, Tenover FC: Molecular Diagnostic Methods for Infectious Diseases: Proposed Guideline. National Committee on Clinical Laboratory Standards Document MM2-P (Vol. 14), No. 4. Lancaster, PA: National Committee on Clinical Laboratory Standards, 1994.

13. Cline MJ: The molecular basis of leukemia. N Engl J Med 330:328–336, 1994.

14. Clark SS, McLaughlin J, Crist WM, Witte ON: Unique forms of the abl tyrosine kinase distinguish Ph-positive CML from Ph-positive ALL. Science 235:85–88, 1987.

15. Kawasaki ES, Clark SS, Coyne MY, Smith SD, Champlin R, Witte ON, McCormick FP: Diagnosis of chronic myeloid and acute lymphocytic leukemia by detection of leukemia-specific mRNA sequences amplified in vitro. Proc Natl Acad Sci USA 85:5698–5702, 1988.

16. Kantarjian H, Talpaz M, Estey E, Ku S, Kurzrock R: What is the contribution of molecular studies to the diagnosis of BCR-ABL-positive disease in adult acute leukemia? Am J Med 96:133–138, 1994.

17. Crisan D, Farkas DH: Bone marrow biopsy imprint preparations: use for molecular diagnostics in leukemias. Ann Clin Lab Sci 23:407–422, 1993.

18. Gehly GB, Bryant EM, Lee AM, Kidd PG, Thomas ED: Chimeric BCR-ABL messenger RNA as a marker for minimal residual disease in patients transplanted for Philadelphia chromosome-positive acute lymphoblastic leukemia. Blood 78:458–465, 1991.

19. Hunger SP, Galili N, Carroll AJ, Crist WM, Link MP, Cleary ML: The t(1;19)(q23;p13) results in consistent fusion of E2A and PBX1 coding sequences in acute lymphoblastic leukemias. Blood 77:687–693, 1991.

20. Izraeli S, Kovar H, Gadner H, Lion T: Unexpected heterogeneity in E2A/PBX1 fusion messenger RNA detected by the polymerase chain reaction in pediatric patients with acute lymphoblastic leukemia. Blood 80:1413–1417, 1992.

21. Devaraj PE, Foroni L, Kitra-Roussos V, Secker-Walker LM: Detection of BCR-ABL and E2A-PBX1 fusion genes by RT-PCR in acute lymphoblastic leukaemia with failed or normal cytogenetics. Br J Haematol 89:349–355, 1995.

22. Chen CS, Sorensen PH, Domer PH, Reaman GH, Korsmeyer SJ, Heerema NA, Hammond GD, Kersey JH: Molecular rearrangements on chromosome 11q23 predominate in infant acute lymphoblastic leukemia and are associated with specific biologic variables and poor outcome. Blood 81:2386–2393, 1993.

23. Biondi A, Rambaldi A, Rossi V, Elia L, Caslini C, Basso G, Battista R, Barbui T, Mandelli F, Masera G, et al.: Detection of ALL-1/AF4 fusion transcript by reverse transcription-polymerase chain reaction for diagnosis and monitoring of acute leukemias with the t(4;11) translocation. Blood 82:2943–2947, 1993.

24. Downing JR, Head DR, Raimondi SC, Carroll AJ, Curcio-Brint AM, Motroni TA, Hulshof MG, Pullen DJ, Domer PH: The der(11)-encoded MLL/AF-4 fusion transcript is consistently detected in t(4;11)(q21;q23)-containing acute lymphoblastic leukemia. Blood 83:330–335, 1994.

25. Nowell PC, Hungerford DA: A minute chromosome in human chronic granulocytic leukemia. Science 132:1497–1501, 1960.

26. Shtivelman E, Lifshitz B, Gale RP, Canaani E: Fused transcript of abl and bcr genes in chronic myelocytic leukemia. Nature 300:765–767, 1985.

27. Maurer J, Janssen JWG, Thiel E, van Denderen J, Ludwig WD, Aydemir U, Heinz B, Fonatsch C, Harbott J, Reiter A, Riehm H, Hoelzer D, Bartram CR: Detection of chimeric BCR-ABL genes in acute lymphoblastic leukemia by the polymerase chain reaction. Lancet 337:1055–1058, 1991.

28. Bloomfield CD, Arthur DC, Frizzera G, Levine EG, Peterson BA, Gajl-Peczalska KJ: Nonrandom chromosome abnormalities in lymphoma. Cancer Res 43:2975–2984, 1983.

29. Yunis JJ, Frizzera G, Oken MM, McKenna J, Theologides A, Arnesen M: Multiple recurrent genomic defects in follicular lymphoma. A possible model for cancer. N Engl J Med 8;316(2):79–84, 1987.

30. Yunis JJ, Mayer MG, Arnesen MA, Aeppli DP, Oken MM, Frizzera G: bcl-2 and other genomic alterations in the prognosis of large-cell lymphoma N Engl J Med 320:1047–1054, 1989.

31. Tsujimoto Y, Gorham J, Cossman J, Jaffe E, Croce CM: The t(14;18) translocation involved in B-cell neoplasms results from mistakes in VDJ joining. Science 229:1390–1393, 1985.

32. Hua C, Zorn S, Jensen JP, et al.: Consequences of the t(14;18) chromosomal translocation in follicular lymphoma: deregulated expression of a chimeric and mutated BCL-2 gene. Oncogene Res 2:263–275, 1988.

33. Hockenberry D, Nunez G, Millman C, Schreiber RD, Korsmeyer S: Bcl-2, an inner mitochondrial membrane protein blocks programmed cell death. Nature 348:334–336, 1990.

34. Bakhshi A, Jensen JP, Goldman P, Wright JJ, McBride OW, Epstein AI, Korsmeyer SJ: Cloning the chromosomal breakpoint to t(14;18) human lymphoma. Clustering around J_H on chromosome 14 and near a transcriptional unit on 18. Cell 41:899–906, 1985.

35. Bakhshi A, Wright JJ, Graninger W, Seto M, Owens J, Cossman J, Jensen JP, Goldman P, Korsmeyer SJ: Mechanism of the t(14;18) chromosomal translocation: structural analysis of both derivative 14 and 18 reciprocal partners. Proc Natl Acad Sci USA 84:2396–2400, 1987.

36. Cleary ML, Sklar J: Nucleotide sequence of a t(14;18) chromosomal breakpoint in follicular lymphoma and demonstration of a breakpoint-cluster region near a transcriptionally active locus on chromosome 18. Proc Natl Acad Sci USA 82:7439–7443, 1985.

37. Cleary ML, Smith SD, Sklar J: Cloning and structural analysis of cDNAs for bcl-2 and a hybrid bcl-2/immunoglobulin transcript resulting from the t(14;18) translocation. Cell 47:19–28, 1986.

38. Weiss LM, Warnke RA, Sklar J, Cleary ML: Molecular analysis of the t(14;18) chromosomal translocation in malignant lymphomas. N Engl J Med 317:1185–1189, 1987.

39. Ngan BY, Nourse J, Cleary ML: Detection of chromosomal translocation t(14;18) within the minor cluster region of bcl-2 by polymerase chain reaction and direct genomic sequencing of the enzymatically amplified DNA in follicular lymphomas. Blood 73:1759–1762, 1989.

40. Ladanyi M, Wang S: Detection of rearrangements of the BCL2 major breakpoint region in follicular lymphomas. Correlation of polymerase chain reaction results with Southern blot analysis. Diagn Mol Pathol 1:31–35, 1992.

41. Stetler-Stevenson M, Raffeld M, Cohen P, Cossman J: Detection of occult follicular lymphoma by specific DNA amplification. Blood 72:1822–1825, 1988.

42. Lee MS, Chang KS, Cabanillas F, Freireich EJ, Trujillo JM, Stass SA: Detection of minimal residual cells carrying the t(14;18) by DNA sequence amplification. Science 237:175–178, 1987.

43. Sklar J: Polymerase chain reaction. The molecular microscope of residual disease. J Clin Oncol 9:1521–1524, 1991.

44. Berinstein NL, Jamal HH, Kuznjiar B, Klock RJ, Reis MD: Sensitive and reproducible detection of occult disease in patients with follicular lymphoma by PCR amplification of t(14;18) both pre- and post-treatment. Leukemia 7:113–119, 1993.

45. Berinstein NL, Reis MD, Ngan BY, Sawka CA, Jamal HH, Kuzniar B: Detection of occult lymphoma in the peripheral blood and bone marrow of patients with untreated early-stage and advanced-stage follicular lymphoma. J Clin Oncol 11:1344–1352, 1993.

46. Lambrechts AC, Hupkes PE, Dorssers LC, van't Veer MB: Translocation (14;18)-positive cells are present in the circulation of the majority of patients with localized (stage I and II) follicular non-Hodgkin's lymphoma. Blood 82:2510–2516, 1993.

47. Gribben JG, Saporito L, Barber M, et al.: Bone marrows of non-Hodgkin's lymphoma patients with a bcl-2 translocation can be purged of polymerase chain reaction-detectable lymphoma cells using monoclonal antibodies and immunomagnetic bead depletion. Blood 80:1083–1089, 1992.

48. Gribben JG, Freedman AS, Neuberg D, et al.: Immunologic purging of marrow assessed by PCR before autologous bone marrow transplantation for B-cell lymphoma. N Engl J Med 325:1525–1533, 1991.

49. Finke J, Slanina J, Lange W, Dolken G: Persistence of circulating t(14;18) positive cells in long-term remission after radiation therapy for localized-stage follicular lymphoma. J Clin Oncol 11:1668–1673, 1993.

50. Price CG, Meerabux J, Murtagh S, Cotter FE, Rohatiner AZ, Young BD, Lister TA: The significance of circulating cells carrying t(14;18) in long remission from follicular lymphoma. J Clin Oncol 9:1527–1532, 1991.

51. Limpens J, de Jong D, van Krieken JH, Price CG, Young BD, van Ommen GJ, Kluin PM: Bcl-2/JH rearrangements in benign lymphoid tissues with follicular hyperplasia. Oncogene 6:2271–2276, 1991.

52. Aster JC, Kobayashi Y, Shiota M, Mori S, Sklar J: Detection of the t(14;18) at similar frequencies in hyperplastic lymphoid tissues from American and Japanese patients. Am J Pathol 141:291–299, 1992.
53. Stetler-Stevenson M, Cush-Stanton S, Cossman J: Involvement of the bcl-2 gene in Hodgkin's disease. J Natl Cancer Inst 82:855–858, 1994.
54. Segal GH, Scott M, Jorgensen T, Braylan RC: Standard polymerase chain reaction analysis does not detect t(14;18) in reactive lymphoid hyperplasia. Arch Pathol Lab Med 118:791–794, 1994.
55. Luthra R, Hai S, Pugh WC: Polymerase chain reaction detection of the t(11;14) translocation involving the bcl-1 major translocation cluster in mantle cell lymphoma. Diagn Mol Pathol 4:4–7, 1995.
56. Williams ME, Swerdlow SH, Meeker TC: Chromosome t(11;14)(q13;q32) breakpoints in centrocytic lymphoma are highly localized at the bcl-1 major translocation cluster. Leukemia 7:1437–1440, 1993.
57. Molot RJ, Meeker TC, Wittwer CT, Perkins SL, Segal GH, Masih AS, Braylan RC, Kjeldsberg CR: Antigen expression and polymerase chain reaction amplification of mantle cell lymphomas. Blood 83:1626–1631, 1994.
58. Rimokh R, Berger F, Delsol G, Digonnet I, Rouault JP, Tigaud JD, Gadoux M, Coiffier B, Bryon PA, Magaud JP: Detection of the chromosomal translocation t(11;14) by polymerase chain reaction in mantle cell lymphomas. Blood 83:1871–1875, 1995.
59. Downing JR, Shurtleff SA, Zielenska M, Curcio-Brint AM, Behm FG, Head DR, Sandlund JT, Weisenburger DD, Kossakowska AE, Thorner P, et al.: Molecular detection of the (2;5) translocation of non-Hodgkin's lymphoma by reverse transcriptase-polymerase chain reaction. Blood 85: 3416–3422, 1995.
60. Waggott W, Lo YM, Bastard C, Gatter KC, Leroux D, Mason DY, Boultwood J, Wainscoat JS: Detection of NPM-ALK DNA rearrangement in CD30 positive anaplastic large cell lymphoma. Br J Haematol 89: 905–907, 1995.
61. Lopategui JR, Sun LH, Chan JK, Gaffey MJ, Frierson Jr HF, Glackin C, Weiss LM: Low frequency association of the t(2;5)(p23;q35) chromosomal translocation with CD30+ lymphomas from American and Asian patients. A reverse transcriptase-polymerase chain reaction study. Am J Pathol 146:323–328, 1995.
62. Orscheschek K, Merz H, Hell J, Binder T, Bartels H, Feller AC: Large-cell anaplastic lymphoma-specific translocation (t[2;5] [p23;q35]) in Hodgkin's disease: indication of a common pathogenesis? Lancet 345:87–90, 1995.
63. Ladanyi M, Cavalchire G, Morris SW, Downing J, Filippa DA: Reverse transcriptase polymerase chain reaction for the Ki-1 anaplastic large cell lymphoma-associated t(2;5) translocation in Hodgkin's disease Am J Pathol 145:1296–1300, 1994.
64. Barr FG, Chatten J, D'Cruz CM, Wilson AE, Nauta LE, Nycum LM, Biegel JA, Womer RB: Molecular assays for chromosomal translocations in the diagnosis of pediatric soft tissue sarcomas. JAMA 273:553–557, 1995.

65. Toretsky JA, Neckers L, Wexler LH: Detection of (11;22)(q24;q12) translocation-bearing cells in peripheral blood progenitor cells of patients with Ewing's sarcoma family of tumors. J Natl Cancer Inst 87:385–386, 1995.
66. Sandberg AA, Bridge JA: The cytogenetics of bone and soft tissue tumors. Austin; TX: Landes, 1994.
67. Stenman G, Kindblom LG, Angervall L: Reciprocal translocation t(12;22)(q13;q13) in clear-cell sarcoma of tendons and aponeuroses. Genes Chromosome Cancer 4:122–127, 1992.
68. Reeves BR, Fletcher CD, Gusterson BA: Translocation t(12;22)(q13;q13) is a nonrandom rearrangement in clear cell sarcoma. Cancer Genet Cytogenet 64:101–113, 1992.
69. Travis JA, Bridge JA: Significance of both numerical and structural chromosomal abnormalities in clear cell sarcoma. Cancer Genet Cytogenet 64:104–116, 1992.
70. Rodriguez E, Sreekantaiah C, Reuter VE, Motzer RJ, Chaganti RS: t(12;22)(q13;q13) and trisomy 8 are nonrandom aberrations in clear-cell sarcoma. Cancer Genet Cytogenet 64:107–110, 1992.
71. Mrozek K, Karakousis CP, Perez-Mesa C, Bloomfield CD: Translocation t(12;22)(q13;q12.2–12.3) in a clear cell sarcoma of tendons and aponeuroses. Genes Chromosom Cancer 6:249–252, 1993.
72. Knight JC, Renwick PJ, Cin PD, Van den Berghe H, Fletcher CD: Translocation t(12;16)(q13;p11) in myxoid liposarcoma and round cell liposarcoma: molecular and cytogenetic analysis. Cancer Res 55:24–27, 1995.
73. Panagopoulos I, Mandahl N, Ron D, Hoglund M, Nilbert M, Mertens F, Mitelman F, Aman P: Characterization of the CHOP breakpoints and fusion transcripts in myxoid liposarcomas with the 12;16 translocation. Cancer Res 15:6500–6503, 1994.
74. Fligman I, Lonardo F, Jhanwar SC, Gerald WL, Woodruff J, Ladanyi M: Molecular diagnosis of synovial sarcoma and characterization of a variant SYT-SSX2 fusion transcript. Am J Pathol 147:1592–1599, 1995.
75. Shipley J, Crew J, Birdsall S, et al: Interphase Fluorescence *in situ* hybridization and reverse transcription polymerase chain reaction as a diagnostic aid for synovial sarcoma. Am J Pathol 148:559–567, 1996.

Part II

Organ and Site-Specific Tumors

Chapter 5

Direct Demonstration of Lineage Specificity in Hematologic Neoplasms

Sakari Knuutila

Introduction

Approximately 150 recurrent chromosomal aberrations have been described in hematologic neoplasms *(1)*. Many are associated with certain morphologic, immunologic, or clinical subtypes of leukemia and lymphoma. Some are of clear-cut biological importance, and about 50 specific translocations and inversions have been shown to cause gene fusions that activate cancer genes *(2)*. To investigate the fundamental biological question of stem cells, and in view of therapeutic considerations, it is essential to identify the malignant cells among the numerous cell types in the hematopoietic system. Chromosomal aberrations are excellent cancer-specific markers. Phenotypic markers can be also used to characterize the cell lineages and stages of differentiation of malignant cells. Hematopoietic cells and malignancies are typically classified according to cell morphology and immunophenotype *(3)*.

A technique known as MAC (morphology, antibody, chromosomes) has been developed that allows genotypic analysis by chromosome banding or *in situ* hybridization and phenotypic analysis by cytochemical and immunocytochemical techniques *(4–11)*. All

From: *Human Cytogenetic Cancer Markers*   Edited by S. R. Wolman and S. Sell
Humana Press Inc., Totowa, NJ

these parameters can be seen simultaneously or sequentially both in single metaphases or interphase cells. This chapter describes the MAC methodology and presents its applications to hematologic neoplasms.

Methodology

MAC Method

The recently published MAC manuals *(10,11)* describe the MAC method fully. MAC yields simultaneous or sequential information on the phenotype (nuclear morphology, cytoplasmic features, immunophenotype) and the genotype (chromosome aberrations, gene/DNA losses) of a single mitotic or interphase cell, from many kinds of cellular material, such as preparations of cell suspensions, tissue sections, smears, or preparations of cells cultured *in situ*.

For the genotype study, chromosome banding and/or molecular cytogenetic nonradioactive *in situ* hybridization (NISH) techniques are employed. For the phenotype study, any cyto/histochemical staining or immunocytochemical techniques can be adopted (Figs. 1–4, pp. 98–100). Genotypic and immunophenotypic features can be studied simultaneously (Figs. 2–3), or sequentially; in the latter instance the phenotype study is followed by chromosome banding or NISH (Figs. 1 and 4).

In sequential analysis the cells are usually photographed before NISH is carried out. They are then relocalized after hybridization, and photographed again. Finally, the results of these two steps are compared. This system yields accurate histological and/or cellular morphological information. For example, sequential analysis is preferred for the detection of basophilic granulocytes, because the NISH procedure destroys this granulation *(12)*. Moreover, a reliable histological analysis is often impossible after NISH. On the other hand, the sequential method is time-consuming; simultaneous analysis is, therefore, the procedure of choice whenever morphological or histological characteristics are of secondary interest.

NISH signals and immunophenotype can be studied using either a fluorescence or nonfluorescence, i.e., enzymatic, system. The nonfluorescence systems we have used are the immunoperoxidase system and the alkaline phosphatase antialkaline phosphatase system. In comparison to fluorescence methods, the nonfluorescent preparations are permanent and easy to photograph.

When metaphase cells are studied, a mild cell-membrane stabilizing hypotonic solution is usually used to obtain sufficient chromosome spreading inside the intact cell membrane. If MAC is applied to interphase cells only, hypotonic treatment should be avoided because it may dramatically change the cell morphology.

Other Direct Techniques

The MAC method was based on the study by Stenman et al. *(13)*, who used immunostaining on cytospin preparations. Several modifications and related techniques have emerged recently *(14–16)*. For phenotypic analysis some employ only cytochemical techniques *(17)*, and others use only immunocytochemical techniques *(18)*. Most of the techniques limit the target to interphase cells.

Applications

Figure 5 (p. 101) is a schematic presentation of cell differentiation and maturation into human blood cells. Traditionally hematologic neoplasms have been classified according to cell morphology and more recently, according to immunophenotype *(3)*. Morphological analysis of most hematologic neoplasms indicates the involvement of one or more cell lineages but rules out the simultaneous involvement of all lineages. Table 1 (pp. 102–103) lists MAC studies giving direct conclusive evidence of the involvement of specific cell lineages in a series of 65 patients with hematologic neoplasms.

Pluripotent Stem Cell Neoplasms

Philadelphia chromosome is a recurrent chromosome aberration, not only in chronic myelocytic leukemia (CML), but also in acute lymphocytic leukemia (ALL). Besides direct evidence of the presence of the abnormality in B-lymphocytes, at least in some cases of CML (Patient 11), there is plenty of indirect evidence, based on

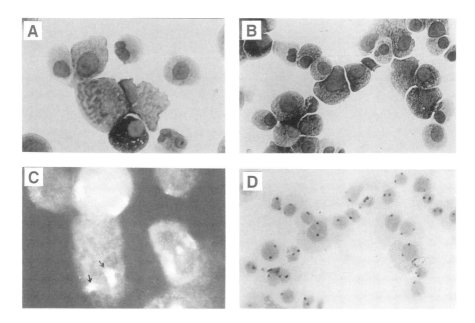

Fig. 1. Sudan black B (SBB) staining (upper parts) followed by *in situ* hybridization (lower parts). Cytospin preparation from bone marrow aspirate of a patient with myelodysplastic syndrome. Lower left: Chromosomal *in situ* suppression hybridization with 8-specific whole chromosome painting probe. Hybridization signals were detected with fluorescein isothiocyanate and chromosomes were counterstained with propidium iodide. Arrows indicate chromosomes 8 in a metaphase cell. Lower right: *In situ* hybridization with 1-specific α-satellite centromeric probe. Signal detection by diaminobenzidine tetrahydrochloride-H_2O_2 precipitation. Hematoxylin nuclear counterstaining. For methodological details, *see* ref. *11*. (*See* color insert following p. 212.)

studies of clonality and cell lines of the involvement of both myeloid and lymphoid cells *(19–22)*. Whether postthymic T-cells have the aberration is still a subject of controversy *(23–25)*. The involvement of mature T-lymphocytes could not be demonstrated, but instead the involvement of large granular lymphocytes was shown, at least in one patient (Patient 11).

The Ph-positive ALL also seems to be a pluripotential stem cell disease. In Patient 30, the presence of Ph chromosome was demonstrated not only in ALL blasts, but also in glycophorin A (GPA)-positive erythroblasts. In this patient the ALL blasts were

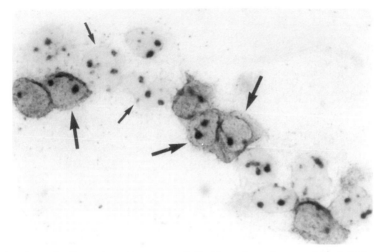

Fig. 2. Alkaline phosphatase antialkaline phosphatase (APAAP) staining followed by *in situ* hybridization. Positive cells, i.e., T lymphocytes have two hybridization signals (large arrows), whereas many of the negative cells have three copies of chromosome 1 (small arrows). For methodological details, *see* ref. *11*. (*See* color insert following p. 212.)

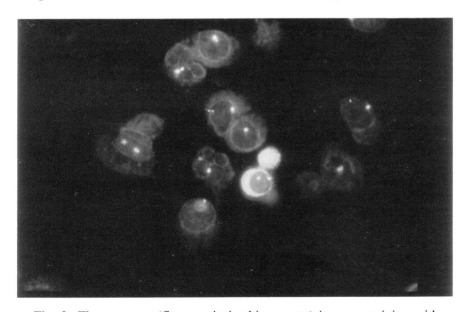

Fig. 3. Fluorescence (fluorescein isothiocyanate) immunostaining with glycophorin A monoclonal antibody (erythroid cells) followed by dual color fluorescence *in situ* hybridization (red X-signal detected with Cy3 fluorochrome and green Y-signal with tetramethylrhodamine. Cytospin preparation from bone marrow aspirate of a healthy bone marrow donor. For methodological details, *see* ref. *10*. XY-cocktail probe provided by Integrated Genetics (Framingham, MA). (*See* color insert following p. 212.)

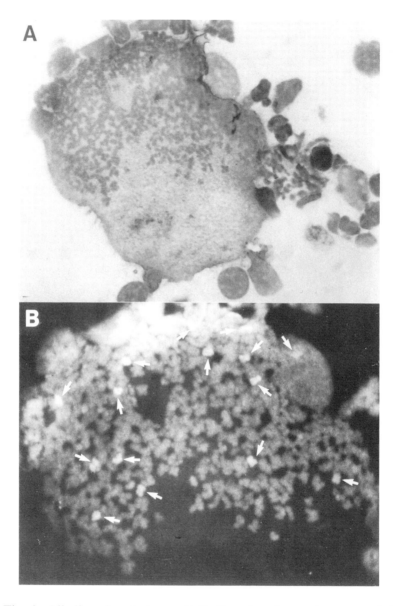

Fig. 4. Alkaline phosphatase antialkaline phosphatase immunostaining with CD61 megakaryocytic antibody (provided by D. Mason, Oxford, UK) (**A**) followed by chromosomal *in situ* suppression hybridization with 20-specific whole chromosome painting probe (American Type Culture Collection, Rockville, MD) (**B**). Signal detection with fluorescein isothiocyanate. Arrows indicate chromosome 20. Cytospin preparation from bone marrow specimen from a patient with a myeloproliferative disease. For methodological details, *see* ref. *10.* (*See* color insert following p. 212.)

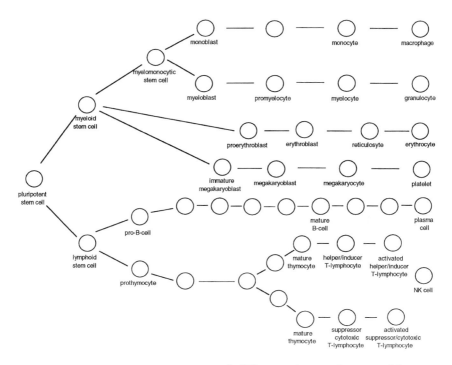

Fig. 5. Schematic presentation of differentation pathways of human blood cells.

not GPA-positive, even though they were CD13 myeloid-antigen positive.

Myeloid cells may also be involved in Ph-negative ALL. Patient 38 had gain of an X chromosome in ALL blasts and, interestingly enough, also in GPA-positive erythroblasts. In this patient the ALL blasts were again GPA-negative, which strongly indicates that erythroid cells were also leukemic.

Might Ostensibly Normal Lymphoid Cells Be Involved in Myeloid Neoplasms?

The answer is yes. In Patient 25 the leukemic cells were morphologically primitive blasts. They were biphenotypic with CD13 myeloid antigen and CD19 lymphoid antigen. Yet they were GPA- and CD22 lymphoid-antigen negative. In addition to leukemic blasts,

Table 1
Lineage Specificity of 65 Patients Studied by Direct MAC Method at the
Department of Medical Genetics, University of Helsinki
(Critical Findings Bordered)

Patient No	Diagnosis/Chromosome aberration (aberration used for ISH underlined)	MAC system	Granulocytic/Monocytic	Polymorphonuclear granul.	Erythroid	Megakaryocytic	Lymphoid stem cells (CD10)	B-lymphocytic	T-lymphocytic	Large granular lymphocytes	CD30-pos.	Ref.
Myeloproliferative disease (MPD) or myelodysplastic syndrome (MDS)												
1	ET/del(20)(q11)	P	+		+	+	+		−			38
2*	PV → MF/ del(20)/	G	−		+	+			−			38
	del(13)(q22)	G	+		−				−			
3	RA/t(1;7)(q10;p10)	Pl	+	+	+		?+	−	−			39
4*	RA/del(5)(q13q33)/	G	+			+						38
	+8	G	+									
5	RA/+8	Pl	+		+	+						39
6	RARS/del(20)(q11)	P	+		+							38
7	RARS-EO/del(5)(q13q33),cx	P	+	EO +	+		+	−	−			32, 33
8	RARS	P	+		+	+						40
9	RAEB/+8	P	−	−	+				−			39
10	RAEBt/del(20)/idem,i(17)(q10)/idem,i(17),+13	I	+		+		+		−			32
Chronic myeloid leukemia (CML)												
11	CML-BC/+i(1)(q10), t(9;22)	Pl	+	+	+	+	+	+	−	+		25
12	CML-BC/+8, t(9;22)	Pl	+		+	+			−	−		25
Acute myeloid leukemia (AML)												
13	AML-M0/cx	Pl	+						−			38
14-15	AML-M2/t(8;21)(q22;q22)	P	+		−				−			38
16	AML-M2/-X	P	+		−				−			38, 41
17-19	AML-M3/t(15;17)(q22;q11-12)	P	+		−				−			38, 41
20	AML-M4/-7		+	SB −					SB −			36
21	AML-M5/+8	Pl	+		−				−			38
22	AML-M6/t(8;12)(p21;p11), del(12)(p11-13)	Pl	+		+				−			38
23-24	AML-M7/t(3;3)(q21;q26)	G	+		+	+			−			38
25	AML-NC/+8	Pl	+	+	+	+	+	+	+	−		32
26	AML-NC/+i(1)(q10),del(13)(q?12q?14)	I	+		+				−			32
Chronic lymphocytic leukemia (CLL)												
27	CLL-B/+12	Pl	−					k +	−			42-44
28	CLL-T/inv(14),cx	G						−	CD4 +			45
Acute lymphoid leukemia (ALL)												
29	ALL-EO/+X,t(5;14)(q31;q32),i(7)(q10)	I	−	Eo,Ba			+	+	−			12
30	ALL-Ph/t(9;22),cx				+		+					46
31	ALL-Ph/t(9;22),cx				−		+					46
32-33	ALL/50-67,+10,cx	I	−				+					47
34-37	ALL/54-59,+12 or +X,cx	I	−		−		+					47
38	ALL/54-56,+X,cx	I	−		+		+					47
NonHodgkin lymphoma (NHL)												
39-42	NHL-B/t(14;18)(q32;q21),cx	G						k or λ +	−			38
43-48	NHL-B/47,cx-90,cx	G						k or λ +	−			48
49-51	NHL-Ki-1/46,cx	G						?k	?−	+		49
52-54	NHL-T/	G						−	+			50
Hodgkin's lymphoma (HL)												
55-65	HL/,cx	G						−	−	+		38, 51

GPA-positive erythroblasts, CD22-positive B-lymphocytes, and CD3-positive lymphocytes had the clonal chromosome aberration. Thus this patient's leukemia was considered to be a pluripotent stem cell disease committed to all myeloid and lymphoid cell lineages. Consequently the present results confirm previous indirect findings *(26–32)*.

Stem Cell Aberrations

In myelodysplastic syndromes (MDS) [del(5) and t(1;7)], myeloproliferative diseases [del(20)], and in acute myeloid leukemias, (AML) [t(3;3) and t(8;12)/subtype M6] the chromosomal aberrations were present in at least two of the myeloid cell lineages (Table 1). Thus, the mutation took place in a pluripotent stem cell capable of maturing into granulocytic/monocytic, erythrocytic, or megakaryocytic cells. In MDS (Patient 3), the abnormality t(1;7) was probably present in B-cells, but not in T-cells.

Single Lineage Aberrations

The highly specific translocations of chromosomes 8;21 and 15;17 in AML subtypes M2 and M3 were seen only in granulocytic/monocytic mitoses, never in erythrocytic mitoses (Patients 14–15 and 17–19). Other diseases where the chromosomal abnormality is only found in one cell lineage include ALL with eosinophilia, t(5;14) in lymphoid stem cells (Patient 29); CLL and non-Hodgkin's lymphoma, trisomy 12 and t(8;14), respectively, in

---

Table 1 *(opposite page):* Abbreviations: Diseases: AML-M0, subtype M0 of acute myeloid leukemia; AML-NC, AML nonclassified; ALL-EO, acute lymphoid leukemia with eosinophilia; CML-BC, CML at blast crisis; ET, essential thrombocytosis; PV→MF, Polycythemia vera changes to myelofibrosis; RA, refractory anemia; RAEB, RA excess of blasts; RAEBt, RAEB blast transformation; RARS, RA with ringed sideroblasts; RARS-EO, RARS with eosinophilia. MAC system: G, G-banding or Giemsa-staining of metaphase chromosomes; I, interphase cytogenetics with repeat sequence alphoid probes; P, chromosome painting of metaphase chromosomes with library probes. Others: *, presence of two companionship clones; k, immunoglobulin kappa light-chain positive cells; λ, lambda light-chain positive cells; Ba, basophils; cx, complex karyotype abnormality; SB, Southern blotting analysis from selected cells.

light chain clonal B-cells (Patients 27 and 39–42); and Hodgkin's lymphoma, CD30-positive Reed-Sternberg cells (Patients 55–65).

Eosinophilia and/or Basophilia in Hematologic Neoplasms—Reaction to Leukemia or Leukemic Process?

It is not rare to see eosinophilia or basophilia in MDS *(33)*. Moreover, it is typically found in ALL with the 5;14 translocation *(12)*. In MDS the clonal chromosome aberration in eosinophils from one patient was demonstrated (Patient 7), whereas the eosinophils and basophils from the ALL patient (Patient 29) were normal indicating that, rather than being a part of the leukemic process, these cells were merely reactive.

In addition, the clonal chromosome aberrations were shown in polymorphonuclear cells from patients with MDS (Patients 3 and 6) or AML (Patient 25). There are also several direct *(15,17,18,34–37)* and indirect studies offering evidence that granulocytes, monocytes, or lymphocytes contain the clonal marker.

Lineage Involvement and Prognosis

The abnormalities del(20), t(1;7), del(5), t(9;22), t(8;12) and t(3;3), which have been interpreted as stem cell abnormalities, are associated with subtypes of leukemia that are highly resistant to chemotherapy. By contrast, the abnormalities restricted to a single lineage, t(8;21) and t(15;17), are associated with subtypes that respond well to chemotherapy. Awareness that pluripotent stem cells are not involved in such cases promises greater confidence and accuracy in the selection of treatment.

Concluding Remarks

The MAC findings presented are of both biological and clinical importance. MAC analysis has revealed the following key findings:

1. Single ostensibly normal erythroblasts in ALL-blast populations have the same clonal chromosome aberration;
2. The Ph chromosome is also present in GPA-positive erythroid cells in ALL;

3. Normal-looking eosinophils or basophils either may or may not have the same chromosome aberration; and
4. Some chromosome aberrations arise in pluripotent stem cells whereas others are found only in stem cells restricted to a single lineage.

In addition, these data are examples of results that can be obtained by an approach that allows simultaneous analysis of the following parameters on a single cell: cellular morphology, immunophenotype, and leukemia-specific chromosome aberration.

Editors' Note

It is essential to develop similar approaches for solid tumors, in many of which we lack the basic cytogenetic data that are generally available and well understood for the leukemias. Although immunophenotyping is usually less relevant, the application of other types of tissue-specific and lineage-specific cytologic markers is necessary to resolve interpretive questions arising out of data from short- and long-term tissue culture of solid tumors.

References

1. Heim S, Mitelman F: Cancer Cytogenetics New York: Liss, 1995.
2. Rabbitts TH: Chromosomal translocations in human cancer. Nature 372:143–149, 1994.
3. Second MIC Cooperative Study Group: Morphologic, immunologic and cytogenetic (MIC) working classification of the acute myeloid leukaemias. Br J Haematol 68:487–494, 1988.
4. Teerenhovi L, Knuutila S, Ekblom M, Rossi L, Borgström GH, Tallman JK, Andersson L, de la Chapelle A: A method for simultaneous study of the karyotype, morphology, and immunologic phenotype of mitotic cells in hematologic malignancies. Blood 64:1116–1122, 1984.
5. Knuutila S, Keinänen M: Chromosome banding techniques for morphologically classified cells. Cytogenet Cell Genet 39:70–72, 1985.
6. Wessman M, Knuutila S: A method for the determination of cell morphology, immunologic phenotype and numerical chromosomal abnormalities on the same mitotic or interphase cell. Genet (Life Sci Adv) 7:127–130, 1988.
7. Knuutila S, Teerenhovi L: Immunophenotyping of aneuploid cells. Cancer Genet Cytogenet 41:1–17, 1989.
8. Tiainen M, Popp S, Parlier V, Emmerich P, Jotterand Bellomo M, Ruutu T, Cremer T, Knuutila S: Chromosomal *in situ* suppression hybridization of

immunologically classified mitotic cells in hematologic malignancies. Genes Chromosom Cancer 4:135–140, 1992.

9. Larramendy ML, Kovanen PE, Knuutila S: MAC (morphology, antibody, chromosomes) method for study of cell proliferation in unfractionated human hematopoietic cell cultures. J Histotechnol 15:31–38, 1992.

10. Knuutila S: Morphology antibody chromosome technique for determining phenotype and genotype of the same cell. Unit 4.7. In: Boyle AL (ed.), Current Protocols in Human Genetics. Madison CT: Wiley, 1996.

11. Knuutila S, Nylund SJ, Wessman M, Larramendy ML: Analysis of genotype and phenotype on the same interphase or mitotic cell. A manual of MAC (morphology antibody chromosomes) methodology. Cancer Genet Cytogenet 72:1–15, 1994.

12. Knuutila S, Alitalo R, Ruutu T: Power of the MAC (morphology antibody chromosomes) method in distinguishing reactive and clonal cells: Report of a patient with acute lymphatic leukemia, eosinophilia and t(5;14). Genes Chromosom Cancer 8:219–223, 1993.

13. Stenman S, Rosenqvist M, Ringertz R: Preparation and spread of unfixed metaphase chromosomes for immunofluorescence staining of nuclear antigens. Exp Cell Res 90:87–94, 1975.

14. van den Berg H, Vossen JM, Langlois van den Bergh R, Bayer J, van Tol MJD: Detection of Y chromosome by *in situ* hybridization in combination with membrane antigens by two-color immunofluorescence. Lab Invest 64:623–628, 1991.

15. Kibbelaar RE, van Kamp H, Dreef EJ, de Groot-Swings G, Kluin-Nelemans JC, Beverstock GC, Fibbe WE, Kluin PM: Combined immunophenotyping and DNA *in situ* hybridization to study lineage involvement in patients with myelodysplastic syndromes. Blood 79:1823–1828, 1992.

16. Weber-Matthiesen K, Winkemann M, Müller-Hermelink A, Schlegelberger B, Grote W: Simultaneous fluorescence immunophenotyping and interphase cytogenetics: a contribution to the characterization of tumor cells. J Histochem Cytochem 40:171–175, 1992.

17. Anastasi J, Vardiman JW, Rudinsky R, Patel M, Nachman J, Rubin CM, Le Beau MM: Direct correlation of cytogenetic findings with cell morphology using *in situ* hybridization: an analysis of suspicious cells in bone marrow specimens of two patients completing therapy for acute lymphoblastic leukemia. Blood 77:2456–2462, 1991.

18. Price CM, Kanfer EJ, Colman SM, Westwood N, Barrett AJ, Greaves MF: Simultaneous genotypic and immunophenotypic analysis of interphase cells using dual-color fluorescence: a demonstration of lineage involvement in polycythemia vera. Blood 80:1033–1038, 1992.

19. Fialkow PJ, Denman AM, Jacobson RJ, Lowenthal MN: Chronic myelocytic leukemia. Origin of some lymphocytes from leukemic stem cells. J Clin Invest 62:815–823, 1978.

20. Martin PJ, Najfeld V, Hansen JA, Penfold GK, Jacobson RJ, Fialkow PJ: Involvement of the B-lymphoid system in chronic myelogenous leukemia. Nature 287:49,50, 1980.

21. Munker R, Miller CW, Berenson J, Dreazen O, Koeffler HP: A Ph[1] chromosome positive B cell line expresses the fusion protein P 210. Nouv Rev Fr Hematol 31:39–43, 1989.

22. Knuutila S, Lindlöf M, Kovanen PE, Ramqvist T, Ruutu T, Andersson LC: Philadelphia chromosome as the sole abnormality and p210 *bcr-abl* chimeric protein expression in an Epstein-Barr virus-transformed B cell line from a patient with chronic myeloid leukemia. Acta Haematol 90:190–194, 1993.

23. Bartram CR, de Klein A, Hagemeijer A, van Agthoven T, van Kessel AG, Bootsma D, Grosveld G, Ferguson-Smith MA, Davies T, Stone M, Heisterkamp N, Stephenson JR, Groffen J: Translocation of c-*abl* oncogene correlates with the presence of a Philadelphia chromosome in chronic myelocytic leukaemia. Nature 306:277–280, 1983.

24. Jonas D, Lübbert M, Kawasaki ES, Henke M, Bross KJ, Mertelsmann R, Herrmann F: Clonal analysis of bcr-abl rearrangement in T lymphocytes from patients with chronic myelogenous leukemia. Blood 79:1017–1023, 1992.

25. Knuutila S, Larramendy M, Ruutu T, Helander T: Involvement of natural killer cells in chronic myeloid leukemia. Cancer Genet Cytogenet 79:21–24, 1995.

26. Ferraris AM, Raskind WH, Bjornson BH, Jacobson RJ, Singer JW, Fialkow PJ: Heterogeneity of B cell involvement in acute nonlymphocytic leukemia. Blood 66:342–344, 1985.

27. Boehm TL, Werle A, Drahovsky D: Immunoglobulin heavy chain and T-cell receptor gamma and beta chain gene rearrangements in acute myeloid leukemias. Mol Biol Med 4:51–62, 1987.

28. Janssen JWG, Buschle M, Layton M, Drexler HG, Lyons J, van den Berghe H, Heimpel H, Kubanek B, Kleihauer E, Mufti GJ, Bartram CR: Clonal analysis of myelodysplastic syndromes: evidence of multipotent stem cell origin. Blood 73:248–254, 1989.

29. Leone R, Lo Coco F, De Rossi G, Diverio D, Frontani M, Spadea A, Testi AM, Cordone I, Mandelli F: Immunoglobulin heavy chain and T-cell receptor beta chain gene rearrangements in acute non lymphoid leukemia. Haematologica 75:125–128, 1990.

30. Buccheri V, Matutes E, Dyer MJ, Catovsky D: Lineage commitment in biphenotypic acute leukemia. Leukemia 7:919–297, 1993.

31. Tsukamoto N, Morita K, Maehara T, Okamoto K, Karasawa M, Omine M, Naruse T: Clonality in myelodysplastic syndromes: demonstration of pluripotent stem cell origin using X-linked restriction fragment length polymorphisms. Br J Haematol 83:589–594, 1993.

32. El-Rifai W, Larramendy ML, Ruutu T, Knuutila S: Lymphoid involvement in a patient with acute myeloid leukemia: a direct phenotypic and genotypic study of single cells. Genes Chromosom Cancer 15:34–37, 1996.

33. El-Rifai W, Pettersson T, Larramendy ML, Knuutila S: Lineage involvement and karyotype in a patient with myelodysplasia and blood basophilia. Eur J Haematol 53:288–292, 1994.

34. Han K, Lee W, Harris CP, Kim W, Shim S, Meisner LF: Quantifying chromosome changes and lineage involvement in myelodysplastic syndrome (MDS) using fluorescent *in situ* hybridization (FISH). Leukemia 8:81–86, 1994.

35. Fugazza G, Bruzzone R, Dejana AM, Gobbi M, Ghio R, Patrone F, Rattenni S, Sessarego M: Cytogenetic clonality in chronic myelomonocytic leukemia studied with fluorescence *in situ* hybridization. Leukemia 9:109–114, 1995.
36. Kere J, Knuutila S, Ruutu T, Leskinen R, de la Chapelle A: Monocytic involvement by monosomy 7 preceded acute myelomonocytic leukemia in a patient with myelodysplastic syndrome. Leukemia 2:69–73, 1988.
37. van Lom K, Hagemeijer A, Smit EME, Löwenberg B: *In situ* hybridization on May-Grünwald-Giemsa-stained bone marrow and blood smears of patients with hematologic disorders allows detection of cell-lineage-specific cytogenetic abnormalities. Blood 82:884–888, 1993.
38. Knuutila S, Teerenhovi L, Larramendy ML, Elonen E, Franssila K, Nylund SJ, Timonen T, Heinonen K, Mahlamäki E, Winqvist R, Ruutu T: Cell lineage involvement of recurrent chromosomal abnormalities in hematologic neo-plasms. Genes Chromosome Cancer 10:95–102, 1994.
39. Nylund SJ, Verbeek W, Larramendy ML, Ruutu T, Heinonen K, Hallman H, Knuutila S: Cell lineage involvement in four patients with myelodysplastic syndrome and t(1;7) or trisomy 8 studied by simultaneous immunopheno-typing and fluorescence in situ hybridization. Cancer Genet Cytogenet 70:120–124, 1993.
40. Parlier V, Tiainen M, Beris P, Miescher PA, Knuutila S, Jotterand Bellomo M: Trisomy 8 detection in granulomonocytic, erythrocytic and megakaryocytic lineages by chromosomal *in situ* suppression hybridization in a case of refrac-tory anaemia with ringed sideroblasts complicating the course of paroxysmal nocturnal haemoglobinuria. Br J Haematol 81:296–304, 1992.
41. Knuutila S, Majander P, Ruutu T: 8;21 and 15;17 translocations. Abnormalities in a single cell lineage in acute granulocytic leukemia. Acta Haematol 92:88–90, 1994.
42. Knuutila S, Larramendy M, Ruutu T, Paetau A, Heinonen K, Mahlamäki E: Analysis of phenotype and genotype of individual cells in neoplasms. Cancer Genet Cytogenet 68:104–113, 1993.
43. Knuutila S, Elonen E, Teerenhovi L, Rossi L, Leskinen R, Bloomfield CD, de la Chapelle A: Trisomy 12 in B cells of patients with B-cell chronic lym-phocytic leukemia. N Engl J Med 314:865–869, 1986.
44. Autio K, Elonen E, Teerenhovi L, Knuutila S: Cytogenetic and immunologic characterization of mitotic cells in chronic lymphocytic leukaemia. Eur J Haematol 39:289–298, 1987.
45. Larramendy ML, Peltomäki P, Salonen E, Knuutila S: Chromosomal abnor-mality limited to T4 lymphocytes in a patient with T-cell chronic lympho-cytic leukaemia. Eur J Haematol 45:52–59, 1990.
46. Knuutila S, El-Rifai W, Larramendy ML, Ruutu T: Direct evidence of involvement of erythroid cells in Ph-positive acute lymphocytic leukemia. Unpublished data.
47. Larramendy ML, El-Rifai W, Saarinen U, Alitalo R, Luomahaara S, Knuutila S: Myeloid lineage involvement in acute lymphoblastic leukemia: A morphology antibody chromosomes (MAC) study. Exp Hematology 23:1563–1567, 1995.

48. Franssila KO, Lindholm C, Teerenhovi L, Knuutila S: A method combining morphological, immunocytochemical and chromosomal examinations of the same cell in the study of lymphoproliferative diseases. Eur J Haematol 40:332–338, 1988.
49. Knuutila S, Lakkala T, Teerenhovi L, Peltomäki P, Kovanen R, Franssila K: t(2;5)(p23;q35)—A specific chromosome abnormality in large cell anaplastic (Ki-1) lymphoma. Leukemia Lymphoma 3:53–59, 1990.
50. Lindholm C, Franssila KO, Teerenhovi L, Elonen E, Peltomäki P, Rapola J, Ruutu T, Saarinen U, Knuutila S: Characterization of neoplastic and reactive cells in T-cell lymphomas with cytogenetic, surface marker, and DNA methods. Br J Haematol 73:68–75, 1989.
51. Teerenhovi L, Lindholm C, Pakkala A, Franssila K, Stein H, Knuutila S: Unique display of a pathologic karyotype in Hodgkin's disease by Reed-Sternberg cells. Cancer Genet Cytogenet 34:305–311, 1988.

Chapter 6

Breast Tumor Cytogenetic Markers

Marilyn L. Slovak

Introduction

Breast cancer is the most frequent neoplasm in women from Western countries *(1)*, with a cumulative lifetime breast cancer risk of about 1 in 10 *(2)*. Most cases are sporadic, but familial clustering is observed in ~20% of breast tumors and at least 5–10% of cases appear to be a result of the inheritance of an autosomal dominant gene *(3–5)*. The exact number and distribution of predisposing genes is currently unknown. The underlying etiology of breast cancer is poorly understood, and only recently have several genetic-based mechanisms emerged *(6,7)*. This lack of essential genetic information is a major limitation to the development of clinical applications in breast cancer.

Recent technological advances in cytogenetics have allowed for a means to overcome the inherent poor growth characteristics of primary breast neoplasias, thus providing new opportunities to study these complex, polygenic diseases *(8)*. This is underscored by the fact that 337 of 5870 (6%) of the solid tumor cytogenetic studies listed in the 1994 *Catalog of Chromosome Aberrations in Cancer (9)*, the major data bank for neoplastic cytogenetic abnormalities, are derived from breast tumors, a figure that has more than tripled from the 1991 edition. The remarkable diversity of chromosomal

From: *Human Cytogenetic Cancer Markers* Edited by S. R. Wolman and S. Sell
Humana Press Inc., Totowa, NJ

aberrations with high intra- and intertumor variability makes interpretation of their clinical and biological significance in breast tumors difficult; nevertheless, these data are beginning to yield insights into epithelial tumor initiation and progression.

Significance of Early Studies

In general, early breast cancer cytogenetic studies were based on advanced stage disease or on cell lines established from pleural effusions. The numerous and complex karyotypic aberrations observed in these studies provided limited information toward the possible primary (initiation) or secondary (progression) genetic events in breast cancer pathogenesis. However, these "historic" studies raised some very important technical and scientific questions regarding the use of in vitro culture methods; the reliability of the resulting cytogenetic data; the significance of diploid tumors, and whether nonrandom cytogenetic aberrations in advanced breast cancers could lead to the identification of genes relevant to mechanisms of origin, progression, and clinical behavior of breast tumors. These critical questions recognize the underlying genetic complexity of breast cancer and the impending need to merge information from several scientific disciplines. Such a multiparameter approach would permit a broad overview of the tumor by incorporating data on the genetic make-up of individual tumor cells, specific gene alterations, clonal evolution of disease, intratumor heterogeneity, and intertumor heterogeneity.

Cytogenetic Research Applications in Breast Cancer

Classic cytogenetic analysis is currently the only genetic method that provides an overview of the complexity of the genetic changes in individual tumor cells, and best illustrates intratumor heterogeneity and clonal evolution. Accordingly, classic or standard cytogenetics is the method of choice to determine overall genetic changes, whereas molecular strategies are needed to investigate individual gene mutations, deletions, and amplifications. To this end, cytogenetic alterations focus attention on areas where putative genes involved in epithelial tumor initiation and progression may be found. Furthermore, karyotypic data provide the basis for a systematic strategy to develop molecular genetic clinical applications in breast cancer.

Recently, two molecular cytogenetic techniques, fluorescence *in situ* hybridization (FISH) and comparative (or competitive) genome hybridization (CGH), were introduced that complement classic cytogenetics. FISH utilizes repetitive DNA probes to detect aneusomy, cosmid probes to detect gene amplification or deletions for specific oncogenes or tumor suppressor genes (e.g., *ERBB2, N-* or *CMYC,* or *TP53*), and whole chromosome paints to define complex chromosomal rearrangements in both interphase nuclei and metaphase spreads. The application of these probes to interphase tumor cells without loss of details of cellular and tissue morphology permits one to associate genetic alterations with specific cell types or areas within a tumor. An extension of this assay, FICTION, or fluorescence immunophenotyping and interphase cytogenetics as a tool for investigation of neoplasms, characterizes karyotypically aberrant cells morphologically and immunophenotypically *(10)*, similar to the MAC (morphology, antibody, chromosomes) approach for leukemias described in Chapter 5 *(6)*.

FISH has been used successfully to determine the genetic alterations in archived paraffin-embedded tumors and freshly prepared touch preparations or fine needle aspirations. This allows for confirmation of the breast tumor cytogenetic results after in vitro cell culture *(11–13)*. FISH using dissociated cells from fresh or frozen tumors has been applied to breast cancers for the detection of aberrations and correlations with other types of genetic alterations (Fig. 1A, and B); however, with dissociated cells is difficult to achieve precise pathologic correlation with the genetic results because contamination by stromal, inflammatory, or nontumor parenchymal cells is inevitable. Touch or imprint preparations in which some geographic representation of the tissue architecture is maintained, have also been useful in defining specific genic alterations in breast tissue.

FISH applied to tissue sections after formalin fixation and paraffin embedding has the advantage of preserving basic tissue details and permitting comparison of the finer structures by examination of serial sections with conventional histologic stains. Although the histological sectioning results in partial nuclear loss, this drawback is offset by maintenance of tissue organization and by

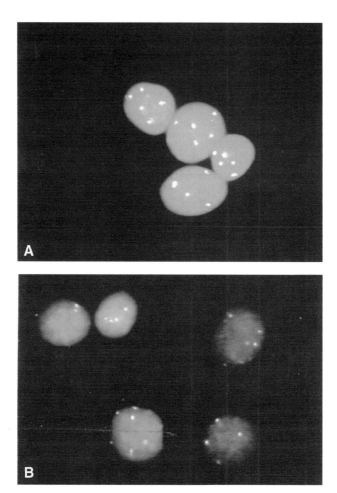

Fig. 1. Detection of numerical chromosomal aberrations in breast tumors by FISH. **(A)** Using an alpha satellite probe for the pericentromeric region of chromosome 1 (D1Z5, Oncor, Gaithersburg, MD), five chromosome signals are identified in dissociated breast tumor cells. The five signals correspond to the five derivative chromosome 1s observed in the karyotype presented in Fig. 2. **(B)** Chromosome 8 intratumor cell heterogeneity detected by FISH using an chromosome 8-specific alpha satellite probe (D8Z2, Oncor). These dissociated tumor cells show a range of two to five chromosome 8 signals/cell. (*See* color insert following p. 212.)

access to lesions otherwise limited by size. The power of paraffin-section based applications is best illustrated by Dhingra et al. *(14)* who demonstrated that different morphologic areas in a metastatic breast tumor corresponded to heterogeneity of centromere 17 signals. Although simultaneous application of FISH with immunohistochemical markers is potentially feasible, many of the antigens currently available are neither highly tumor-specific nor breast-specific and some are not suitable for study in formalin-fixed, paraffin-embedded material. Nevertheless, FISH analysis holds promise for identifying genetically-defined subgroups that may predict tumor behavior.

The HER-2/*neu ERBB2* oncogene itself is detectable by FISH and is especially powerful in distinguishing between increased signal because of extra chromosome copies and that related to true gene amplification *(15)*. FISH in imprint preparations from fresh or frozen breast tissues can also aid in diagnosis when morphology is ambiguous *(13)*. An added advantage when cosmid or regional probes such as the HER-2/*neu* oncogene are employed is that the frequency of three- and four-signal cells reflects the fraction of G2M cells present and, thus, bears an approximation of the DNA-synthetic fraction in the tumor cell population *(16)*.

CGH, the second molecular cytogenetic approach, allows for the detection and localization of DNA sequence copy-number variation over the entire tumor genome without the use of specific probes or prior knowledge of aberrations. The large size of affected regions may reflect simultaneous activation/alteration of many, possibly related functions. The extent and number of sites involved may also provide a rough measure of comparative genetic instability among tumors of similar histotype, grade, and stage. The chief advantage of CGH is its ability to identify the overall gains and amplifications, with the caveat that heterogeneity within the sampled tissue (both within the tumor and from adjacent normal cells) may dilute such identification. The main limitations of CGH are twofold: It provides little information regarding individual tumor cells and requires amplification levels of greater than five- to sevenfold for detection. Today, these cytogenetic-based approaches can be combined to identify genetic alterations associated with individual risk assessment and risk factors in breast cancer.

Diploid Tumors

Diploid or cytogenetically normal primary breast tumors have been reported by several investigators *(17–21)*. Despite the fact that some of these investigators supported their findings by monoclonal antibody testing for cytokeratins, invasion assays, growth in agar, and morphology *(22)*, others suggest they failed to capture the tumor cell population *(23,24)*. Addressing this issue, Pandis et al. *(21)* argued that their findings of normal karyotypes in 4 of 20 primary breast cancers should be interpreted as either subvisible genetic changes present in the tumors, or as nondividing tumor cells in the presence of dividing normal epithelial cells. In support of this latter suggestion, estimates of the frequency of normal karyotypes after direct preparation of malignant solid tumors have been reported to be <1% *(25)*. Bullerdiek et al. *(20)* found a high proportion of diploid tumors (11/16), but attributed this result to culture conditions that favored fibroblast growth. Lastly, the observation of both normal and abnormal karyotypes appeared to be more common in breast tumors with numerous infiltrating lymphocytes *(26)*. Cummulatively, the diploid tumor dispute appears to be confounded by culture conditions, suboptimal banding, infiltrating lymphocytes, or normal stromal cells, and by the fact that a "normal" karyotype at the 400–550 band level of resolution does not exclude the possibility of relatively small changes in DNA content that might not be visible by standard cytogenetics. In the future, sequential FISH/immunohistochemistry or FICTION *(10)* studies should provide insight into the clinical significance of "diploid" karyotypes in breast tumors.

Benign Proliferative Breast Disorders (PBDs)

An increased risk of developing breast cancer has been associated with the benign PBDs. These disorders include diffuse epithelial hyperplasia with or without atypia, papillomas, and fibroadenomas *(27–31)*. In a recent study by Dietrich et al. *(32)*, recurrent clonal karyotypic aberrations were described in 16/30 (>50%) cases of PBD. Consistent abnormalities included der(1;16)(q10;p10), del(1)(q12), del(3)(p12–14), r(9)(p24q34), and alterations of chromosomes 1 and 12, especially regions 12p11–13 and 12q13–15. Similar clonal aberrations have been reported by others in smaller subsets of breast fibroadenomas *(33,34)*. Of interest, the cyclin D2 and *CDK-4* genes map to 12p13 and 12q13, respectively, and may play a role in aberrant cell proliferation in PBD. In addition, the *MDM2* gene, which also maps to 12q13–14, enhances the tumorigenic potential of cells when it is overexpressed and can form a tight complex with p53 to escape p53-regulated growth control *(35)*. Additional genetic alterations appear to be necessary for malignant transformation. Follow-up studies of women with fibroadenomas characterized by clonal cytogenetic aberrations in conjunction with careful clinical and mammographic evaluation should reveal whether these women are at increased risk to develop breast cancer.

FISH-based studies will be key in the genetic evaluation of pre-neoplastic and proliferative lesions of the breast. These discrete small lesions must first be defined histologically and, therefore, are not amenable to conventional metaphase analysis. In a recent study by Micale et al. *(36)* using centromeric probes selected for their relevance to previously described breast cancer cytogenetic aberrations, an increase in frequency and extent of chromosomal aberrations with malignant progression was shown. Similarities of specific losses of chromosomes 16, 17, or 18 in hyperplastic and malignant breast lesions from the same individual provided evidence that some hyperplasias contribute to the sequence of progression to malignancy. Proliferative lesions were characterized mainly by borderline chromosome losses whereas advanced lesions (lobular carcinomas *in situ* [CIS], ductal CIS, invasive ductal cancer) were characterized by unequivocal losses and gains. Gains of chromosome 1 were noted in both *in situ* and invasive carcinoma, but were absent from proliferative lesions, consistent with the interpretation that this trisomy is probably not an early cytogenetic change in breast cancer tumorigenesis as suggested by others *(24,37–39)*.

Single Trisomies in Primary Breast Tumors

Trisomy as the sole aberration in breast cancer has been suggested as an early cytogenetic change *(21,40)*. Trisomy 7 was the only recurrent, solitary numerical finding in 5/20 cases *(21)* and in two tumors reported by Thompson et al. *(24)*. Near-diploid clones were associated with simple numerical changes caused by nondisjunction resulting in monosomy 17, monosomy 19, and trisomy 7 *(24)*. However, trisomy 7 as the sole aberration in solid tumors has been challenged as a neoplasia-specific aberration, with evidence that it may occur in stromal elements, inflammatory cells, or tumor-infiltrating lymphocytes *(41,42)*. Alternatively, trisomy may indicate a general tendency of diploid tumor stem cells to undergo mitotic nondisjunction *(43)*.

In a study of 185 primary breast carcinomas, trisomy 8 was the most frequent clonal chromosomal gain (10 invasive ductal carcinomas and 1 invasive lobular carcinoma) *(43)*. Gains of 8q are also frequently reported *(9,24,38,44)*. Because trisomy 8 occurs in benign as well as malignant tumors, it may endow the cells with a growth advantage, contributing to the phenotype, but not directly responsible for malignancy that in turn may depend on other cytogenetically visible or invisible mutations. Genes on chromosome 8 include the *CMYC* oncogene (8q24) that has been associated with proliferation and unfavorable prognosis *(45,46)*, and the fibroblast growth factor (FGF) receptor *FGFR/FLG* (8p12) that is amplified in ~15% of breast cancers and has been associated with small, low grade, estrogen-positive tumors *(47)*. These and other unknown genes could affect selection for trisomy 8 as either a primary or a secondary cytogenetic aberration in breast cancer.

Trisomy 18 as the primary or sole cytogenetic aberration has been described in breast tumors of varied morphology *(19,21,38, 43,48)*. Genes such as *BCL-2* (18q21), an inhibitor of apoptosis *(49)* or *DCC* (deleted in colon cancer) (18q21), are potential sources of growth advantage in the development of breast cancer *(50)*.

Common Cytogenetic Changes in Primary Breast Disease

This chapter attempts to describe the current status of genetic alterations in breast tumors in a "user friendly" manner for clinical scientists. Examination of cytogenetic data from five recent breast cancer investigations and their correlation with published molecular studies are emphasized. These studies described recurring karyotypic aberrations in primary breast cancers utilizing either direct or short-term cultures and confirm earlier reports as well as more recent anecdotal information. The cases cover a broad range in numbers, case selection, and focus of interpretation. The series selected for this review were:

1. A study of 30 near-diploid or para-diploid cases with the presumption that near-diploid cases were more likely to reveal primary chromosomal events (39);

2. A study reporting clonal cytogenetic anomalies in 24/26 (92%) breast tumors with many tumors in the triploid to tetraploid range *(51)*;
3. An investigation describing clonal cytogenetic aberrations in 28 human breast cancers almost all derived from ductal carcinomas *in situ* (DCIS), presumably an earlier stage of disease (24);
4. A large series by Pandis et al. who focused on methodological modifications for short-term culturing of 122 breast tumors *(21,37,38,44, 52–54)*; and
5. Data from 40 primary breast cancers analyzed by short-term culture from my laboratory (26), including data from 10 near-diploid, 7 near-triploid, 1 tetraploid, and 10 bimodal cytogenetically aberrant cases are presented.

A representative hyperdiploid karyotype exhibiting the common numerical and structural aberrations in breast cancer is presented in Fig. 2. It is clear that significant improvements in methodology and banding have resulted in new and more precise data on the cytogenetics of primary breast cancers in these studies and others *(55)*.

Chromosome 1 was the most frequently altered chromosome among the five studies and in the published literature *(9,56)*. Despite the vast intercellular variability and unbalanced rearrangements resulting in losses, gains of 1q (and 8q) appear to be the most frequent *(24,26,38,44)*. The der(1;16)(q10;p10), resulting in gain of 1q and loss of 16q, was described frequently as a sole karyotypic anomaly *(24,37–39,44)*. This 1;16 translocation, however, is not unique to breast cancer. Pericentromeric rearrangements of chromosome 1 have also been noted in benign proliferative disorders of epithelial and stromal breast tissue *(32)*. The unbalanced 1;16 translocation has been described in multiple myeloma, plasma cell leukemia, myelodysplastic syndrome, Ewing's sarcoma, and other solid tumors *(57–59)*. Interestingly, the classical and alphoid DNA sequences localized to secondary constrictions (or constitutive heterochromatin regions) of chromosomes 1 and 16 could result in uncoiling, elongation, and excess breakage (chromosome instability), leading to exchanges between homologous or near-homologous sequences *(60)*.

The recurrent nature of these chromosomal aberrations resulting in gain of 1q and loss of 16q indicates that they may serve as instability markers with functional significance in breast disease evolution. The proposed causal relations among hypomethylation,

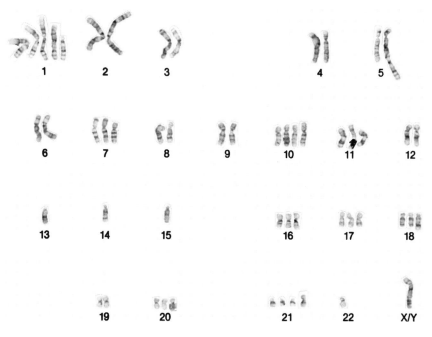

Fig. 2. Representative karyotype of a grade III, poorly differentiated, infiltrating ductal breast tumor. This hyperdiploid breast tumor karyotype is characterized by 54 chromosomes, gains of chromosome 1 or 1q, ?der(2), dic(1;2)(q10;p?23), der(6)t(6;11)(q21;q13), partial trisomy 7, del(8)(p11.2p2?1), +10 +10, add(10)(p13), +11, −13, −14, −15, +16, +17, +add(18)(q21), +20, +21 +21, −22, −X, +der(X). Please refer to Fig. 1A for corresponding FISH analysis.

repetitive DNA sequences, and resultant pericentromeric exchanges in tumors should be investigated in depth.

Collectively, the chromosomal banding results of 231 primary breast cancers from five independent studies indicate the most common numerical aberrations include gains of chromosomes 7, 8, 18, and 20 and losses of X, 8, 9, 13, 14, 17, and 22. Structural aberrations have defined nonrandom gains of 1q, 3q, 6p, and 8q and losses of 1p, 3p, 6q, 8p, 9p, 11p, 11q, 16q, 17p, 19p, and 19q. The non-random occurrence of these chromosomal alterations suggests they may house genes critical to the basic pathobiology of the disease.

Numerous sites of breakage resulting in either loss or rearrangement were common among the five studies. Their rank order varied especially when one considers the possibility of a two-band interval on either side of the designated breakpoint in suboptimal banded studies and the limited contribution of one study that described whole chromosome arm anomalies instead of specific breakpoints *(39)*. More than 25 "hot spots" of breakage and rearrangement were identified but, other than those just noted, only a few (many different sites on chromosome 1, 3p11–21, 6q21–22, 11q21–25, 19q13) were cited in more than one of these studies. For the sake of brevity, these "hotspot" breakpoints are described in the Structural Abnormalities and their Molecular Associations and in Table 1.

Structural Abnormalities and their Molecular Associations

Consistent karyotypic deletions are highly suggestive of inactivation of putative tumor suppressor genes (TSG), yet few of the altered target genes have been identified. As indicated, cytogenetic rearrangements and deletions in breast cancer range from single bands to whole arms *(26,39,61)*. Moreover, cytogenetic alterations are expected to support loss of heterozygosity (LOH) studies for these chromosomal arms (1p, 1q, 3p, 6q, 7q, 8p, 9q, 11p, 13q, 14q, 15q, 16q, 17p, 17q, 18q, 22q, and Xp) (for review of allelotype studies *see* refs. *6* and *7*). Although cytogenetic losses of chromosome 1 are complemented by many LOH studies *(62–64)*, the correspondence of location of the lesions is imperfect. Limitations of both karyotyping techniques (e.g., the inability to detect genetic inactivating events such as microdeletions and homologous recombination with a defective allele) and molecular genetic methods (e.g., probe variation, sensitivity of the various molecular assays used, breast tumor heterogeneity, and lack of tumor cell enrichment) most likely account for many of the discrepancies in the literature. A genetic dissection strategy that combines the known smallest commonly deleted karyotypic region with molecular assays in precursor or *in situ* lesions will be the most constructive in defining the specific critical events in the early stages of breast tumorigenesis. An introduction and example of this powerful strategy follows.

Deletions of the short arm of chromosome 1 appear to be associated with poor prognosis *(61,64–66)* and at least one common region of LOH, 1p35–36, was correlated with the presence of lymph node

Table 1
Genetic Alterations in Breast Cancer

Chromosome region	Associations	Refs.
del(1p)	Poor prognosis	*(61,64–66)*
del(1)(p35–36)	Lymph node metastases; large tumor size; nondiploid tumor; common in DCIS; ?*PK58*	*(65,67,70)*
gain of 1q	36% of breast tumors; observed in both primary and metastatic disease	*(36,37,39, 72,73,150)*
del(1)(q21–31)	?TSG	*(73)*
gain 1q41–44	?Oncogene	*(73)*
del(3p)	Early event; three LOH regions identified: 3p11–14, 3p14–23, 3p24–26	*(9,51,54, 74–76)*
del(6)(q13–27)	No relationship with ER status	*(79,80)*
+7	Early event	*(21,24,40)*
del(7)(q31)	Early event, poor prognosis; metastatic potential; *TP53* alterations	*(76,81,83,84)*
+8/gain of 8q abn of 8q24	33% of breast tumors; observed in both primary and metastatic disease; tumor proliferative anomaly (*CMYC*); invasive disease	*(9,24,25,38, 39,43,44, 47,143)*
del(8)(p21–22)	Early event; invasive/metastatic potential	*(86,87)*
del(11)(p15.5)	Observed in 25% breast tumors; familial association; independent of 11q loss	*(89,90,93)*
del(11)(q13)	Early event in sporadic tumors; ?*MEN-1* TSG, invasion/ metastatic potential	*(95)*
Amplification of 11q13	4–17% of breast tumors; poor prognosis; invasive; recurrence in node negative tumors; ?*CCND* and *EMS1*	*(96–100)*
del(11)(q23–24)	No correlation with PR status; aggressive, postmetastatic	*(72,89,102, 103,105,106)*

Table 1 *(continued)*

Chromosome region	Associations	Refs.
	course; poor prognosis; familial/predisposition association; LOH of 17p13.1 with metastatic disease	
LOH 13q12–13	Breast cancer susceptibility gene (BRCA2); autosomal dominant; early onset; male breast cancer	*(87,158,159)*
del(16)(q12.1) and del(16)(q24.2)	Early, preinvasive event	*(87,103)*
del(16)(q21), del(16)(q22–23), del(16)(q24.3)	Invasive disease; distant metastases	*(24,51, 108–111)*
del(17p)	Two sites identified: 17p13.3 and *TP53*; common early event; invasive disease; LOH with 17q and 13q; LOH 1p or amplification of 8p and progression	*(11,87,94, 114–118, 125)*
abn 17p13.1/ TP53	Early event; more common in medullary, ductal invasive disease; mutations frequent in ER/ PR negative tumors; germline mutations in Li-Fraumeni syndrome; poor prognosis; increased chromosomal instability	*(85,121–124, 140,141,160)*
amplification of 17q12	HER2/*neu* (*ERBB2*); 20% of invasive breast tumors; observed in all stages (initiation and early progression); high-grade tumors; ER/PR negative tumors; short survival	*(97,135–138)*
LOH 17q21	Breast cancer susceptibility gene *BRCA1*; early onset; autosomal dominant; mutations observed in sporadic tumors; increased risk of ovarian cancer	*(132,133,158)*

(continued)

Table 1 *(continued)*

Chromosome region	Associations	Refs.
	Possible second site associated with aberrant expression of plakoglobin gene	*(134)*
amplification of 17q21–24	Distal to HER2/*neu*	*(145,150)*
LOH 17q25	?unknown TSG	*(119)*
amplification of 20q13.2	Aggressive tumors	*(145,150,152)*
Xq11–13	Germline mutation of androgen receptor gene; male breast tumors; Reifenstein syndrome	*(162,163)*

metastasis, large tumor size, and nondiploid tumors *(67)*. Karyotypic aberrations involving 1p36 *(26,39)* were consistent with LOH studies in ductal carcinomas *(65)*. Because distal chromosome 1 aberrations are reported frequently in other malignancies, genic alterations of 1p36 may imply changes associated with tumor progression. Genes localized to 1p36 appear to control cell division *(68–70)* and perhaps control amplification of the *MYC* genes *(71)*. These findings suggest that a possible mechanism for intratumor heterogeneity may be related to aberrant expression of the cell cycle regulatory genes.

Similarly, the common 1q alterations described in primary tumors *(37,39)* and metastases *(72)* have been further refined by molecular analysis. Two 1q subgroups have been defined: loss of the entire 1q and/or gain of multiple copies of chromosome 1q (because of mitotic nondisjunction usually within the constitutive heterochromatin) and structural rearrangements resulting in partial deletions and partial gains of 1q *(73)*. Deletions defined by molecular and cytogenetics approaches narrowed the location of a putative TSG to within a 16 c*M* region of 1q21–31, whereas the smallest region of over-representation localized to 1q41–44 implied activation of an oncogene(s) in this region *(73)*.

Deletions of 3p have been reported as the sole abnormality in breast cancer, thus implying an early or primary event in breast tumorigenesis *(54)*. Interstitial deletions of the short arm of chromosome 3 were noted in more than one study *(39,51,54)* but another study reported over-representation of 3q *(24)* implying an unbalanced 3p:3q ratio. The smallest deleted segment of the short arm of chromosome 3 among these studies was narrowed to 3p11–21. Cooperatively, classic cytogenetics, FISH, and LOH studies have identified three independent deletion clusters: 3p11–14 *(9,54,74)*, 3p14–23 *(51)*, and 3p24–26 (74–76). These data coincide with breakpoints observed in lung and renal adenocarcinoma suggesting that the putative TSGs are not specific for breast cancer.

Rearrangements of chromosome 6 were common but highly variable with a reported frequency as high as 44% *(24)*, but less commonly observed by others *(26,38,39,51)*. Chromosome 6 aberrations were represented by 6q losses *(39)*, 6q22–27 breaks in triploid tumors *(51)*, 6p11–13 breaks and 6p gains *(24)*, deletions of 6q21–22 *(38)*, and 6p23 and 6q13–21 breaks *(26)*. Allelic losses in three distinct regions of 6q, namely 6q13–21, 6q23–24, and 6q27 *(77,78)*, have failed to support relationships between LOH (6q24–27) and the estrogen receptor (ER) gene (mapped to 6q25.1) or ER content *(79,80)*.

Deletions of 7q were an infrequent cytogenetic finding *(26)*, although 27–41% of breast tumors exhibit LOH at the *MET* locus on 7q31 *(76,81–84)*. Using a highly polymorphic (C-A)n microsatellite repeat, the putative TSG has been localized to within a 2-c*M* segment distal to *MET* near 7q31.1–31.2 *(83)*. Allele loss of 7q31 has been reported to be an early event in breast cancer *(83,84)*, associated with a poor prognosis *(81)*. By restriction fragment length polymorphism (RFLP) analysis, Champeme et al. *(84)* observed a similar frequency of 7q loss in primary and relapse tumor samples. These data suggest LOH on 7q31 may inactivate a TSG with metastatic potential as a relatively early event. An association between *TP53* mutations and 7q31 LOH may reflect a cooperative partnership toward either the generation or progression of breast cancer *(76)* and an overall poor survival *(81,85)*.

Chromosome 8 abnormalities occur in approx 33% of human breast tumors *(39)*. These abnormalities include whole chromosome gains and losses, isochromosome 8q, translocations, homogeneously staining region (HSR) bearing chromosomes, and, the most frequent, deletion of 8p. Molecular studies for 8p LOH are highly variable, ranging from <10–55% *(6,86,87)*. The more sensitive microsatellite assays have identified two LOH sites to the short arm of chromosome 8, 8p22, and 8p21 *(86)*. The authors found no correlation with several pathological features of breast cancer (size, grade, ER or progesterone receptor [PR] status, ploidy, S-phase, and the presence of metastases). However, based on 8p loss in small breast lesions that gain the ability to metastasize, the authors suggested loss of the putative 8p TSG may be an early event in breast carcinogenesis and tumor invasion.

Nonrandom abnormalities of chromosome 11 were common with preferential involvement of 11p15, 11q13, and 11q23 *(26,38, 88)*. Microsatellite markers for chromosome 11 have defined three regions associated with allelic imbalance in breast cancer (11p15.5, 11q13, and 11q22–q23) *(89,90)* and demonstrated loss within 11p15 independent of 11q loss *(89)*. In general, about 25% of breast cancers develop LOH at 11p15. Allelic deletion of the Harvey-*RAS* gene (11p15) is controversial *(91,92)*, and other putative TSGs at 11p15.5 within the *TH-HBB* region are being actively investigated *(90,93)*.

The initial lack of concordance for 11q loss observed between cytogenetic and molecular studies was related to use of molecular probes that mapped proximal to the chromosomal deletions *(39,94)*. With improved technology, two classes of breast cancer have been recognized with respect to 11q13 alterations. The first group is characterized by LOH within the *INT2* and *PYGM* region, pinpointing loss of the multiple endocrine tumor (*MEN-1*) TSG in breast cancer *(95)*. Micro-dissected *in situ* and invasive human breast cancer lesions provided evidence for 11q13 loss early in development of sporadic human breast cancer and gave molecular support to the hypothesis that invasive breast cancer arises from *in situ* lesions *(95)*. The second group shows amplification for 11q13 in ~4–17% of breast tumors *(96,97)* that has been associated with decreased survival *(96,98,99)*, and within the subgroup of node-negative patients, with an increased probability of tumor recurrence *(100)*. The 11q13 amplicon extends between 800 and 1,500 kb and houses several genes that may contribute to tumor development: *CCND1/PRAD1/BCL-1*, *EMS1*, *HSTF1/FGF4*, *INT2/FGF3 (96,97, 99,101)*. Of these, *EMS1* and *CCND1* are the only genes shown to be overexpressed with or without amplification, indicating several potential mechanisms for oncogene activation *(101)*.

Irrespective of the reported 40–50% LOH reported at 11q23–q24 *(89,90,102)*, there appears to be no statistically significant relationship between the PR gene (at 11q22–23) content or expression and loss of 11q *(103)*. At least two TSGs have been proposed for this chromosomal region *(90)*. Candidate genes of interest include the ataxia telangiectasia gene (11q22.3), Fanconi anemia group D locus, and *NCAM (104)*. The *MLL* gene is not included in either of the two 11q23 LOH regions defined for breast cancer *(90)*. Of interest, LOH of 11q23 (either alone or in conjunction with LOH of 11p15) in the primary tumor appears to be predictive of aggressive postmetastatic disease course and poor prognosis *(105)*. A significant increase of breast cancer in families carrying the constitutional t(11;22)(q23;q11) translocation is further evidence favoring a susceptibility gene on 11q23 (or 22q11) for breast cancer *(106)*.

Both Hainsworth et al. *(51)* and Thompson et al. *(24)* found rearrangements of 16q22–24 in near-diploid cases, suggesting that this region may contain genes important in the early stages of breast cancer. Allelic loss of 16q24.2-qter has been reported in up to 60% of sporadic breast tumors irrespective of invasion, metastasis, differences in clinical stage, tumor size, histological grade, or ER status *(107–109)*. LOH of 16q12.1 and 16q24.2 in the noninvasive DCIS precursor lesions imply loss of putative TSGs localized to these chromosome bands that may play an early, preinvasive role in the oncogenesis of breast cancer *(87)*. These data are supported by the finding of the der(1;16)(q10;p10), resulting in gain of 1q and loss of 16q, as a sole karyotypic anomaly in primary breast tumors *(24,37–39,44)*. Conversely, in invasive breast cancer, three regions on chromosome 16 may contain loci for TSGs: 16q24.3-qter, 16q22–23, and 16q21 *(108–110)*. These results are in agreement with two of the del(16q) cases reported by Hainsworth et al. *(51)* with marked invasive ductal cancers, and with reports associating 16q abnormalities with distant metastases *(110,111)*. Interestingly, genes associated with cancer invasion have been mapped to this chromosomal region (i.e., E-cadherin, M-cadherin, cell adhesion regulator gene *[CAR]) (112)* as well as a gene relevant to metastasis *(113)*. Taken together, multiple loci on 16q may be involved in the development of breast cancer. Alterations of

other candidate genes in this region such as *BBC1* (breast basic con-
served-1 gene) and *DPEP1* (dipeptidase-1 gene) may also be relevant
to breast cancer development.

Karyotypic alterations of chromosome 17 are very frequent in
breast cancer, but complete loss of chromosome 17 by nondisjunction appears uncommon. With at least five distinct breakage and
reunion "hotspots" localized to this chromosome, it is not surprising
that many molecular breast cancer studies have focused on chromosome 17. FISH investigations of Matsumura et al. *(11)* and
Rosenberg et al. *(114)* indicate that loss from distal 17p is more common than is loss of *TP53*. These results are in agreement with two
putative, mutually independent, molecularly defined TSG sites on
17p localized to 17p13.3 and within *TP53 (94,115–118)*. Deletion of
a 17p13.3 locus has been reported in ~60% of breast tumors as a possible early event *(94,117–119)*, whereas mutations in *TP53* have
been found in 17–46% of the investigated tumors *(85,119,120)*.
TP53 alterations appear to be more common in medullary and ductal
invasive breast carcinoma *(121,122)*, have been observed frequently
in ER negative or PR negative tumors *(122)*, and have been strongly
associated with poor survival regardless of nodal involvement
(85,122,123). An evaluation of 119 breast tumors with *TP53* mutations revealed that ~50% of the missense mutations clustered within
the L2 and L3 domains, the zinc binding domains; by univariate
analysis, mutations in these domains in primary tumors were significantly associated with shorter disease-free survival and overall survival *(85)*. Moreover, LOH on 17p was correlated with high nuclear
grade and with comedo subtype of DCIS *(87)*, lending support to the
speculation that alterations of *TP53* may occur in the earliest phase
of breast cancer. This alteration is conserved during progression
from intraductal to infiltrating carcinoma to metastatic disease *(124)*.
LOH on 17p has been correlated with LOH on 17q and 13q *(87)*. A
cooperative effect of the alteration between LOH at 17p with amplification of the *FLG* gene (8p12) or LOH of 1p has been hypothesized
for tumor progression *(125)*. These results suggest that more extensive study of the relationship between *TP53* mutations and treatment
outcome is warranted in breast cancer.

Allele loss patterns on the long arm of chromosome 17 define
three distinct regions of interest: proximal 17q21 corresponding to

BRCA1, the gene predisposing to hereditary breast and ovarian cancer; 17q21.3–q22; and the distal band 17q25 *(119,126–131)*. Mutations of *BRCA1* have been described in a small subset of sporadic primary breast and ovarian cancers *(132,133)*, but the gene is large and the mutations appear widely distributed. LOH of the human plakoglobin gene, a component of the cadherin-catenin complex that maps to 17q21, may indicate that it represents a putative TSG in this location *(134)*; other relevant genes in the more distal regions have not yet been defined.

Amplification of HER-2/*neu* (*ERBB2*) is found in 15–60% of investigated breast tumors. In general, *ERBB2* amplification correlates with high grade, negative ER and PR status, and is an independent predictor of shorter disease-free survival in both node-negative and node-positive patients *(97,135–137)*. *ERBB2* alterations are present at all clinical stages with equivalent expression in the noninvasive and invasive components of breast tumors. Such data are consistent with a role of *ERBB2* in the initiation or early progression of a subset of breast tumors *(138)*.

Cumulatively, molecular alterations of chromosome 17 have been reported in 80% of breast tumor studies *(119)*, a frequency substantially higher than that of cytogenetic aberrations. Primary breast tumors with *TP53* abnormalities exhibited a significantly higher proportion of complex chromosome aberrations *(139)*, and were more likely to show allelic loss of chromosome 17 and amplification of *ERBB2* compared to tumors with wild-type *TP53 (122,139)*. Cells with abnormal p53 do not show normal G_1 arrest in response to DNA damage, leading to accumulation of multiple unrepaired lesions *(140,141)*. The resultant chromosomal instability and concomitant intratumor heterogeneity are consistent with presumed roles of p53 in cancer predisposition, spontaneous tumorigenesis, disease progression, and perhaps therapy-related disease.

Gene Amplification

Gene amplification receives much attention because of its association with a poor prognosis in cancer. Cytogenetic studies on primary (untreated) breast cancers have indicated the presence of HSRs or abnormally banding regions (ABRs) *(37,142,143)*, and the

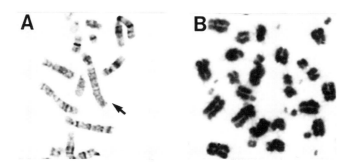

Fig. 3. Cytogenetic evidence of gene amplification in breast cancer. (**A**) An HSR localized to the long arm of chromosome 11 (arrow). (**B**) dmin chromosomes, an infrequent finding in breast tumors.

less frequent double minutes (dmins) chromosomes *(26,144)* in 4–60% of tumors studied (Fig. 3). Although HSRs have been localized to many chromosome arms (8p, 19p, 11q, 15p, 16p, 8q, 9p, and 20q) *(26,38,39,142,143,145,146)*, there is little agreement on frequency, type of aberration (HSR vs dmin), or localization of amplification sites among the studies reviewed.

Differences in amplification frequency range from reports of HSRs in 60% of 84 primary breast cancers *(143)* to averages of <10% *(21,51,144,147)* to absent *(24)*. These discrepancies may result from an inexact interpretation of HSRs or ABRs, especially in the presence of complex karyotypes, poor or suboptimal banding, numerous marker chromosomes, or selection biases of the different cell culturing methods used *(52)*. Correlations with diagnostic or prognostic factors in breast cancer remain to be determined, although one study suggested that HSRs correlated with young age (<50 yr) ($p < 0.05$), but failed to show statistical significance with other clinico-pathological features of the disease (tumor size, histologic grade, metastatic axillary nodes, or loss of hormonal receptors) *(143)*.

The genes most frequently amplified in breast cancer include *MYC, ERBB2, CCND1*, and *INT2/FGF3*, (for reviews *see* refs. 6 and 7), but these molecular amplifications have correlated poorly if at all with cytogenetic evidence. Southern blot analyses of 16 proto-oncogenes failed to reveal association with HSRs, even though low-level amplified sequences of *HST* and *INT2* (×3), *CMYC* (×2–3), and *FES* (>10) were observed *(148)*. Collectively, these data indicate that both chromosome rearrangements and gene amplification can be regarded as frequent biologic markers of breast cancers; a precise definition of HSRs/ABRs is needed, perhaps based on molecular cytogenetics (FISH) using whole chromosome paints or CGH; and amplifications observed by classic cytogenetics that are not identified by molecular assays suggest the existence of unknown genes of potential importance in breast carcinogenesis. The latter may be investigated using a combination of CGH, FISH, and chromosome microdissection studies *(149)*.

CGH evidence from two independent groups indicates that other yet unknown genes play a role in breast cancer *(145,150)*. Using cell lines as reference for studies of 33 fresh primary surgical breast cancers, Kallioniemi et al. *(150)* reported common regional increases in 17q and 20q in breast cancer. The extent of the abnormalities found in the primary tumors is remarkable, especially in light of the comment that amplification in the range of two- to five-fold was insufficient for detection, and that evidence of losses was not presented. Sixty-four percent of the cases in this study showed greater than fivefold gains of whole chromosomes or whole chromosome arms with the most common increases being 1q and 8q, 36 and 27%, respectively. These results compare well with classic cytogenetic studies. Regional increases were most frequent in sequences originating from 17q21–24 and 20q13 in cell lines, and to a lesser extent in the primary cancers. The amplified region on 17q was distal to the HER-2/*neu* (ERBB2) locus and was amplified independently of it in cell lines with known amplification of the gene by Southern blot. The relatively high (5–10× copy numbers suggest that unknown genes important in breast cancer are present in these regions. Extended studies have narrowed the region of greatest amplification to a 1.5-Mb length in 20q13.2 *(151)*. The importance of amplification at this site was emphasized because of association with aggressive tumors *(152)*.

The other group utilized a modified CGH to study breast cancer tumors already assumed to have gene amplification based on prior recognition of HSRs by conventional karyotyping *(142,145,146)*. Their findings are very similar to those cited *(150–152)* with whole chromosome arm over-representations more frequent than regional amplifications and with minor distinctions as to which sites were

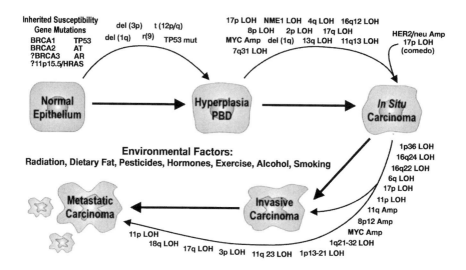

Fig. 4. Breast cancer genetic alterations. Molecular and cytogenetic studies have identified multiple and complex genetic alterations in breast cancer and thus support the epidemiological hypothesis that 3–8 genetic hits accumulate for a malignancy to develop. No single common genetic alteration is common to all breast cancer. The role of environmental and lifestyle factors remains unknown. Therefore, it appears to be unreasonable to assume a single pattern of sequential changes will account for all breast tumors.

most common (especially with respect to 20q13 and 8p). Interestingly, they also observed HER-2/*neu* (ERBB2) gene amplification in association with CGH of a more distal locus on chromosome 17. The discrepancies between their CGH and HSR results were explained as possible heterogeneity or karyotypic misinterpretation. In a substantial number of cases, the CGH results indicated nonnative origin of the observed HSRs.

Genic Interactions

The heterogeneity of karyotypic findings in breast cancer may reflect the many different mechanisms or routes associated with breast cancer tumorigenesis (Fig. 4). In combination, molecular and cytogenetic studies identify complexity and multiplicity of genetic alterations that correspond with evidence of intratumor heterogeneity, variable phenotypes, and perhaps polyclonality in breast cancer. Karyotypic and molecular studies support the epidemiological hypothesis that three to eight genetic abnormalities must accumulate for a malignancy to develop *(153)*. Positional cloning studies are needed to identify the candidate TSGs and oncogene genes in targeted chromosomal regions. Follow-up clinico-pathological correlations of these proposed cancer genes may become the basis for genetically based prognostic subgroups.

Several studies have focused on interactive cooperating genetic alterations in breast cancer. Tumors carrying a combination of 11p and 17p LOH may have increased metastatic potential *(154)*, and LOH on 11p in association with amplification of either *MYC* or *ERBB2* has been linked with recurrent disease *(125)*. Both LOH and cytogenetic deletions of the 11q22–q23.3 region appear more common in metastatic breast cancers and are significantly correlated with LOH at 17p13.1 *(72,89,102)*. To determine if chromosomal regions that appear to be preferentially involved in breast cancer network with one another, correlations of LOH, and specific gene amplification with histopathological and clinical parameters in a large series of tumors are needed.

Clonality

Over 90% of the cases reported by Thompson et al. *(24)*, Hainsworth et al. *(51)*, and Slovak et al. *(26)*, were clonally aberrant. However, three independent reports by Pandis et al. *(21,38,40)* described the presence of unrelated clones in at least 34% of their primary tumors, suggesting a polyclonal origin in a significant subset (one third) of breast tumors. This provocative result may be supported by the vast heterogeneity observed within these tumors. However, the effects of environmental influences and other chromosome instability mechanisms (e.g., faulty DNA repair), such as that described after radiation exposure *(155)*, may have an underlying detrimental effect on mitosis and segregation, leading to apparent cytogenetic polyclonality. Because most complex breast tumor karyotypes are described as composite karyotypes, the question of unicellular vs multiclonal origin needs to be addressed using a sequential molecular-cytogenetic, FISH/immunohistochemistry or FICTION *(10)* approach to determine whether karyotypically unrelated clones contain common genic alterations in pathologically defined breast tumor cells. Alternatively, LOH studies have proven to be of merit in determining a muticentric vs monocentric origin of breast tumors *(156)*.

Metastatic Disease and Clonal Evolution of Disease

One may argue there is limited utility for cytogenetic studies in metastatic disease because of their complex genetic make-up. However, karyotypic data from metastases may provide constructive information for an understanding of tumor progression. In a selected series of 34 samples from various metastatic sites, Trent et al. *(72)* indicated over-representation of 1q, 6p, 7, 11, and losses of 1p, 6q, 7, and 11q were common. Gain of chromosome 20 was a consistent finding in near-triploid tumors. Structural abnormalities clustered to 1p11–q21, 7pter, 11p12–q12, and 6q11–21. In comparison with primary breast tumors cultured in the same laboratory *(24)*, the primary cancers were more commonly associated with near-diploid tumors, whereas metastatic disease was characterized by an increase in karyotypic complexity and cytogenetic evidence of gene amplification.

Stages of breast cancer evolution have been proposed *(72,157)*. One paradigm suggests that cytogenetic evidence for breast cancer begins with unbalanced rearrangements, followed by chromosomal loss and endoreduplication events leading to formation of hyperdiploid clones. Next, the near-diploid cells are eliminated and additional cycles of chromosomal loss with an occasional endoreduplication event lead to the selection of a polyploid tumor population *(157)*. This model suggests that the rate by which chromosomes are lost and rearranged chromosomes appear is an indicator of tumor progression. Gene amplification has been proposed as a late-stage (tumor progression) event *(72)*.

Inherited Breast Disease

Lynch et al. *(3)* were the first to recognize a dominant pattern of inheritance in breast cancer in a small subgroup (~4–5%) of patients, suggesting the existence of one or more breast cancer susceptibility genes. Recently, two breast cancer susceptibility genes have been localized, *BRCA1* to 17q21 and *BRCA2* to 13q12–13 *(158,159)*. Mutations of these genes confer a high risk of early onset breast cancer. *BRCA1* confers an increased risk of ovarian cancer, which is not associated with *BRCA2 (132)*. *BRCA2* mutations have been associated with male breast cancer, whereas no male breast cancers have been observed in *BRCA1* families *(159)*. These genes confer risk, not 100% expression, to a carrier, but loss of function of the *BRCA1* gene may also be modulated by other risk factors and exposures.

The Li-Fraumeni syndrome is a familial autosomal dominant disorder characterized by an inherited (germline) mutation of *TP53* and an increased risk of developing various types of cancer, predominately soft tissue sarcomas, brain tumors, and breast cancers *(160)*. As mentioned earlier, Lindblom et al. *(106)* studied families in which the inheritance of a t(11;22)(q23;q11) may be associated with a predisposition to hereditary/familial breast cancer. Additionally, a familial association of breast cancer with rhabdomyosarcoma and the finding of concordance between the minimal shared region of LOH for the Beckwith-Wiedemann syndrome/rhabdomyosarcoma region and breast tumors on 11p15.5 raises the possibility that the hereditary predisposing factors among these diseases and syndrome may involve the same predisposing pleiotropic TSG *(93,161)*. Lastly, germline mutation of the androgen receptor gene (most notably of amino acids 607 and 608) localized to proximal Xq has been reported in two brothers and in a second independent case with partial androgen insensitivity (Reifenstein syndrome) *(162,163)*.

Summary

The development of breast cancer is associated with multiple genetic abnormalities resulting in alterations of normal mechanisms of growth control that lead to genomic instability and ultimately to a malignant phenotype. Most of the genetic alterations are not inherited, but rather are acquired somatically in breast epithelium. Genetic studies are in agreement with the proposed epidemiological hypothesis that three to eight genetic abnormalities should accumulate for a malignancy to develop *(153)*. A productive route to detect genes that are causal of or contributory to cancer is the recognition of frequent and specific chromosome aberrations associated with particular tumors or tumor-prone individuals. Collectively, the data gleaned from cytogenetics, FISH, CGH, and molecular genetic assays have pinpointed locations or have identified specific gene alterations in breast tumors. However, no single common genetic alteration is unique or common to all breast cancers. Although ordering and/or determining the number of genetic alterations in development and progression of specific solid tumors is desirable, many of the changes described in this chapter occur in 10–40% of breast cancers. Thus, genetic events in breast cancer are likely to involve a diverse range of genes in different subsets of tumors.

Current studies suggest early genetic alterations of primary breast cancer that appear to involve losses on 3p, 7q31, 11q13, 16q12.1, 16q24.2, 17p13.3, 17p13.1, 8p21–22, 13q12–13, 17q, and perhaps gain of 1q. With clonal evolution, breast cancers show preferential loss of 1p36, 6q24–27, 11q22–23, 16q21, 16q22–23 and/or 16q24.3-qter, and perhaps the presence of HSRs/ABRs or dmins. A poor prognosis has been reported in the presence of mutations of *TP53*, loss within bands 7q31 and 11q13, or amplification of 11q13. Breast cancer susceptibility loci have been mapped to 11p15.5, 13q12–13, 17q21, 17p13.1, and mutations of the androgen receptor gene localized to Xq11–13. Alterations affecting 1p36 and 17p13.1 and other DNA cell cycle regulatory repair genes appear to affect intra- and intertumor heterogeneity resulting from genetic instability. Of course, the potential interactions of environmental influences on this multifactorial (polygenic) disease remain to be determined, especially in light of the alarming increased risk of young patients for developing breast cancer 10–15 yr after being treated for Hodgkin's disease *(164)*.

Therapeutic trials are just beginning to incorporate this genetic information. A proposal to treat patients with multiple genetic (≥ 3) alterations as high risk for purposes of postoperative management and long-term outcome is designed to measure recurrence and survival rates over 5–10 yr *(111)*. This novel treatment strategy may prove the value of genetic markers as routine prognostic indicators for clinical breast cancer management. Hormonal therapy appears advantageous in p53 negative/*bcl-2* positive breast tumors *(165)*. *ERBB2* antisense olignucleotides have been shown to inhibit the proliferation of *ERBB2*-amplified breast tumor cell lines, indicating uses for a new class of potential pharmacological agents in those breast tumors (~25%) overexpressing *ERBB2 (166)*. In cases of TSG loss or mutation, gene replacement therapy may be an attractive possibility, assuming a functional TSG can be introduced successfully and expressed stably to retard tumor growth.

Genetic alterations in precursor lesions such as atypical hyperplasia or PBD and the later stages of DCIS and lobular carcinoma *in situ* are lacking. Links between inherited predisposition and the increasing risk of breast cancer are still poorly understood, but will provide critical clues for the application of genetics to diagnosis and prevention of disease. Thus, without effective prevention measures, an efficacious approach for control of breast cancer may be the development of genetic diagnostic tools that recognize predisposing genes and early genetic alterations; these may provide means to reverse the first steps of tumorigenesis.

References

1. Wingo PA, Tong T, Bolden S: Cancer statistics, 1995. Canadian Cancer J Clin 45:8–30, 1995.
2. King M, Rowell S, Love SM: Inherited breast and ovarian cancer: What are the risks? What are the choices? JAMA 269:1975–1980, 1993.
3. Lynch HT, Albano WA, Danes BS, Layton MA, Kimberling WJ, Lynch JF, Cheng SC, Costello KA, Mulchahy GM, Wagner CA, Tindall SL: Genetic predisposition to breast cancer. Cancer 53:612–622, 1984.
4. Wolman SR, Dawson PJ: Genetic events in breast cancer and their clinical correlates. Crit Rev Oncogene 2:277–291, 1991.
5. Rowell S, Newman B, Boyd J, King MC: Inherited predisposition to breast and ovarian cancer. Am J Hum Genet 55:861–865, 1994.
6. Devilee P, Cornelisse CJ: Somatic genetic changes in human breast cancer. Biochem Biophys Acta 1198:113–130, 1994.
7. Devilee P, Schuuring E, van de Vijver MJ, Cornelisse CJ: Recent developments in the molecular genetic understanding of breast cancer. Oncogene 5:247–270, 1994.
8. Callahan R, Cropp CS, Merlo GR, Liscia DS, Cappa APM, Lidereau R: Somatic mutations and human breast cancer. Cancer 69:1582–1588, 1992.
9. Mitelman F: Catalog of Chromosome Aberrations in Cancer. Johansson B, Mertens F (eds.), New York: Wiley-Liss, 1994.
10. Weber-Matthiesen K, Winkemann M, Muller-Hermelink A, Schegelberger B, Grote W: Simultaneous fluorescence immunophenotyping and interphase

cytogenetics: a contribution to the characterization of tumor cells. J Histochem Cytochem 40:171–175, 1992.

11. Matsumura K, Kallioniemi A, Kallioniemi O, Chen L, Smith HS, Pinkel D, Gray J, Waldman FM: Deletion of chromosome 17p loci in breast cancer cells detected by fluorescence *in situ* hybridization. Cancer Res 52: 3474–3477, 1992.

12. Cajulis RS, Frias-Hidvegi D: Detection of numerical chromosomal abnormalities in malignant cells in fine needle aspirates by fluorescence *in situ* hybridization of interphase cell nuclei with chromosome-specific probes. Acta Cytologica 37:391–396, 1993.

13. Abati A, Sanford JS, Fetsch P, Marincola FM, Wolman SR: Fluorescence *in situ* hybridization (FISH): a user's guide to optimal preparation of cytologic specimens. Diagn Cytol 13:485–492, 1995.

14. Dhingra K, Sahin A, Supak J, Kim SY, Hortobagyi G, Hittelman WN: Chromosome *in situ* hybridization on formalin-fixed mammary tissue using non-isotopic, non-fluorescent probes: technical considerations and biological implications. Breast Cancer Res Treat 23:201–210, 1992.

15. Kallioniemi O, Kallioniemi A, Kurisu W, Thor A, Chen L, Smith HS, Waldman FM, Pinkel D, Gray JW: *ERBB2* amplification in breast cancer analyzed by fluorescence *in situ* hybridization. Proc Natl Acad Sci USA 89:5321–5325, 1992.

16. Wolman SR, Sanford JS, Flom K, Feiner H, Abati A, Bedrossian C: Genetic probes in cytology: principles and practice. Diagn Cytol 13:429–435, 1995.

17. Wolman SR, Smith HS, Stampfer M, Hackett AJ: Growth of diploid cells from breast cancers. Cancer Genet Cytogenet 16:49–64, 1985.

18. Zhang R, Wiley J, Howard SP, Meisner LF, Gould MN: Rare clonal karyotypic variants in primary cultures of human breast carcinoma cells. Cancer Res 49:444–449, 1989.

19. Geleick D, Muller H, Matter A, Torhorst J, Regenass U: Cytogenetics of breast cancer. Cancer Genet Cytogenet 46:217–219, 1990.

20. Bullerdiek J, Leuschner E, Taquia E, Bonk U, Bartnitzke S: Trisomy 8 as a recurrent clonal abnormality in breast cancer? Cancer Genet Cytogenet 65:64–67, 1993.

21. Pandis N, Heim S, Bardi G, Idvall I, Mandahl N, Mitelman F: Chromosome analysis of 20 breast carcinomas: cytogenetic multiclonality and karyotypic-pathologic correlations. Genes Chromosom Cancer 6:51–57, 1993.

22. Smith HS, Liotta LA, Hancock MC, Wolman SR, Hackett AJ: Invasiveness and ploidy of human mammary carcinomas in short-term culture. Proc Natl Acad Sci USA 82:1805–1809, 1985.

23. Trent J: Cytogenetic and molecular biologic alterations in human breast cancer: a review. Breast Cancer Res Treat 5:221–229, 1985.

24. Thompson F, Emerson J, Dalton W, Yang JM, McGee D, Villar H, Knox S, Massey K, Weinstein R, Bhattacharyya A, Trent J: Clonal chromosome abnormalities in human breast carcinomas. I. Twenty-eight cases with primary disease. Genes Chromosom Cancer 7:185–193, 1993.

25. Atkin NB, Baker MC: Are human cancers ever diploid—or often trisomic? Conflicting evidence from direct preparations and cultures. Cytogenet Cell Genet 53:58–60, 1990.

26. Slovak ML, Ho J, Simpson JF: Cytogenetic studies of 46 human breast carcinomas. Proc Am Assoc Cancer Res 33:40, 1992.

27. Dupont WD, Page DL, Parl FF, Vnencak-Jones CL, Plummer WD, Rados MS, Schuyler PA: Long-term risk of breast cancer in women with fibroadenoma. N Engl J Med 331:10–15, 1994.

28. Dupont WD, Page DL: Risk factors for breast cancer in women with proliferative breast disease. N Engl J Med 312:146–151, 1985.

29. Dupont WD, Parl FF, Hartmann WH, Brinton LA, Winfield AC, Worrell JA, Schuyler PA, Plummer WD: Breast cancer risk associated with proliferative breast disease and atypical hyperplasia. Cancer 71:1258–1265, 1993.

30. Levi F, Randimbison L, Van-Cong T, La Vecchia C: Incidence of breast cancer in women with fibroadenoma. Int J Cancer 57:681–683, 1994.

31. McDivitt RW, Stevens JA, Lee NC, Wingo PA, Rubin GL, Gersell D: Histologic types of benign breast disease and the risk for breast cancer. The Cancer and Steroid Hormone Study Group. Cancer 69:1408–1414, 1992.

32. Dietrich CY, Pandis N, Teixeira MR, Bardi G, Gerdes A, Andersen JA, Heim S: Chromosome abnormalities in benign hyperproliferative disorders of epithelial and stromal breast tissue. Int J Cancer 60:49–53, 1995.

33. Ozisik YY, Meloni AM, Stephenson CF, Peier A, Moore GE, Sandberg AA: Chromosome abnormalities in breast fibroadenomas. Cancer Genet Cytogenet 77:125–128, 1994.

34. Calabrese G, Di Virgilio C, Cianchett E, Guanciali Franchi P, Stuppia L, Parruti G, Bianchi PG, Palka G: Chromosome abnormalities in breast fibroadenomas. Genes Chromosom Cancer 3:202–204, 1991.

35. Momand J, Zambetti GP, Olson DC, George DL, Levine AJ: The *mdm-2* oncogene product forms a complex with the p53 protein and inhibits p53-mediated transactivation. Cell 69:1237–1245, 1992.

36. Micale MA, Visscher DW, Gulino SE, Wolman SR: Chromosomal aneuploidy in proliferative breast disease. Hum Pathol 25:29–35, 1994.

37. Pandis N, Heim S, Bardi G, Idvall I, Mandahl N, Mitelman F: Whole-arm t(1;16) and i(1q) as sole anomalies identify gain of 1q as a primary chromosomal abnormality in breast cancer. Genes Chromosom Cancer 5:235–238, 1992.

38. Pandis N, Jin Y, Gorunova L, Petersson C, Bardi G, Idvall I, Johansson B, Ingvar C, Mandahl N, Mitelman F, Heim S: Chromosome analysis of 97 primary breast carcinomas: identification of eight karyotypic subgroups. Genes Chromosom Cancer 12:173–185, 1995.

39. Dutrillaux B, Gerbault-Seureau M, Zafrani B: Characterization of chromosomal anomalies in human breast cancer: a comparison of 30 paradiploid cases with few chromosome changes. Cancer Genet Cytogenet 49:203–217, 1990.

40. Pandis N, Teixeira MR, Gerdes A, Limon J, Bardi G, Andersen JA, Idvall I, Mandahl N, Mitelman F, Heim S: Chromosome abnormalities in bilateral breast carcinomas. Cancer 76:250–258, 1995.

41. Johansson B, Heim S, Mandahl N, Mertens F, Mitelman F: Trisomy 7 in nonneoplastic cells. Genes Chromosom Cancer 6:199–205, 1993.
42. Dal Cin P, Aly MS, Delabie J, Ceuppens JL, van Gool S, van Damme B, Baert L, van Poppel H, van den Berghe H: Trisomy 7 and trisomy 10 characterize subpopulations of tumor-infiltrating lymphocytes in kidney tumors and in the surrounding kidney tissue. Proc Natl Acad Sci USA 89:9744–9748, 1992.
43. Rohen C, Meyer-Bolte K, Bonk U, Ebel T, Staats B, Leuschner E, Gohla G, Caselitz J, Bartnitzke S, Bullerdiek J: Trisomy 8 and 18 as frequent clonal and single-cell aberrations in 185 primary breast carcinomas. Cancer Genet Cytogenet 80:33–39, 1995.
44. Pandis N, Bardi G, Jin Y, Dietrich C, Johansson B, Andersen J, Mandahl N, Mitelman F, Heim S: Unbalanced t(1;16) as the sole karyotypic abnormality in a breast carcinoma and its lymph node metastasis. Cancer Genet Cytogenet 75:158–159, 1994.
45. Kreipe H, Feist H, Fischer L, Felgner J, Heidorn K, Mettler L, Parwaresch R: Amplification of c-*myc* but not of c-*erb*B-2 is associated with high proliferative capacity in breast cancer. Cancer Res 53:1956–1961, 1993.
46. Pertschuk LP, Feldman JG, Kim DS, Nayeri K, Eisenberg KB, Carter AC, Thelmo WT, Rhong ZT, Benn P, Grossman A: Steroid hormone receptor immunohistochemistry and amplification of c-*myc* protooncogene. Cancer 71:162–171, 1993.
47. Theillet C, Adelaide J, Louason G, Bonnet-Dorion F, Jacquemier J, Adnane J, Longy M, Katsaros D, Sismondi P, Gaudray P, Birnbaum D: *FGFR1* and *PLAT* genes and DNA amplifcation at 8p12 in breast and ovarian cancers. Genes Chromosom Cancer 7:219–226, 1993.
48. Bullerdiek J, Bonk U, Staats B, Leuschner E, Gohla G, Ebel T, Bartnitzke S: Trisomy 18 as the first chromosome abnormality in a medullary breast cancer. Cancer Genet Cytogenet 73:75–81, 1994.
49. Haldar S. Negrini M, Monne M, Sabbioni S. Croce CM: Down-regulation of *bcl-2* by *p53* in breast cancer cells. Cancer Res 54:2095–2097, 1994.
50. Thompson AM, Morris RG, Wallace M, Wyllie AH, Steel CM, Carter DC: Allele loss from 5q21 (APC/MCC) and 18q21 (DCC) and DCC mRNA expression in breast cancer. Br J Cancer 68:64–68, 1993.
51. Hainsworth PJ, Raphael KL, Stillwell RG, Bennett RC, Garson OM: Cytogenetic features of twenty-six primary breast cancers. Cancer Genet Cytogenet 52:205–218, 1991.
52. Pandis N, Bardi G, Heim S: Interrelationship between methodological choices and conceptual models in solid tumor cytogenetics. Cancer Genet Cytogenet 76:76–84, 1994.
53. Pandis N, Heim S, Bardi G, Limon J, Mandahl N, Mitelman F: Improved technique for short-term culture and cytogenetic analysis of human breast cancer. Genes Chromosom Cancer 5:14–20, 1992.
54. Pandis N, Jin Y, Limon J, Bardi G, Idvall I, Mandahl N, Mitelman F, Heim S: Interstitial deletion of the short arm of chromosome 3 as a primary

chromosome abnormality in carcinomas of the breast. Genes Chromosom Cancer 6:151–155, 1993.

55. Steinarsdottir M, Petursdottir I, Snorradottir S, Eyfjord JE, Ogmundsdottir HM: Cytogenetic studies of breast carcinomas: different karyotypic profiles detected by direct harvesting of short-term culture. Genes Chromosom Cancer 13:239–248, 1995.

56. Mitchell ELD, Santibanez-Koref MF: 1p13 is the most frequently involved band in structural chromosomal rearrangements in human breast cancer. Genes Chromosom Cancer 2:278–289, 1990.

57. Mugneret F, Sidaner I, Favre B, Manone L, Maynadie M, Caillot D, Solary E: der(16) t(1;16)(q10;p10) in multiple myeloma: a new non-random abnormality that is frequently associated with Burkitt's type translocations. Leukemia 9:277–281, 1995.

58. Mugneret F, Dastugue N, Favre B, Sidaner I, Salles B: der(16)t(1;16)(q11;q11) in myelodysplastic syndromes: a new non-random abnormality characterized by cytogenetic and fluorescence *in situ* hybridization studies. Br J Haematol 90:119–124, 1995.

59. Douglass EC, Rowe ST, Valentine M, Parham D, Meyer WH, Thompson E: A scond nonrandom translocation, der(16)t(1;16)(q21;q13), in Ewing sarcoma and peripheral neuroectodermal tumor. Cytogenet Cell Genet 53:87–90, 1990.

60. Almeida A, Kokalj-Vokac N, Lefrancois D, Viegas-Pequignot E, Jeanpierre M, Dutrillaux B, Malfoy B: Hypomethylation of classical satellite DNA and chromosome instability in lymphoblastoid cell lines. Hum Genet 91:538–546, 1993.

61. Hainsworth PJ, Raphael KL, Stillwell RG, Bennett RC, Garson OM: Rearrangement of chromosome 1p in breast cancer correlates with poor prognostic features. Br J Cancer 66:131–135, 1992.

62. Devilee P, van Vliet M, Bardoel A, Kievitis T, Kuipers-Dijkshoorn N, Pearson PL, Cornelisse CJ: Frequent somatic imbalance of parental chromosomes 1 in human primary breast carcinoma. Cancer Res 51:1020–1025, 1991.

63. Larsson C, Bystrom C, Skoog L, Rotstein S, Nordenskjold M: Genomic alterations in human breast carcinomas. Genes Chromosom Cancer 2:191–197, 1990.

64. Bieche I, Champeme M, Matifas F, Cropp CS, Callahan R, Lidereau R: Two distinct regions involved in 1p deletion in human primary breast cancer. Cancer Res 53:1990–1994, 1993.

65. Genuardi M, Tsihira H, Anderson DE, Saunders GF: Distal deletion of chromosome 1p in ductal carcinoma of the breast. Am J Hum Genet 45:73–82, 1989.

66. Bieche I, Champeme M, Merlo G, Larsen C, Callahan R, Lidereau R: Loss of heterozygosity of the L-myc oncogene in human breast tumors. Hum Genet 85:101–105, 1990.

67. Borg A, Zhang Q, Olsson H, Wenngren E: Chromosome 1 alterations in breast cancer: allelic loss on 1p and 1q is related to lymphogenic metastases and poor prognosis. Genes Chromosom Cancer 5:311–320, 1992.

68. Bunnell B, Heath LS, Adams DE, Lahti JM, Kidd VJ: Elevated expression of a p58 protein kinase leads to changes in the CHO cell cycle. Proc Natl Acad Sci USA 87:7467–7471, 1987.

69. Bunnell B, Adams DE, Kidd VJ: Transient expression of a p58 protein kinase cDNA enhances mammalian glycosyltransferase activity. Biochem Biophys Res Commun 171:196–203, 1990.

70. Eipers PG, Barnoski BL, Han J, Carroll AJ, Kidd VJ: Localization of the expressed human p58 protein kinase chromosomal gene to chromosome 1p36 and a highly related sequence to chromosome 15. Genomics 11:621–629, 1991.

71. Bieche I, Champeme M, Lidereau R: A tumor suppressor gene on chromosome 1p32-pter controls the amplification of *MYC* family genes in breast cancer. Cancer Res 54:4274–4276, 1994.

72. Trent J, Yang J, Emerson J, Dalton W, McGee D, Massey K, Thompson F, Villar H: Clonal chromosome abnormalities in human breast carcinomas II. Thirty-four cases with metastatic disease. Genes Chromosom Cancer 7:194–203, 1993.

73. Bieche I, Champeme M, Lidereau R: Loss and gain of distinct regions of chromosome 1q in primary breast cancer. Clin Cancer Res 1:123–127, 1995.

74. Chen L, Matsumura K, Deng G, Kurisu W, Ljung B, Lerman MI, Waldman FM, Smith HS: Deletion of two separate regions on chromosome 3p in breast cancers. Cancer Res 54:3021–3024, 1994.

75. Sato T, Akiyama F, Sakamoto G, Kasumi F, Nakamura Y: Accumulation of genetic alterations and progression of primary breast cancer. Cancer Res 51:5794–5799, 1991.

76. Deng G, Chen L, Schott DR, Thor A, Bhargava V, Ljung B, Chew K, Smith HS: Loss of heterozygosity and *p53* gene mutations in breast cancer. Cancer Res 54:499–505, 1994.

77. Devilee P, van Vliet M, van Sloun P, Dijkshoorn NK, Hermans J, Pearson PL, Cornelisse CJ: Allelotype of human breast carcinoma: a second major site for loss of heterozygosity is on chromosome 6q. Oncogene 6:1705–1711, 1991.

78. Orphanos V, McGrown G, Hey Y, Boyle JM, Santibanez-Koref M: Proximal 6q, a region showing allele loss in primary breast cancer. Br J Cancer 71:290–293, 1995.

79. Magdelenat H, Gerbault-Seureau M, Dutrillaux B: Relationship between loss of estrogen and progesterone receptor expression and of 6q and 11q chromosome arms in breast cancer. Int J Cancer 57:63–66, 1994.

80. Iwase H, Greenman JM, Barnes DM, Bobrow L, Hodgson S, Mathew CG: Loss of heterozygosity of the oestrogen receptor gene in breast cancer. Br J Cancer 71:448–450, 1995.

81. Bieche I, Champeme M, Matifas F, Hacene K, Callahan R, Lidereau R: Loss of heterozygosity on chromosome 7q and agressive primary breast cancer. Lancet 339:139–143, 1992.

82. Larsson C, Bystrom C, Skoog L, Rotstein S, Nordenskjold M: Genomic alterations in human breast carcinomas. Genes Chromosom Cancer 2:191–197, 1990.

83. Zenklusen JC, Bieche I, Lidereau R, Conti CJ: $(C-A)_n$ microsatellite repeat D7S522 in the most commonly deleted region in human primary breast cancer. Proc Natl Acad Sci USA 91:12,155–12,158, 1994.

84. Champeme M, Bieche I, Beuzelin M, Lidereau R: Loss of heterozygosity on 7q31 occurs early during breast tumorigenesis. Genes Chromosom Cancer 12:304–306, 1995.

85. Borresen A, Andersen TI, Eyfjord JE, Cornelis RS, Thorlacius S, Borg A, Johansson U, Theillet C, Scherneck S, Hartman S, Cornelisse CJ, Hovig E, Devilee P: *TP53* mutations and breast cancer prognosis: particularly poor survival rates for cases with mutations in the zinc-binding domains. Genes Chromosom Cancer 14:71–75, 1995.

86. Yaremko ML, Recant WM, Westbrook CA: Loss of heterozygosity from the short arm of chromosome 8 is an early event in breast cancers. Genes Chromosom Cancer 13:186–191, 1995.

87. Radford DM, Fair KL, Phillips NJ, Ritter JH, Steinbrueck T, Holt MS, Donis-Keller H: Allelotyping of ductal carcinoma in situ of the breast: deletion of loci on 8p, 13q 16q, 17p, and 17q. Cancer Res 55:3399–3405, 1995.

88. Ferti-Passantonopoulou A, Panani AD, Raptis S: Preferential involvement of 11q23–24 and 11p15 in breast cancer. Cancer Genet Cytogenet 51: 183–188, 1991.

89. Carter SL, Negrini M, Baffa R, Gillum DR, Rosenberg AL, Schwartz GF, Croce CM: Loss of heterozygosity at 11q22–q23 in breast cancer. Cancer Res 54:6270–6274, 1994.

90. Negrini M, Rasio D, Hampton GM, Sabbioni S, Rattan S, Carter SL, Rosenberg AL, Schwartz GF, Shiloh Y, Cavenee WK, Croce CM: Definition and refinement of chromosome 11 regions of loss of heterozygosity in breast cancer: identification of a new region at 11q23.3. Cancer Res 55:3003–3007, 1995.

91. Theillet C, Lidereau R, Escot C, Hutzell P, Brunet M, Gest J, Schlom J, Callahan R: Loss of a c-H*ras*-1 allele and agressive human primary breast carcinomas. Cancer Res 46:4776–4781, 1986.

92. Rochlitz CF, Scott GK, Dodson JM, Liu E, Dollbaum C, Smith HS, Benz CC: Incidence of activating ras oncogene mutations associated with primary metastatic human breast cancer. Cancer Res 49:357–360, 1989.

93. Winqvist R, Mannermaa A, Alavaikko M, Blanco G. Taskinen PJ, Kiviniemi H, Newsham I, Cavenee W: Refinement of regional loss of heterozygosity for chromosome 11p15.5 in human breast tumors. Cancer Res 53:4486–4488, 1993.

94. Mackay J, Elder PA, Steel CM, Forrest APM, Evans HJ: Allele loss on short arm of chromosome 17 in breast cancers. Lancet ii:1384–1385, 1988.

95. Zhuang Z, Merino MJ, Chuaqui R, Liotta LA, Emmert-Buck MR: Identical allelic loss on chromosome 11q13 in microdissected *in situ* and invasive human breast cancer. Cancer Res 55:467–471, 1995.

96. Schuuring E, Verhoeven E, vanTinteren H, Peterse JL, Nunnink B, Thunnissen FBJM, Devilee P, Cornelisse CJ, van de Vijver MJ, Mooi WJ,

Michalides RJAM: Amplification of genes within the chromosome 11q13 region is indicative of poor prognosis in patients with operable breast cancer. Cancer Res 52:5229–5234, 1992.

97. Gaffey MJ, Frierson HF, Williams ME: Chromosome 11q13, c-*erb*B-2, and c-*myc* amplification in invasive breast carcinoma: clinicopathologic correlations. Modern Pathol 6:654–659, 1993.

98. Tsuda HS, Hirohashi Y, Shimosato T, Hirota S, Tsugane H, Yamamoto N, Miyajima K, Toyoshima T, Yamamoto J, Yokota T, Yoshida H, Sakamoto H, Terada M, Suigmura T: Correlation between long-term survival in breast cancer patients and amplification of two putative oncogene-coamplification units: hst-1/int-2 and c-erbB2/ear-1. Cancer Res 49:3104–3108, 1989.

99. Champeme M, Bieche I, Lizard S, Lidereau R: 11q13 amplification in local recurrence of human primary breast cancer. Genes Chromosom Cancer 54 12:128–133, 1995.

100. Borg A, Sigurdsson H, Clark GM, Ferno M, Fuqua SAW, Olsson H, Killander D, McGurie WL: Association of int-2/hst-1 coamplification in primary breast cancer with hormone-dependent phenotype and poor prognosis. Br J Cancer 63:136–142, 1991.

101. Brookes S, Lammie GA, Schuuring E, de Boer C, Michalides R, Dickson C, Peters G: Amplified region of chromosome band 11q13 in breast and squamous cell carcinomas encompasses three CpG island telomeric of *FGF3*, including the expressed gene *EMS1*. Genes Chromsom Cancer 6:222–231, 1993.

102. Hampton GM, Mannermaa A, Winquist R, Alavaikko M, Blanco G, Taskinen PJ, Kiviniemi H, Newsham I, Cavenee WK, Evans GA: Loss of heterozygosity in sporadic human breast carcinoma: a common region between 11q22 and 11q23.3. Cancer Res 54:4586–4589, 1994.

103. Singh S, Simon M, Meybohm I, Jantke I, Jonat W, Maass H, Goedde HW: Human breast cancer: frequent p53 allele loss and protein overexpression. Hum Genet 90:635–640, 1993.

104. Tomlinson IPM, Stickland JE, Lee ASG, Bromley L, Evans MF, Morton J, O'D McGee J: Loss of heterozygosity on chromosome 11q in breast cancer. J Clin Pathol 48:424–428, 1995.

105. Winqvist R, Hampton GM, Mannermaa A, Blanco G, Alavaikko M, Kiviniemi H. Taskinen PJ, Evans GA, Wright FA, Newsham I, Cavenee WK: Loss of heterozygosity for chromosome 11 in primary human breast tumors is associated with poor survival after metastasis. Cancer Res 55: 2660–2664, 1995.

106. Lindblom A, Sandelin K, Iselius I, Dumanski J, White I, Nordenskjold M, Larsson C: Predisposition for breast cancer in carriers of constitutional translocation 11q;22q. Am J Hum Genet 54:871–876, 1994.

107. Cornelisse CJ, Kuipers-Dijkshoorn N, van Vliet M, Hermans J, Devilee P: Fractional allelic imbalance in human breast cancer increases with tetraploidization and chromosome loss. Int J Cancer 50:544–548, 1992.

108. Cleton-Jansen A, Moerland EW, Kuipers-Dijkshoorn JJ, Callen DF, Sutherland GR, Hansen B, Devilee P, Cornelisse CJ: At least two different

regions are involved in allelic imbalanced on chromosome arm 16q in breast cancer. Genes Chromosom Cancer 9:101–107, 1994.

109. Tsuda H, Callen DF, Fukutomi T, Nakamura Y, Hirohashi S: Allele loss on chromosome 16q24.2-qter occurs frequently in breast cancers irrespectively of differences in phenotype and extent of spread. Cancer Res 54:513–517, 1994.

110. Lindblom A, Rotstein S, Skoog L, Nordenskjold M, Larsson C: Deletions on chromosome 16 in primary familial breast carcinomas are associated with development of distant metastases. Cancer Res 53:3707–3711, 1993.

111. Harada Y, Katagiri T, Ito I, Akiyama F, Sakamoto G, Kasumi F, Nakamura Y, Emi M: Genetic studies of 457 breast cancers. Clinicopathologic parameters compared with genetic alterations. Cancer 74:2281–2286, 1994.

112. Doggett NA, Callen DF: Report of the third international workshop on human chromosome 16 mapping 1994. Cytogenet Cell Genet 68: 166–177, 1995.

113. Silletti S, Yao J, Sanford J, Mohamed AN, Otto T, Wolman SR, Raz A: Autocrine motility factor receptor in human bladder cancer: gene expression, loss of cell-contact regulation, and chromosomal mapping. Int J Oncol 3:801–807, 1993.

114. Rosenberg C, Andersen TI, Nesland JM, Lier ME, Brogger A, Borresen A: Genetic alterations of chromosome 17 in human breast carcinoma studied by fluorescence in situ hybridization and molecular DNA technigues. Cancer Genet Cytogenet 75:1–5, 1994.

115. Merlo GR, Venesio T, Bernardi A, Cropp CS, Diella F, Cappa APM, Callahan R, Liscia DS: Evidence for a second tumor suppressor gene on 17p linked to high S-phase index in primary human breast carcinomas. Cancer Genet Cytogenet 76:106–111, 1994.

116. Coles C, Thompson AM, Elder PA, Cohen BB, Mackenzie IM, Cranston G, Chetty U, Mackay J, Macdonald M, Nakamura Y, Hoyheim B, Steel CM: Evidence implicating at least two genes on chromosome 17p in breast carcinogenesis. Lancet 336:761–763, 1990.

117. Cornelis RS, van Vliet M, Vos CBJ, Cleton-Jansen A, van de Vijver MJ, Peterse JL, Khan PM, Borresen A, Cornelisse CJ, Devilee P: Evidence for a gene on 17p13.3, distal to *TP53*, as a target for allele loss in breast tumors without p53 mutations. Cancer Res 54:4200–4206, 1994.

118. Radford DM, Fair K, Thompson AM, Ritter JH, Holt M, Steinbrueck T, Wallace M, Wells SA, Donis-Keller HR: Allelic loss on chromosome 17 in ductal carcinoma *in situ* of the breast. Cancer Res 53:2947–2950, 1993.

119. Kirchweger R, Zeillinger R, Schneeberger C, Speiser P, Louason G, Theillet C: Patterns of allele losses suggest the existence of five distinct regions of LOH on chromosome 17 in breast cancer. Int J Cancer 56:193–199, 1994.

120. Coles C, Condie A, Chetty U, Steel CM, Evans HJ, Prosser J: *p53* mutations in breast cancer. Cancer Res 52:5291–5298, 1992.

121. Marchetti A, Buttitta F, Pellegrini S, Campani D, Diella F, Cecchetti D, Callahan R, Bistocchi M: *p53* mutations and histological type of invasive breast carcinoma. Cancer Res 53:4665–4669, 1993.

122. Andersen TI, Holm R, Nesland JM, Heimdal KR, Ottestad L, Borresen AL: Prognostic significance of *TP53* alterations in breast carcinoma. Br J Cancer 68:540–548, 1993.
123. Cunningham JM, Ingle JN, Jung SH, Cha SS, Wold LE, Farr G, Witzig TE, Krook JE, Wieand HS, Kovach JS: p53 gene expression in node-positive breast cancer: relationship to DNA ploidy and prognosis. J Natl Cancer Inst 86:1871–1873, 1994.
124. Davidoff AM, Kerns BM, Iglehart JD, Marks JR: Maintenance of *p53* alterations throughout breast cancer progression. Cancer Res 51:2605–2610, 1991.
125. Cheickh MB, Rouanet P, Louason G, Jeanteur P, Theillet C: An attempt to define sets of cooperating genetic alterations in human breast cancer. Int J Cancer 51:542–547, 1992.
126. Cornelis RS, Devilee P, van Vliet: M, Kuipers-Dijkshoorn N. Kersenmaeker A, Bardoel A, Khan PM, Cornelisse CJ: Allele loss patterns on chromosome 17q in 109 breast carcinomas indicate at least two distinct target regions. Oncogene 8:781–785, 1993.
127. Saito H, Inazawa J, Saito S, Kasumi F, Koi S, Sagae S, Kudo R, Saito J, Noda K, Nakamura Y: Detailed deletion mapping of chromosome 17q in ovarian and breast cancers: 2-cM region on 17q21.3 often and commonly deleted in tumors. Cancer Res 53:3382–3385, 1993.
128. Cropp CS, Champeme M, Lidereau R, Callahan R: Identification of three regions on chromosome 17q in primary human breast carcinomas which are frequently deleted. Cancer Res 53:5617–5619, 1993.
129. Cropp CS, Nevanlinna HA, Pyrhonen S, Stenman U, Salmikangas P, Albertsen H, White R, Callahan R: Evidence for involvement of BRCA1 in sporadic breast carcinomas. Cancer Res 54:2548–2551, 1994.
130. Futreal PA, Soderkvist P, Marks JR, Iglehart JD, Cochran C, Barrett JC, Wiseman RW: Detection of frequent allelic loss on proximal chromosome 17q in sporadic breast carcinoma using microsatellite length polymorphisms. Cancer Res 52:2624–2627, 1992.
131. Nagai MA, Yamamoto L, Salaorni S, Pacheco MM, Brentani MM, Barbosa EM, Brentani RR, Mazoyer S, Smith SA, Ponder BAJ, Mulligan LM: Detailed deletion mapping of chromosome segment 17q12–21 in sporadic breast tumours. Genes Chromosom Cancer 11:58–62, 1994.
132. Futreal PA, Liu Q, Shattuck-Eidens D, Cochran C, Harshman K, Tavtigian S, Bennett LM, Haugen-Strano A, Swensen J, Miki Y, Eddington K, McClure M, Frye C, Weaver-Feldhaus J, Ding W, Gholami Z, Soderkvist P, Terry L, Jhanwar S, Berchuck A, Iglehart JD, Marks J, Ballinger DG, Barrett JC, Skolnick MH, Kamb A, Wisemen R: *BRCA1* mutations in primary breast and ovarian carcinomas. Science 266: 120–122, 1994.
133. Meravjer SD, Pham TM, Caduff RF, Chen M, Poy EL, Cooney KA, Weber BL, Collins FS, Johnston C, Frank TS: Somatic mutations in the *BRCA1* gene in sporadic ovarian tumours. Nature Genet 9:439–443, 1995.
134. Aberle H, Bierkeamp C, Torchard D, Serova O, Wagner T, Natt E, Wirsching J, Heidkamper C, Montagna M, Lynch HT, Lenoir GM, Scherer G,

Feunteun J, Kemler R: The human plakoglobin gene localizes on chromosome 17q21 and is subjected to loss of heterozygosity in breast and ovarian cancers. Proc Natl Acad Sci USA 92:6384–6388, 1995.

135. Slamon DJ, Gogolphin W, Jones LA, Holt JA, Wong SG, Keith DE, Levin WJ, Stuart SG, Udove J, Ullrich A, Press MF: Studies of the HER-2/neu proto-oncogene in human breast cancer and ovarian cancer. Science 244: 707–712, 1989.

136. Seshadri R, Firgaira FA, Horsfall DJ, McCaul K, Setlur V, Paul Kitchen for the South Australian Breast Cancer Study Group: Clinical significance of HER-2/*neu* oncogene amplification in primary breast cancer. J Clin Oncol 11:1936–1942, 1993.

137. Lonn U, Lonn S, Nilsson B, Stenkvist B: Prognostic value of *erb*-B2 and *myc* amplification in breast cancer imprints. Cancer 75:2681–2687, 1995.

138. Iglehart JD, Kraus MH, Langton BC, Huper G, Kerns BJ, Marks JR: Increased erbB-2 gene copies and expression in multiple stages of breast cancer. Cancer Res 50:6701–6707, 1990.

139. Eyfjord JE, Thorlacius S, Steinarsdottir M, Valgardsdottir R, Ogmundsdottir HM, Anamthawat-Jonsson K: *p53* abnormalities and genomic instability in primary human breast carcinomas. Cancer Res 55:646–651, 1995.

140. Hartwell L: Defects in a cell cycle checkpoint may be responsible for the genomic instability of cancer cells. Cell 71:543–546, 1992.

141. Yin Y, Tainsky MA, Bischoff FZ, Strong LC, Wahl GM: Wild-type *p53* restores cell cycle control and inhibits gene amplification in cells with mutant *p53* alleles. Cell 70:937–948, 1992.

142. Saint-Ruf C, Gerbault-Seureau M, Viegas-Pequignot E, Zafrani B, Malfoy B, Dutrillaux B: Recurrent homogeneously staining region in 8p1 in breast cancer and lack of amplification of POLB, LHRH, and PLAT genes. Cancer Genet Cytogenet 52:27–35, 1991.

143. Zafrani B, Gerbault-Sseureau M, Mosseri V, Dutrillaux B: Cytogenetic study of breast cancer: clinicopathologic significance of homogeneously staining regions in 84 patients. Hum Pathol 23:542–547, 1992.

144. Gebhart E, Bruderlein S, Augustus M, Siebert E, Feldner J, Schmidt W: Cytogenetic studies on human breast carcinomas. Breast Cancer Res Treat 8:125–138, 1986.

145. Muleris M, Almeida A, Gerbault-Seureau M, Malfoy B, Dutrillaux B: Detection of DNA amplification in 17 primary breast carcinomas with homogeneously staining regions by a modified comparative genomic hybridization technique. Genes Chromosom Cancer 10:160–170, 1994.

146. Almeida A, Muleris M, Dutrillaux B, Malfoy B: The insulin-like growth factor I receptor gene is the target for the 15q26 amplicon in breast cancer. Genes Chromosom Cancer 11:63–65, 1994.

147. Bello MJ, Rey JA: Cytogenetic analysis of metastatic effusions from breast tumors. Neoplasma 36:71–81, 1989.

148. Saint-Ruf C, Gerbault-Seureau M, Viegas-Pequignot E, Zafrani B, Cassingena R, Dutrillaux B: Proto-oncogene amplification and homogeneously

staining regions in human breast carcinomas. Genes Chromosom Cancer 2:18–26, 1990.

149. Trent JM, Weber B, Guan XY, Zhang J, Collins F, Abel K, Diamond A, Meltzer P: Microdissection and microcloning of chromosomal alterations in human breast cancer. Breast Cancer Res Treat 33:95–102, 1995.

150. Kallioniemi A, Kallioniemi O, Piper J, Tanner M, Stokke T, Chen L, Smith HS, Pinkel D, Gray JW, Waldman FM: Detection and mapping of amplified DNA sequences in breast cancer by comparative genomic hybridization. Proc Natl Acad Sci USA 91:2156–2160, 1994.

151. Tanner MM, Tirkkonen M, Kallioniemi A, Collins C, Stokke T, Karhu R, Kowbel D, Shadravan F, Hintz M, Kuo W, Waldman FM, Isola JJ, Gray JW, Kallioniemi O: Increased copy number at 20q13 in breast cancer: defining the critical region and exclusion of candidate genes. Cancer Res 54: 4257–4260, 1994.

152. Berns EMJJ, Klijn JGM, van Staveren IL, Portengen H, Foekens JA: Sporadic amplification of the insulin-like growth factor I receptor gene in human breast tumors. Cancer Res 52:1036–1039, 1992.

153. Klein G, Klein E: Evolution of tumors and the impact on molecular oncology. Nature 315:190–195, 1985.

154. Takita K, Sato T, Miyagi M, Watatani M, Akiyqmq F, Sakmoto G, Kasumi F, Abe R, Nakamura Y: Correlation of loss of alleles on the short arms of chromosomes 11 and 17 with metastasis of primary breast cancer to lymph nodes. Cancer Res 52:3941–3917, 1992.

155. Holzlsouer KJ, Harris EL, Parshad R, Fogel S, Bigbee WL, Sanford KK: Familial clustering of breast cancer: possible interaction between DNA repair proficiency and radiation exposure in the development of breast cancer. Int J Cancer 64:14–17, 1995.

156. Tsuda H, Hirohashi S: Identification of multiple breast cancers of multicentric origin by histological observations and distribution of allele loss on chromosome 16q. Cancer Res 55:3395–3398, 1995.

157. Magdelenat H, Gerbault-Seureau M, Laine-Bidron C, Prieur M, Dutrillaux B: Genetic evolution of breast cancer: II. Relationship with estrogen and progesterone receptor expression. Breast Cancer Res Treat 22:119–127, 1992.

158. Miki Y, Swensen J, Shattuck-Eidens D, Futreal PA, Harshman K, Tavtigian S, Liu Q, Cochran C, Bennett LM, Ding W, Bell R, Rosenthal J, Hussey C, Tran T, McClure M, Frye C, Hattier T, Phelps R, Haugen-Strano A, Katcher H, Yakumo K, Gholami Z, Shaffer D, Stone S, Bayer S, Wray C, Bogden R, Dayananth P, Ward J, Tonin P, Narod S, Bristow PK, Norris FH, Helvering L, Morrison P, Rosteck P, Lai M, Barrett JC, Lewis C, Neuhausen S, Cannon-Albright L, Goldgar D, Wiseman R, Kamb A, Skolnick MH: A strong candidate for the breast and ovarian cancer susceptibility gene *BRCA1*. Science 266:67–71, 1994.

159. Wooster R, Neuhausen SL, Mangion J, Quirk Y, Ford D, Collins N, Nguyen K, Seal S, Tran T, Averill D, Fields P, Marshall G, Narod S, Lenoir GM, Lynch H, Feunteun J, Devilee P, Cornelisse CJ, Menko FH, Daly PA,

Ormiston W, McManus R, Pye C, Lewis CM, Cannon-Albright LA, Peto J, Ponder BAJ, Skolnick MH, Easton DF, Goldgar DE, Stratton MR: Localization of a breast cancer susceptibility gene, *BRCA2*, to chromosome 13q12–13. Science 265:2088–2090, 1994.

160. Li FP, Fraumni JF, Mulvihill JJ, Blattner WA, Dreyfus MG, Tucker MA, Miller RW: A cancer family syndrome in twenty-four kindreds. Cancer Res 48:5358–5362, 1988.

161. Weksberg R, Teshima I, Williams BRG, Greenberg CR, Pueschel SM, Chernos JE, Fowlow SB, Hoyme E, Anderson IJ, Whiteman DAH, Fisher N, Squire J: Molecular characterization of cytogenetic alterations associated with the Beckwith-Wiedemann syndrome (BWS) phenotype refines the localization and suggests the gene for BWS is imprinted. Human Mol Genet 2:549–556, 1993.

162. Wooster R, Mangion J, Eeles R, Smith S, Dowsett M, Averill D, Barrett-Lee P, Easton DF, Ponder BAJ: A germline mutation in the androgen receptor gene in two brothers with breast cancer and Reifenstein syndrome. Nature Genet 2:132–134, 1992.

163. Lobaccaro J, Lumbroso S, Belon C, Galtier-Dereure F, Bringer J, Lesimple T, Heron J, Pujol H, Sultan C: Male breast cancer and the androgen receptor gene. Nature Genet 5:109–110, 1993.

164. Yahalom J, Petrek JA, Biddinger PW, Kessler S, Dershaw DD, McCormick B, Osborne MP, Kinne DA, Rosen PP: Breast cancer in patients irradiated for Hodgkin's disease: a clinical and pathologic analysis of 45 events in 37 patients. J Clin Oncol 10:1674–1681, 1992.

165. Hurlimann J, Larrinaga B, Vala DLM: *bcl-2* protein in invasive ductal breast carcinomas. Virchows Archiv 426:163–168, 1995.

166. Colomer R, Lupu R, Bacus SS, Gelmann EP: *erb*B-2 antisense oligonucleotides inhibit the proliferation of breast carcinoma cells with *erb*B-2 oncogene amplification. Br J Cancer 70:819–825, 1994.

Chapter 7

Karyotypic Characteristics of Colorectal Tumors

Georgia Bardi, Nikos Pandis, Felix Mitelman, and Sverre Heim

Introduction

Colorectal cancer is not only one of the most common human malignancies, but one with a high mortality rate. A variety of mechanisms have been implicated in the development of colorectal cancer, including dietary and other environmental as well as genetic factors, especially somatic cell mutations. In spite of the utilization of numerous histopathologic and other tumor markers *(1–3)*, the management of patients with this disease is difficult and prognostication remains notoriously unreliable.

One investigative approach promising to yield information, not only about the pathogenetic events of tumorigenesis in general, but also about the inherent aggressiveness of individual neoplasms, is the analysis of the tumor cells' acquired genetic abnormalities. The search for such changes can proceed, at least, at three different levels of resolution: at the cellular level by classic cytological methods or flow cytometric measurement of total nuclear DNA, at the cytogenetic level by microscopic examination of metaphase chromosomes, and at the gene or primary DNA structure level utilizing molecular

From: *Human Cytogenetic Cancer Markers*   Edited by S. R. Wolman and S. Sell
Humana Press Inc., Totowa, NJ

genetic techniques. The latter approach has been the most popular in recent years and has led to several exciting discoveries, e.g., the identification of the pathogenetic role of the *APC (4)* and *MCC (5)* genes in 5q, *TP53* in 17p *(6)*, and *DCC* in 18q *(7)*. When the new DNA-level knowledge was forged into a genetic model of large bowel carcinogenesis by Fearon and Vogelstein *(8)*, for the first time, the sequential events of multistage tumor development *(9)* could be rephrased in molecular terms.

However powerful the DNA recombinant techniques may be, they entail certain inherent limitations compared with cytological screening techniques such as classical cytogenetics with banding *(10)*, especially when it comes to detecting previously unsuspected abnormalities and clonal heterogeneity within the tumor parenchyma. As we see, the systematic cytogenetic study of colorectal tumor cells has not only yielded information corroborating and extending the molecular genetic model of carcinogenesis, but has also provided a host of new and unexpected discoveries. Yet again it underscores how essential it is for a balanced picture of the genetic mechanisms of tumorigenesis that investigations should focus on both the microscopic and submicroscopic resolution levels.

Colorectal Carcinomas Have Nonrandom Chromosome Aberrations

Nearly 300 karyotypically abnormal carcinomas of the large bowel, almost all of them sporadic adenocarcinomas, have been reported *(11)*. The value of the published information is somewhat diminished by the fact that as many as 50% of these cases had one or more unidentified chromosomal markers or otherwise incompletely described karyotypes. In spite of this, the main conclusion, that carcinomas of the large intestine display characteristic patterns of acquired chromosomal abnormalities, can now be said to have been established beyond doubt.

In all major published series of cytogenetically investigated colorectal carcinomas, clonal chromosome aberrations (Fig. 1) were found in the vast majority of cases. However, a small fraction of the tumors, on average 10% *(12–14)*, appear to have a normal chromosome complement. This does not constitute conclusive evidence

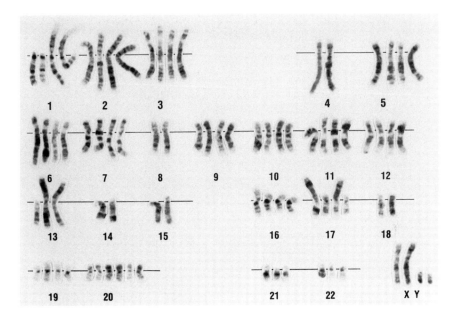

Fig. 1. Karyogram of a colon adenocarcinoma with 81 chromosomes and several aberrations.

against the somatic mutation theory of cancer. Some tumors with a normal karyotype may have only submicroscopic genomic rearrangements or the examined cells may have been of stromal origin; once a cell enters mitosis and is taken through the steps necessary for chromosome analysis, it is no longer possible to determine its phenotype. That stromal admixture in primary cultures of colorectal carcinomas may represent a real problem is evident from the fact that the growth fraction of tumor parenchyma cells may be as low as 2% *(15,16).* At least to some extent this problem can be overcome, however, as demonstrated by the increase in the percentage of cytogenetically abnormal cases experienced when the culturing techniques are optimized *(14).* Whatever the explanation for the finding of normal tumor karyotypes may be, they seem to reflect some kind of biologically important reality, inasmuch as patient survival in these cases tends to be longer *(17).*

The modal chromosome number of colorectal carcinomas with clonal chromosome aberrations varies from near-diploid to near-pentaploid (Fig. 1). More than half of the cases have had near-diploid

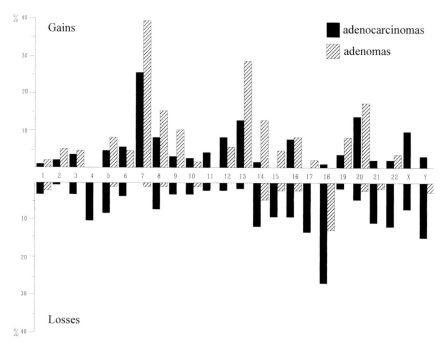

Fig. 2. Histogram showing the frequencies of numerical chromosomal changes in the colorectal adenomas (88 cases) and adenocarcinomas (220 cases) reported in the cytogenetic literature.

or pseudodiploid karyotypes, which is consistent with the finding in several DNA flow cytometry studies that a high percentage of colorectal carcinomas are diploid *(18,19)*. Evidently, among the flow cytometrically normal cases may be not only tumors with normal karyotypes or one or a few numerical and/or structural changes, but also tumors with massive chromosomal rearrangements leading to no or only small changes in the total DNA content. Carcinomas with a near-triploid chromosome number usually have both numerical and structural rearrangements, although a few such tumors with numerical abnormalities only have recently been described *(14)*.

The most common numerical aberrations (Fig. 2) have been the loss of one chromosome 18 (detected in 26% of all examined cases), gain of chromosome 7 (25%), loss of the Y (15%), gain of chromosome 20 (14%), loss of chromosome 17 (13%), gain of chromosome 13, and loss of chromosomes 14 and 22 (each seen in 12% of all tumors with abnormalities).

With the exception of the Y, all chromosomes have now been involved recurrently in structural rearrangements in colorectal carcinomas. The most common aberrations have been i(8)(q10), i(17)(q10), del(17)(p11), i(13)(q10), i(1)(q10), and del(1)(p13). The net outcomes of these rearrangements are loss of 1p and gain of 1q, loss of 8p and gain of 8q, loss of 13p and gain of 13q, and loss of 17p and gain of 17q. The consistent losses presumably exert their influence through loss of tumor suppressor genes, but the effect of the gains remains elusive. Although the aforementioned anomalies were seen repeatedly in all major series of cytogenetically characterized colorectal carcinomas published until now *(12–14,17,20–22)*, the reported frequency at which they occur has varied considerably. Technical and stochastic factors undoubtedly play a role in bringing about this variability *(23)*, but systematic differences related to the composition of the series examined could also be important.

Colorectal Adenomas Have Nonrandom Chromosome Aberrations

The large bowel offers unique possibilities to evaluate all stages of carcinogenesis inasmuch as the earliest benign precursor lesions, the adenomas, also can be identified and sampled with ease. Approximately 100 such adenomas with chromosome aberrations have now been reported *(11)*. The first studies *(24,25)* left the impression that gains of whole chromosomes were the only, or at least the predominant, aberrations. As data from new and larger series were added *(26–31)*, the consensus picture of the karyotypic characteristics of benign colorectal tumors has undergone considerable refinements.

In our experience, based on published *(27,30)* as well as unpublished data, up to 80% of large bowel polyps carry clonal chromosomal abnormalities. Other investigators have reported lower percentages of abnormal tumors, 30 *(28)* to 50% *(29,31)*. In all series, however, most karyotypically abnormal polyps, 90% in our material, have had only few cytogenetic abnormalities yielding a pseudo- or near-diploid karyotype. The remainder have been near-triploid or near-tetraploid with massive chromosome changes, often anomalies that are recurrent in colorectal adenocarcinomas as well. At present, therefore, one cannot point to any single karyotypic feature that is capable of distinguishing unequivocally between benign and malignant colorectal tumors. In groupwise comparisons, however, the adenomas come across as karyotypically much more simple than their malignant counterparts.

The most frequent chromosome abnormality in colorectal polyps is +7 (Fig. 3A), found in approx 40% of all reported cases (Fig. 2), mostly as the sole anomaly *(11)*. Although the pathogenetic relevance of +7 in both large bowel neoplasms *(32)* and tumors of other tissues *(33)* has been questioned, the recent finding of this trisomy in the epithelial component of adenomatous polyps (Fig. 3B) by chromosome banding analysis of metaphase cells *(34)* and by *in situ* hybridization with centromere-specific probes in interphase cells *(35)* supports the early suggestion *(36,37)* that it plays a primary role in some colorectal neoplasms. A gene called *DRA*, from *down*regulated in *a*denomas, has been localized to 7q22–q31.1 and shown to be specifically expressed in colon mucosa *(38,39)*. Overexpression of this gene could be an important outcome of trisomy 7. Among other candidate genes are the *MUC3* and *MET* oncogenes that map to 7q22 *(40)*. The actual pathogenetic involvement of any of these gene loci is still entirely speculative, however, as is indeed the very mechanism by which the presence of an extra copy of any particular chromosome might translate into a shift in growth potential sufficient to precipitate neoplastic transformation.

Gain of chromosome 13 is the second most common numerical abnormality (Fig. 2) in large bowel adenomas and has been found in almost 30% of the cases. Then, in descending frequency, follow gain of chromosome 20 (17%), gain of chromosome 8 (15%), gain of chromosome 14, and loss of chromosome 18 (each 13%). Each of these changes has occasionally been detected as the only anomaly. Whereas loss of chromosome 18 might work through loss of one *DCC* allele *(7)*, the important molecular result of the other wholechromosome imbalances is unknown.

A deletion of the short arm of one chromosome 1 is the most common structural rearrangement in intestinal polyps (Fig. 4) *(26,27,29–31,41)*. We have seen it in 30% of all cases with an abnormal karyotype, often as the only anomaly, which led us to suggest that it is an early, possibly primary, genetic change in the development of large bowel tumors *(27)*. Although the deletion has varied in

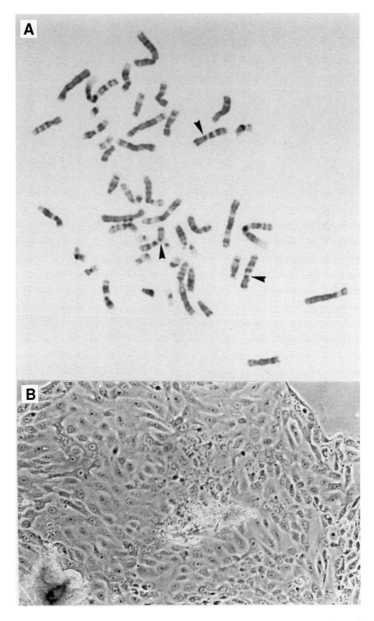

Fig. 3. (A) Metaphase from a colon adenoma with trisomy 7 as the only cytogenetic anomaly. Arrowheads indicate the three copies of chromosome 7. (B) Inverted microscope picture showing the epithelial morphology of an adenoma with +7 as the only chromosomal change.

Deletion of 1p36

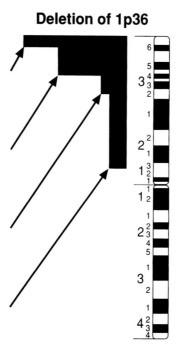

Fig. 4. 1p36 is the minimal common deleted part of the short arm of chromosome 1 in various 1p deletions seen in intestinal polyps. The arrows point to breakpoints recurrently involved.

size from tumor to tumor, band 1p36 was always lost *(27)*, indicating that the putative tumor suppressor locus maps to this band. Corroborative evidence to the same effect came from the study by Tanaka et al. *(42)*, who showed that the introduction of a normal 1p36 segment into a colorectal carcinoma cell line made it nontumorigenic. Relevant in this context may be the finding in a mouse model of colorectal tumorigenesis *(43)* that loss at a site on chromosome 4, which is homologous to 1p36 in humans, is an early tumorigenic event; this may be a clue to the putative gene of importance. Finally, allelic imbalance or loss of one distal allele in 1p was found by DNA analysis in 20% of the polyps investigated by Lothe et al. *(44)*.

Among the benign colorectal tumors with loss of 1p36 are not only adenomas, but also hyperplastic polyps, i.e., lesions without any cellular atypia. Whether they too have a tendency to progress toward carcinomas is not yet clear *(45–47)*. The cytogenetic data indicate that they are genuine neoplasms, however, with karyotypic features similar to those of small tubular adenomas *(30)*.

Deletions of the short arm of chromosome 1 are also seen in large bowel carcinomas *(see above)*, although relatively speaking, not as frequently and often with a larger segment lost than in adenomas. Usually the del(1p) in carcinomas is accompanied by several other anomalies, but cases also exist in which it was the only karyotypic change. Rests of adenomatous tissue were then often found in the tumors, and it has been suggested that these remnants could harbor the cells with 1p as the sole change *(14)*.

Karyotype and Tumor Site

The correlation analysis between tumor karyotype and site performed by Bardi et al. *(14)* showed statistically significant differences. Rectal carcinomas more often had abnormal karyotypes than carcinomas of the colon, and carcinomas in the distal colon were more often cytogenetically normal than those in the proximal colon (Fig. 5). The modal chromosome number was found to correlate with tumor site in a parallel manner. Whereas in the distal colon near-diploid and near-triploid to near-tetraploid tumors were seen equally often, tumors with massive chromosomal aberrations were less common in the proximal colon and rectum. Reichmann et al. *(48)* and Muleris et al. *(13)* also reported more abnormal tumors in the rectum than in the colon. Flow cytometric DNA analyses have shown that proximal large bowel carcinomas more often are diploid than distal ones *(49–52)*. The combined evidence, therefore, indicates that carcinogenesis occurs by different mechanisms in different segments of the large bowel. This could be a result of systematic variation in the carcinogenic effect of the bowel content. Alternatively, differences in susceptibility to fecal carcinogens based on the different embryologic origin of various large bowel segments could be of the essence *(53)*.

Karyotype and Tumor Histology

A statistically significant association was found between the karyotype of colorectal carcinomas and their degree of differentiation when cytogenetically abnormal tumors were divided into those

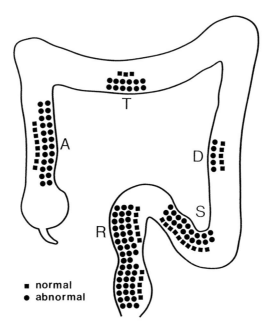

Fig. 5. Site distribution of the 146 colorectal adenocarcinomas examined by us. Squares denote karyotypically normal tumors and circles
denote karyotypically abnormal tumors. A, ascending colon; T, transverse
colon; D, descending colon; S, sigmoid; and R, rectum.

with only numerical changes and those also having structural
aberrations *(14,54)*. Carcinomas carrying structural chromosomal
rearrangements were more often poorly differentiated, whereas
well- and moderately differentiated tumors more often had only
numerical aberrations or normal karyotypes.

In large bowel adenomas, Bomme et al. *(30)* found an association
between cytogenetic pattern and the tumors' degree of dysplasia, histologic type, and size. All villous and tubulovillous adenomas, i.e., the
adenomas most likely to progress to carcinomas *(55)*, had structural
chromosome aberrations. Adenomas with numerical changes only
were mildly dysplastic. Whereas all but one of the adenomas with
structural rearrangements showed either moderate or severe dysplasia.
Furthermore, polyps with a normal karyotype had either mild or moderate, but never severe, dysplasia. Polyps with structural aberrations
were on average larger than polyps with only numerical changes or
those with a normal karyotype. The data strongly indicate that the

accumulation of chromosomal changes in adenomas correlates with pathologic features: The more malignancy-like the phenotype, the more complex the karyotype. Presumably, this correlation reflects a causal relationship, with the acquired genetic changes enabling the cells to assume an increasingly malignant growth pattern.

Karyotype and Prognosis

In a relatively small study performed by Bardi et al. *(17)*, a statistically significant correlation between tumor karyotype and patient survival was demonstrated. Patients with complex tumor karyotypes had shorter survivals than those whose tumors had no or only few and simple chromosome anomalies. It is currently unknown whether the karyotype represents an independent indicator of survival or, if it is not, which of the more conventional prognostic factors it covaries with. Very little is known about the prognostic impact of particular aberrations or aberration patterns. Laurent-Puig et al. *(56)* used multivariate analysis to show that loss of heterozygosity on the short arm of chromosome 17 was independently associated with shorter survival. They concluded that loss of 17p alleles was a marker of tumor aggressiveness.

Initiation and Progression of Colorectal Tumors: Genetic Models of Carcinogenesis

Recent data from cytogenetic and molecular genetic investigations of benign and malignant large bowel tumors indicate that the existing picture of colorectal carcinogenesis should be modified. Among the genetic regions not included in the early Fearon and Vogelstein *(8)* model, but now known to be nonrandomly involved, are 1p and 8p, mostly lost through deletions or isochromosome formation, and 13q, which is typically gained through addition of whole chromosome copies or isochromosome formation. Cytogenetic studies have shown that aberrations leading to loss of chromosome 18 and the short arm of chromosome 17, changes that were formerly thought to be malignancy-specific *(8,57)*, can also be detected occasionally in colorectal adenomas *(30)*. Similar results have been obtained with DNA recombinant techniques in studies showing loss of the *DCC* and

TP53 genes not only in malignant tumors, but in a proportion of benign polyps as well *(58–60)*. In addition, a high frequency of deletions on the short arms of chromosomes 1 and 8 and on the long arm of chromosome 22 were found in these molecular genetic investigations *(58–60)*.

Although one cannot at present identify any particular genetic abnormality as marking a colorectal epithelial cell as malignant, this should not be allowed to obscure the fact that fairly distinct group-wise genetic differences exist, corresponding to the various phenotypic stages of carcinogenesis in this tissue. In typical cases, more and more microscopically identifiable genetic changes are acquired as adenomas transform into carcinomas. Although some aberrations (deletions of 1p, numerical changes such as +7, +8, +13, −18, and +20) are likely to occur at a very early stage, by and large it seems that the sequential order of the changes is less important than their eventual sum. As far as *de novo* colorectal carcinomas that do not evolve from a preceding adenoma are concerned, no cytogenetic evidence is at hand to evaluate whether they differ in their genetic constitution in any way from the more typical, exophytic carcinomas. Nor have so-called "flat adenomas" *(47)* been subjected to systematic cytogenetic scrutiny. To determine the karyotypic characteristics of these lesions will be one of the main goals of cytogenetic analysis of colorectal tumors in the future, as will be the elucidation of which changes characterize metastatic and other multilesional large bowel cancers.

Genetic Heterogeneity in Sporadic
and Hereditary Forms of Colorectal Cancer

In spite of the distinct karyotypic nonrandomness that characterizes tumorigenesis in the large bowel, it cannot be denied that considerable genetic heterogeneity does exist even among tumors at the same phenotypic stage; for example, some carcinomas have very simple cytogenetic changes, whereas others have complex karyotypes. We have interpreted the data as compatible with the existence of two main colorectal adenocarcinoma cytogenetic subgroups: Near-triploid or near-tetraploid tumors with complex chromosome aberrations, both numerical and structural. These tumors are preferentially located in the distal colon, are often poorly differentiated, and are associated with short patient survival. The second subgroup consists of near-diploid tumors with simple, mostly numerical, chromosomal aberrations and often cytogenetically unrelated clones. These tumors are typically located in the proximal colon or rectum, they are moderately or well differentiated, and the patient survival is longer. Flow cytometric and DNA recombinant data are consistent with this dichotomy. Kouri et al. *(61)* showed that hereditary carcinomas with an aneuploid DNA content were more frequently located in the distal colon, whereas carcinomas in the proximal colon typically were near-diploid. Other investigators have reached the same conclusion in studies of sporadic cancers *(50–52)*. Delattre et al. *(49)* found that allelic losses were common in tumors in the distal colon, but rare in those located more proximally.

Several interesting correlations suggest themselves when this karyotype-based division is collated with the molecular genetic information recently obtained on the two main hereditary forms of colorectal cancer, familial adenomatous polyposis (FAP) and hereditary nonpolyposis colorectal cancer (HNPCC). The former disease is brought about by germ line mutations in the *FAP* gene in 5q21 *(4)*. HNPCC is brought about by germ line mutations of mismatch repair genes in 2p or 3p, mutations that give rise to widespread dinucleotide microsatellite instability, the RER+ phenotype *(62–65)*. It turns out that whereas the carcinomas of FAP demonstrate loss of heterozygosity and other aberration features indistinguishable from the group of massively rearranged tumors recognized karyotypically *(53)*, those of HNPCC seem to have undergone only minor genetic alterations. Similar degrees of heterogeneity as far as acquired changes are concerned, therefore, characterize both hereditary and sporadic colorectal tumors, with similar site distributions of genetically simple and complex carcinomas in the two settings. When more cases of both sporadic and hereditary cancer of the large bowel are examined both cytogenetically and using molecular techniques, it should be possible to find out the extent to which the seeming parallelism is valid; and whether the presence or absence of the RER+ phenotype influences the choice of transformation pathway as colorectal cells move from a benign but neoplastic state and then to increasing degrees of malignancy.

References

1. Jass JR, Atkin WS, Cuzick J, Bussey HJR, Morson BC, Northover JMA, Todd IP: The grading of rectal cancer: historical perspective and a multivariate analysis of 447 cases. Histopathology 10:437–459, 1986.
2. O'Brien MJ, O'Keane CJ, Zauber A, Gottlieb LS, Winawer SJ: Precursors of colorectal carcinoma. Biopsy and biologic markers. Cancer 70: 1317–1327, 1992.
3. Cohen AM, Minsky BD, Schilsky RL: Colon cancer. In: DeVita VT, Hellman S, Rosenberg SA (eds.), Cancer Principles and Practice of Oncology, 4th ed. Philadelphia: Lippincott, pp. 929–977, 1993.
4. Groden J, Thliveris A, Sanowitz W, Carlson M, Gelbert L, Albertsen H, Joslyn G, Stevens J, Spirio L, Robertson M, Sargeant L, Krapcho K, Wolff E, Burt R, Hughes JP, Warrington J, McPherson J, Le Paslier D, Abderrahim H, Cohen D, Leppert M, White R: Identification and characterization of the familial adenomatous polyposis gene. Cell 66: 587–600, 1991.
5. Nishisho I, Nakamura Y, Miyoshi Y, Miki Y, Ando H, Horii A, Koyama K, Utsunomiya J, Baba S, Hedge P, Markham A, Krush AJ, Petersen G, Hamilton SR, Nilbert MC, Levy DB, Bryan TM, Preisinger AC, Smith KJ, Su L-K, Kinzler KW, Vogelstein B: Mutations of chromosome 5q21 genes in FAP and colorectal cancer patients. Science 253:665–669, 1991.
6. Hollstein M, Sidransky D, Vogelstein B, Harris CC: P53 mutations in human cancers. Science 253:1366–1370, 1991.
7. Fearon ER, Cho KR, Nigro JM, Kern SE, Simons JW, Ruppert JM, Hamilton SR, Preisinger AC, Thamas G, Kinzler KW, Vogelstein B: Identification of a chromosome 18q gene that is altered in colorectal cancers. Science 247:49–56, 1990.
8. Fearon ER, Vogelstein B: A genetic model for colorectal tumorigenesis. Cell 61:759–767, 1990.
9. Foulds L: The natural history of cancer. J Chronic Dis 8:2–37, 1958.
10. Heim S: Is cancer cytogenetics reducible to the molecular genetics of cancer cells? Genes Chromosome Cancer 5:188–196, 1992.
11. Mitelman F: Catalog of Chromosome Aberrations in Cancer, 5th ed. New York: Wiley-Liss, 1994.
12. Reichmann A, Martin P, Levin B: Chromosomal banding patterns in human large bowel cancer. Int J Cancer 28:431–440, 1981.
13. Muleris M, Salmon R-J, Duttrillaux B: Cytogenetics of colorectal adenocarcinomas. Cancer Genet Cytogenet 46:143–156, 1990.
14. Bardi G, Sukhikh T, Pandis N, Fenger C, Kronborg O, Heim S: Karyotypic characterization of colorectal adenocarcinomas. Genes Chrom Cancer 12:97–109, 1995.
15. Shroy P, Cohen A, Winawer S, Friedman E: New chemotherapeutic drug sensitivity for colon carcinomas in monolayer culture. Cancer Res 48: 3236–3244, 1988.

16. Friedman E, Isaksson P, Rafter J, Marian B, Winawer S, Newmark H: Fecal diglycerides as selective endogenous mitogens for premalignant and malignant human colonic epithelial cells. Cancer Res 49:544–548, 1988.

17. Bardi G, Johansson B, Pandis N, Bak-Jensen E, Örndal C, Heim S, Mandahl N, Andrén-Sandberg Å, Mitelman F: Cytogenetic aberrations in colorectal adenocarcinomas and their correlation with clinicopathologic features. Cancer 71:306–314, 1993.

18. Bauer KD, Lincoln ST, Vera-Roman JM, Wallemark CB, Chmiel JS, Madurski ML: Prognostic implication of proliferative activity and DNA aneuploidy in colonic adenocarcinomas. Lab Invest 57:329–335, 1987.

19. Halvorsen TB, Johannesen E: DNA ploidy, tumor site, and prognosis in colorectal cancer: A flow cytometric study of parafin-embedded tissue. Scand J Gastroenterol 25:141–148, 1990.

20. Ferti AD, Panani AD, Raptis S: Cytogenetic study of rectosigmoidal adenocarcinomas. Cancer Genet Cytogenet 34:101–109, 1988.

21. Konstantinova LN, Fleishman EW, Knisch VI, Perevozchikov AG, Kopnin BP: Karyotype peculiarities of human colorectal adenocarcinomas. Hum Genet 86:491–496, 1991.

22. Wang L, Li L, Zhou HY, Gao XK, Li SJ: t(13q;17p) and del(5q): possibly specific changes in Chinese patients with colorectal cancers. Cancer Genet Cytogenet 62:191–196, 1992.

23. Pandis N, Bardi G, Heim S: Interrelationship between methodological choices and conceptual models in solid tumor cytogenetics. Cancer Genet Cytogenet 76:77–84, 1994.

24. Mitelman F, Mark J, Nilsson PG, Dencker H, Norryd C, Tranberg K-G: Chromosome banding pattern in human colonic polyps. Hereditas 78: 63–68, 1974.

25. Reichmann A, Martin P, Levin B: Chromosomal banding patterns in human large bowel adenomas. Hum Genet 70:28–31, 1985.

26. Couturier-Turpin M-H, Esnous C, Louvel A, Poirier Y, Couturier D: Chromosome 1 in human colorectal tumors. Hum Genet 88:431–438, 1992.

27. Bardi G, Pandis N, Fenger C, Kronborg O, Bomme L, Heim S: Deletion of 1p36 as a primary chromosomal aberration in intestinal tumorigenesis. Cancer Res 53:1895–1898, 1993.

28. Griffin CA, Lazer S, Hamilton SR, Giardiello FM, Long P, Krush AJ, Booker SV: Cytogenetic analysis of intestinal polyps in polyposis syndromes: Comparison with sporadic adenomas. Cancer Genet Cytogenet 67:14–20, 1993.

29. Longy M, Saura R, Dumas F, Leseve J-F, Taine L, Goussot J-F, Couzigou P: Chromosome analysis of adenomatous polyps of the colon: possible existence of two differently evolving cytogenetic groups. Cancer Genet Cytogenet 67:7–13, 1993.

30. Bomme L, Bardi G, Pandis N, Fenger C, Kronborg O, Heim S: Clonal karyotypic abnormalities in colorectal adenomas: clues to the early events in the adenoma–carcinoma sequence. Genes Chrom Cancer 10:190, 1994.

31. Muleris M, Zafrani B, Validire P, Girodet J, Salmon R-J, Dutrillaux B: Cytogenetic study of 30 colorectal adenomas. Cancer Genet Cytogenet 74:104–108, 1994.

32. Bardi G, Johansson B, Pandis N, Heim S, Mandahl N, Andrén-Sandberg Å, Hägerstrand I, Mitelman F: Trisomy 7 in short-term cultures of colorectal adenocarcinomas. Genes Chrom Cancer 3:149–152, 1991.

33. Johansson B, Heim S, Mandahl N, Mertens F, Mitelman F: Trisomy 7 in non-neoplastic cells. Genes Chrom Cancer 6:199–205, 1993.

34. Bardi G, Pandis N, Heim S: Trisomy 7 as the sole cytogenetic aberration in the epithelial component of a colonic adenoma. Cancer Genet Cytogenet 82:82–84, 1995.

35. Herbergs J, de Bruine AP, Marx PTJ, Vallinga MIJ, Stockbrugger RW, Ramaekers FCS, Arends JW, Hopman AHN: Chromosome aberrations in adenomas of the colon. Proof of trisomy 7 in tumor cells by combined interphase cytogenetics and immunocytochemistry. Int J Cancer 57:781–785, 1994.

36. Becher R, Gibas Z, Sandberg AA: Involvement of chromosome 7 and 12 in large bowel cancer: trisomy 7 and 12q-. Cancer Genet Cytogenet 9:329–332, 1983.

37. Ochi H, Takeuchi J, Holyoke D, Sandberg AA: Possible specific changes in large bowel cancer. Cancer Genet Cytogenet 10:121,122, 1983.

38. Schweinfest CW, Henderson KW, Suster S, Kondoh N, Papas TS: Identification of a colon mucosa gene that is down regulated in colon adenomas and adenocarcinomas. Proc Natl Acad Sci USA 90:4166–4170, 1993.

39. Tagushi T, Testa JR, Papas TS, Schweinfest C: Localization of a candidate colon tumor suppressor gene (DRA) to 7q22–q31.1 by fluorescence *in situ* hybridization. Genomics 20:146,147, 1994.

40. Fox M, Lahib F, Pratt W, Attwood J, Gum J, Kim Y, Swallow DM: Regional localization of MUC3 to chromosome 7q22. Cytogenet Cell Genet 58:1920,1921, 1991.

41. Couturier-Turpin MH, Louvel A, Couturier D, Esnous C, Poirier Y, Nepveux P: Tubulovillous adenoma of the colon with hyperdiploidy, double minute chromosomes, and inversion of chromosome 1. Cancer Genet Cytogenet 32:253–262, 1988.

42. Tanaka K, Yanoshita R, Konishi M, Oshimura M, Maeda Y, Mori T, Miyaki M: Suppression of tumorigenicity in human colon carcinoma cells by introduction of normal chromosome 1p36 region. Oncogene 8:2253–2258, 1993.

43. Dietrich WF, Lander E, Smith JS, Moser AR, Gould K, Luongo C, Borenstein N, Dove W: Genetic identification of Mom-1, a major modifier locus affecting Min-induced intestinal neoplasia in the mouse. Cell 75:631–639, 1993.

44. Lothe RA, Andersen SN, Hofstad B, Meling GI, Peltomäki P, Heim S, Brøgger A, Vatn M, Rognum TO, Børresen A-L: Deletion of 1p loci and microsatellite instability in colorectal polyps. Genes Chrom Cancer 14:182–188, 1995.

45. Jass JR, Path MRC: Do all colorectal carcinomas arise in preexisting adenomas? World J Surg 13:45–51, 1989.
46. Longacre TA, Fenoglio-Preiser CM: Mixed hyperplastic adenomatous polyps/serrated adenomas. A distinct form of colorectal neoplasia. Am J Surg Pathol 14:524–537, 1990.
47. Hamilton SR: The adenoma–adenocarcinoma sequence in the large bowel: variations on a theme. J Cell Biochem 6G (Suppl 1):41–46, 1992.
48. Reichmann A, Levin B, Martin P: Human large-bowel cancer: correlation of clinical and histological features with banded chromosomes. Int J Cancer 29:625–629, 1982.
49. Delattre O, Olschwang S, Law DJ, Melot T, Remvikos Y, Salmon RJ, Sastre X, Validire P, Feinberg AP, Thomas G: Multiple genetic alterations in distal and proximal colorectal cancer. Lancet II:353–355, 1989.
50. Barretton G, Gille J, Oevermann E: Flow cytometric analysis of the DNA content in paraffin-embedded tissue from colorectal carcinomas and its prognostic significance. Virchows Arch B Cell Pathol 60:123, 1991.
51. Costa A, Faranda A, Scalmati A: Autoradiographic and flow cytometric assessment of cell proliferation in primary colorectal cancer: relationship to DNA ploidy and clinicopathologic features. Int J Cancer 50:719, 1992.
52. Lanza G, Maestri I, Ballotta MR, Dubini A, Cavazzini L: Relationship of nuclear DNA content to clinicopathologic features in colorectal cancer. Modern Pathol 7:161–165.
53. Bufill JA: Colorectal cancer: evidence for distinct genetic categories based on proximal or distal tumor location. Ann Intern Med 113:779–788, 1990.
54. Bardi G, Johansson B, Pandis N, Mandahl N, Bak-Jensen E, Lindström C, Törnqvist A, Frederiksen H, Andrén-Sandberg Å, Mitelman F, Heim S: Cytogenetic analysis of 52 colorectal carcinomas: non-random aberration pattern and correlation with pathologic parameters. Int J Cancer 55:422–428, 1993.
55. Jass JR: The large intestine. In: Morson BC (ed.), Alimentary Tract. Edinburgh; UK: Churchill Livingstone, pp. 313–395, 1987.
56. Laurent-Puig P, Olschwang S, Delattre O, Remvikos Y, Asselain B, Melot T, Validire P, Muleris M, Girodet J, Salmon R, Thomas G: Survival and acquired genetic alterations in colorectal cancer. Gastroenterol 102:1136–1141, 1992.
57. Baker SJ, Preisinger AC, Jessup JM, Paraskeva C, Markowitz S, Willson JKV: p53 gene mutations occur in combination with 17p allelic deletions as late events in colorectal tumorigenesis. Cancer Res 50:7717–7722, 1990.
58. Hamilton SR: Molecular genetics of colorectal cancer. Cancer 70:1216–1221, 1992.
59. Cho KR, Vogelstein B: Genetic alterations in the adenoma–carcinoma sequence. Cancer 70:1727–1731, 1992.
60. Bodmer W, Bishop T, Karran P: Genetic steps in colorectal cancer. Nature Genet 6:217–219, 1994.
61. Kouri M, Laasonen A, Mecklin JP, Jarvinen H, Franssila K, Pyrhonen S: Diploid predominance in hereditary nonpolyposis colorectal carcinoma evaluated by flow cytometry. Cancer 65:1825–1829, 1990.

62. Aaltonen LA, Peltomäki P, Leach FS, Sistonen P, Pylkkanen L, Mecklin J-P, Jarvinen H, Powell SM, Jen J, Hamilton SR, Petersen GM, Kinzler KW, Vogelstein B, de la Chapelle A: Clues to the pathogenesis of familial colorectal cancer. Science 260:812–816, 1993.

63. Bronner CE, Baker SM, Morrison PT, Warren G, Smith LG, Lescoe MK, Kane M, Earabino C, Lipford J, Lindblom A, Tannergarg P, Bollag RJ, Godwin AR, Ward DC, Nordenskiold M, Fishel R, Kolodner R, Liskay RM: Mutation in the DNA mismatch repair gene homologue hMLH1 is associated with hereditary non-polyposis colon cancer. Nature 368:258–261, 1994.

64. Nicolaides NC, Papadopoulos N, Liu B, Wei Y-F, Carter KC, Ruben S, Rosen CA, Haseltine WA, Fleischmann RD, Fraser CM, Adams MD, Venter JC, Dunlop MG, Hamilton SR, Petersen GM, de la Chapelle A, Vogelstein B, Kinzler KW: Mutations of two PMS homologues in hereditary nonpolyposis colon cancer. Nature 371:75–80, 1994.

65. Papadopoulos N, Nicolaides NC, Wei Y-F, Ruben SM, Carter KC, Rosen CA, Haseline WA, Fleischmann RD, Fraser CM, Adams MD, Venter JC, Hamilton SR, Petersen GM, Watson P, Lynch HT, Peltomäki P, Mecklin J-P, de la Chapelle A, Kinzler KW, Vogelstein B: Mutation of a mutL homolog in hereditary colon cancer. Science 263:1625–1629, 1994.

Chapter 8

Renal and Bladder Cancers

Jonathan A. Fletcher

Introduction

The cytogenetic features of renal and bladder cancers have been defined only over the past 10 yr, but it is already clear that these parameters have substantial diagnostic and prognostic relevance. In fact, the clinical ramifications of chromosome aberrations in genitourinary tumors are in many respects a paradigm for the potential uses of cytogenetics in other types of solid tumors. Very characteristic chromosome aberrations have been identified in different histologic types of renal cancer, and these distinctive cytogenetic profiles are discussed at some length in this chapter (Table 1). Of particular note are the ubiquitous deletion of chromosome 3 short-arm material in nonpapillary clear cell and granular carcinomas (1–3), extra copy number—particularly trisomies—of several chromosomes in renal adenomas and papillary carcinomas (4–7), and hypodiploid karyotypes in chromophobe carcinomas (8). Likewise, many of the common pediatric renal tumors contain characteristic cytogenetic aberrations. Deletion of 11p is a very well-studied and well-publicized aberration in Wilms tumors, but several other aberrations are more frequent and might have greater prognostic relevance (9–13). Another pediatric renal tumor with extremely consistent cytogenetic aberrations is the cellular variant

From: *Human Cytogenetic Cancer Markers*   Edited by S. R. Wolman and S. Sell
Humana Press Inc., Totowa, NJ

Table 1
Cytogenetic and Molecular Aberrations in Renal Tumors

Histologic findings	Cytogenetic events	Molecular events	Frequency %	Diagnostic utility?
Clear cell carcinoma (grade I–II)	Deletion 3p14–21 Trisomy 7		>90 20	Yes ?
		VHL mutation/ deletion	>75	Yes
Clear cell carcinoma (grade II–III)	Deletion 3p14–21 with complex karyotype		>50	?
Papillary renal cell carcinoma	Extra copy number (usually trisomies) of two or more of the following chromosomes: 3, 7, 16, 17, and 20		>80	Yes
	Translocation (X;1)		?	Yes
Papillary renal cell adenoma	–Y, +7, +17		>50	?
Chromophobe carcinoma	Monosomy 1, 2, 6, 10, 13, 17, and 21		>75	Yes
		Deletion of 3p and 17q	50	?

Tumor	Genetic alteration	Comment		Diagnostic marker
Oncocytoma	Monosomies for chromosomes X and 1		30	Yes
	Translocation at 11q13		<50	Yes
		Altered restriction pattern for mitochondrial DNA	<20	Yes
Wilms tumor	Deletion of 11p13	*WT1* deletion and/or point mutation	<20	Yes
	Deletion of 11p15	?Deletion of Beckwith-Wiedemann gene	30	Yes
	Deletion of 16q		>25	No
	Trisomy 12		>30	No
Mesoblastic nephroma (cellular type)	Trisomies 8, 11, and/or 17		>50	Yes
Rhabdoid tumor	Insufficient data			
Clear cell sarcoma	Insufficient data			

(continued)

Table 1 *(continued)*

Histologic findings	Cytogenetic events	Molecular events	Frequency %	Diagnostic utility?
Bladder: transitional cell carcinoma (superficial and invasive tumors)	Trisomy 1q		30	(FISH)[a]
	Deletion 3p		20	(FISH)[a]
	Deletion 4p		20	(FISH)[a]
	Trisomy 7		50	(FISH)[a]
	Trisomy 8q		25	(FISH)[a]
	Deletion 8p		25	(FISH)[a]
	Deletion 9q	?Gelsolin gene deletion	75	FISH[a]
	Deletion 9p	*p16* gene deletion	75	(FISH)[a]
	Trisomy 10		30	(FISH)[a]
	Deletion 11p		30	(FISH)[a]
Bladder: transitional cell carcinoma (invasive tumors only)	Deletion 13q	*RB* mutation	20	(FISH)[a]
	Deletion 17p	*p53* mutation/deletion	50	(FISH)[a]
		C-*erb*B-2 amplification	20	(FISH)[a]

[a]Potential diagnostic utility as a probe target in FISH analyses of urine or bladder washings.

of mesoblastic nephroma: Virtually all such tumors are notable for trisomy 11, often accompanied by extra copy number of other chromosomes *(14,15)*. The cytogenetic profiles in bladder cancer are less well-defined than those in the different histologic types of renal cancer. However, trisomy 7 and deletions of several chromosome regions, e.g., 8p, 9q, 9p, and 17p, are found in substantial numbers of bladder tumors *(16–28)*. Several genetic aberrations are associated with histologic progression in bladder cancer, and these parameters appear to be useful prognosticators *(29–33)*. A particularly exciting development in bladder cancer cytogenetics is the application of fluorescence *in situ* hybridization (FISH) probes for detection of clonal chromosome aberrations in exfoliated cells obtained from urine specimens. The FISH approach holds real promise as an effective means for diagnosis and monitoring of patients with well-differentiated superficial transitional cell carcinomas.

Renal Tumors

The architecture of renal cell carcinomas is quite variable. Most renal cell carcinomas contain solid sheets of cells arranged in trabecular or tubular patterns, but a minority of cases are predominantly papillary. Nonpapillary renal cell carcinomas are generally composed of clear cells having an abundant, clear, cytoplasm. In addition to the classic "clear cell" subtype, there are several other histologies that each account for 5–15% of nonpapillary renal cell carcinomas. These are the granular, sarcomatoid, and chromophobe histologies *(33)*. Both nonpapillary and papillary renal cell carcinomas are associated with distinctive genetic aberrations, and the following discussion addresses the various histologic subtypes separately.

Papillary Renal Tumors

Papillary Renal Cell Tumors: General Considerations

Papillary renal tumors include both benign cortical adenomas and malignant carcinomas. Approximately 10% of all renal carcinomas are predominantly papillary, and the cytogenetic profiles or papillary renal cell carcinomas are different from those in the various nonpapillary renal cell carcinomas. Diagnosis of papillary renal tumors is not always straightforward, and several considerations require particular attention. One consideration is the distinction between papillary renal adenoma and carcinoma. Renal cortical adenomas are extremely common and are generally discovered incidentally by radiography, angiography, or at autopsy. It has been suggested that papillary renal neoplasms smaller than 3 cm be regarded as benign adenomas, whereas those larger than 3 cm be regarded as carcinomas, but the present consensus is that size alone does not permit reliable determination of malignant potential. Another important diagnostic consideration is the distinction between papillary and nonpapillary renal cell carcinoma. Most papillary renal cell carcinomas contain some nonpapillary components, and an arbitrary cut-off of 50% is often used to define the minimal percentage of papillary component required for diagnosis of true papillary renal cell carcinoma. However, there are almost certainly true "papillary" renal cell carcinomas in which the papillary components comprise less than 50% of the total architecture. Reliable distinction between papillary and nonpapillary renal cell carcinoma is important clinically because papillary carcinomas appear to have a better prognosis, stage for stage, than do nonpapillary carcinomas (35,36).

Papillary Renal Adenoma Vs Papillary Renal Cell Carcinoma

Kidneys involved by papillary renal cell carcinoma often contain papillary renal (cortical) adenomas, and the suspicion that papillary renal cell carcinomas arise from the adenomas has been reinforced by cytogenetic studies. Clonal chromosome aberrations were first described in papillary renal cell adenomas by Dal Cin et al. (37) who found an identical group of chromosome aberrations (–Y, +7, +7, +17) in three cases. The cytogenetic motif of –Y, +7, +17 is also found in many papillary renal cell carcinomas, but papillary carcinomas generally contain a number of additional clonal chromosome aberrations (Figs. 1 and 2) (5–7,38). Thus, cytogenetic studies indicate a continuum of chromosome aberrations in papillary renal cell tumors, with extra copy number of chromosomes 7 and 17 contributing to the early phases of nonmalignant neoplastic progression. Kovacs et al. (38) recommended that all renal papillary tumors in which trisomy/tetrasomy 7 and trisomy 17 are the sole autosomal karyotypic aberrations be regarded as papil-

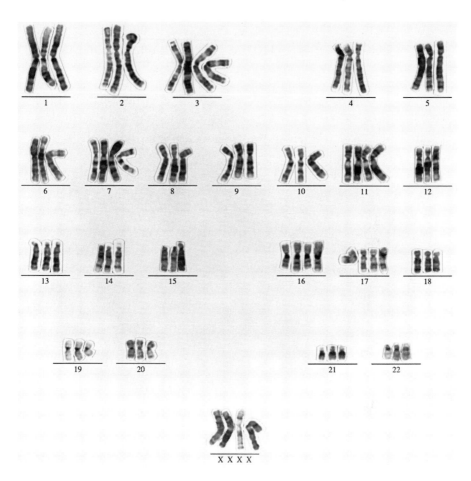

Fig. 1. Hyperdiploid karyotype of a papillary renal cell carcinoma with extra copy number (in relationship to ploidy) of chomosomes 3, 7, 11, 16, 17, and X.

lary renal cell adenomas, irrespective of size. The same investigators recommended that papillary renal cell tumors with complex karyotypic aberrations be regarded as carcinomas, even when small in size *(38)*. Karyotypic complexity appears to be a useful parameter for distinction of papillary renal cell adenoma from carcinoma, but published studies provide little or no clinical follow-up data, and it is not yet known whether karyotypic complexity predicts patient outcome.

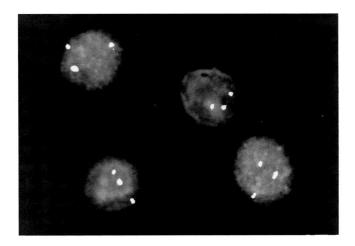

Fig. 2. FISH with a chromosome 7 centromere probe in cells obtained by fine needle aspirate of a renal mass. All cells are trisomic for chromosome 7. Cell block and cytology were consistent with high-grade papillary renal cell carcinoma.

Papillary Vs Nonpapillary Renal Cell Carcinoma

Nonrandom chromosome aberrations in papillary renal cell carcinoma include extra copy number of chromosomes 7, 16, and 17, and loss of the Y chromosome: Each of these aberrations is found in at least 50% of papillary renal cell carcinomas (Figs. 1 and 2) (5–38). Nonrandom chromosome aberrations found in 10–50% of papillary renal cell carcinomas include trisomies 3, 8, 12, and 20 (38). Loss of the Y chromosome and trisomies 7, 12, 16, and 17 have also been described in at least 10% of nonpapillary renal cell carcinomas (1,3,39–41), but several of the other nonrandom papillary renal cell carcinoma aberrations (trisomies 3, 8, 16, and 20) are uncommon in nonpapillary renal cell carcinomas (39,40). Another potential diagnostic parameter is cytogenetic deletion of 3p14–21, which is found in more than 80% of clear cell/granular nonpapillary renal cell carcinomas, but in fewer than 10% of papillary renal cell carcinomas (1,3).

Papillary Renal Cell Carcinomas with Translocations Involving Xp11

Renal carcinomas are uncommon in children and young adults, but a growing number of case reports indicate that most such tumors contain a balanced translocation involving chromosome band Xp11. Balanced translocation t(X;1)(p11.2;q21.2) was described initially in a papillary renal cell carcinoma from a 2-yr-old child *(42)*, and subsequent reports confirmed t(X;1), as well as other translocations at Xp11, in pediatric renal adenocarcinomas *(43–45)*. Interestingly, each of these cases had papillary components that were either focal or widespread. Translocation t(X;1) is not restricted to pediatric carcinomas, but has also been reported in four papillary renal cell carcinomas from adult patients *(46)*. The t(X;1) translocation breakpoint at chromosome band Xp11 has been isolated within a yeast artificial chromosome, and this breakpoint corresponds to the more centromeric (*OATL2* region) of two Xp11 breakpoints characterized in synovial sarcoma *(47–49)*.

Nonpapillary Renal Cell Carcinomas

Clear Cell and Granular Nonpapillary Renal Cell Carcinomas

Chromosome 3p deletion is the most frequent cytogenetic aberration in clear cell and granular nonpapillary renal cell carcinomas. This deletion was found in 70–90% of nonpapillary tumors in some series, and loss of heterozygosity has been confirmed for several regions of 3p in a similar percentage of cases *(2,50–53)*. One target of the 3p deletions is the von Hippel Lindau tumor suppressor gene (*VHL*), located near the telomeric aspect of 3p *(54,55)*. Von Hippel Lindau syndrome results from inheritance of a defective *VHL* allele, and individuals with VHL syndrome often develop bilateral and multifocal renal cell carcinomas. It is now clear that the *VHL* gene is also deleted and/or point mutated in at least 50% of sporadic nonpapillary renal cell carcinomas *(56–59)*. Another target of the 3p deletions in sporadic renal cell carcinomas is a more centromeric tumor suppressor locus in band 3p14 or 3p21 *(51)*. It is unknown whether this second locus corresponds exactly to any of the loci deleted nonrandomly in bronchogenic carcinoma *(60–63)*, but clues to potential locations of the 3p14–p21 renal cancer tumor suppressor derive from both deletion mapping studies *(2)* and from studies of several kindreds in which increased risk of renal cell carcinoma is inherited in autosomal dominant manner. The increased cancer risk in these kindreds is associated with inheritance of a constitutional balanced chromosome translocation involving bands 3p14–p21. Affected individuals in the best described kindred have a constitutional balanced translocation t(3;8) involving chromosome band 3p14: This 3p14 translocation breakpoint has been cloned and one candidate gene identified *(64,65)*. The various 3p tumor suppressor genes are of particular therapeutic relevance, because most nonpapillary renal cell carcinomas appear to result, in part, from inactivation of one or more of these genes. Novel therapeutic approaches based on functional replacement of these tumor suppressor genes might, therefore, be effective across the board in nonpapillary clear cell/granular renal cell carcinomas. Evaluation of 3p deletions might also be relevant diagnostically in the distinction of papillary vs nonpapillary renal cell carcinoma. More than 80% of clear cell and granular nonpapillary renal cell carcinomas have deletion of 3p, whereas cytogenetic deletions of this chromosome arm are found in fewer than 10% of papillary renal cell carcinomas.

Although deletion 3p is the most frequent cytogenetic aberration in clear cell and granular nonpapillary renal cell carcinoma, several other nonrandom cytogenetic aberrations participate in the genesis of these tumors. Nonrandom cytogenetic aberrations found in at least 10% of cases include extra copy number of 5q, trisomy 7, deletion of 17p, and loss of the Y chromosome *(3,8,39)*. Nonrandom deletion of 17p has been confirmed by loss of heterozygosity studies *(3,53,66)*, and other regions with nonrandom loss of heterozygosity include 6q, 9p, 9q, 10q, 11q, and 19p *(3,53,66–68)*. The relevance of trisomy 7 and loss of the Y chromosome has been a matter of contention, because these same aberrations have been detected, primarily after tissue culture, in nonneoplastic kidney tissues *(69–71)*. However, FISH studies of uncultured renal specimens have confirmed trisomy 7 and loss of the Y chromosome in carcinoma populations *(40,72)*. Although the *p53* tumor suppressor gene is located within the 17p deletion region, fewer than 10% of nonpapillary renal cell carcinomas have demonstrable *p53* mutations. Thus, it is possible that a second tumor suppressor gene in the *p53* region is the target of most 17p deletions in renal cell carcinomas. Nonetheless, it is likely that *p53* mutations contribute to neoplastic progression in a subset of renal cell carcinomas. In one study *(73)*, *p53* mutations were found in only 3 of 53 renal cell carcinomas

(6%), but each of these three cases was either a grade III or Robson stage III tumor. In another study *(74) p53* mutations were evaluated separately in the carcinomatous and sarcomatoid components of 14 mixed carcinomatous–sarcomatoid renal cell cancers. Mutations were found in the carcinomatous and sarcomatoid components of 2 and 11 cases, respectively. These studies suggest a role for *p53* mutations in neoplastic progression, particularly in sarcomatoid transformation of renal cell carcinoma. However, *p53* mutations are detected in few renal cancers prior to overt histologic progression, and it is unlikely that evaluation of *p53* status will be useful prognostically in renal cell carcinoma.

Chromophobe Carcinoma

Chromophobe carcinomas are a recently described group that account for approx 5% of renal cell carcinomas. These carcinomas are defined by pale reticular cytoplasm, positive reaction with Hale's acid iron colloid, and ultrastructural presence of cytoplasmic microvesicles and dysmorphic mitochondria *(75)*. Cases that lack Hale's colloidal iron staining, particularly in the absence of ultrastructural evaluation, can be difficult to distinguish from oncocytomas or clear cell/granular renal cell carcinomas. Kovacs et al. *(76)* reported the striking finding of altered mitochondrial DNA restriction patterns in 3 of 10 chromophobe renal cell carcinomas, whereas no such mitochondrial aberrations were detected in a companion group of 10 oncocytomas, 10 papillary renal cell carcinomas, and 5 nonpapillary, nonchromophobe, renal cell carcinomas. Kovacs and colleagues *(77,78)* also described mitochondrial DNA rearrangements in a subset of oncocytomas, and it is interesting that abundant mitochondria— often dysmorphic—are a prominent feature in both oncocytic and chromophobe renal cell tumors. In fact there is substantial histologic overlap between oncocytomas and chromophobe cell carcinomas, and many believe that renal tumors reported as "metastasizing oncocytoma" are actually eosinophilic chromophobe carcinomas. Initially, it was difficult to establish the cytogenetic profile of chromophobe renal cell carcinomas, because they are relatively uncommon neoplasms. However, cytogenetic analyses of two cases revealed hypodiploid karyotypes. The stem-lines in these tumors had 34 and 37 chromosomes, respectively, and both tumors were monosomic for chromosomes 1, 2, 6, 10, 13, 17, and 21 *(1,79)*. Speicher et al. *(80)* extended these observations by evaluating clonal chromosome aberrations in 19 chromophobe cell carcinomas using comparative genomic hybridization. Seventeen of the tumors had losses of whole chromosomes, including chromosome 1 (17 cases); chromosomes 2, 10, and 13 (16 cases each); chromosomes 6 and 21 (15 cases each), and chromosome 17 (13 cases). Extremely hypodiploid karyotypes, particularly those with chromosome counts <40, are uncommon in solid tumors generally, and the characteristic group of monosomies found in chromophobe cell carcinomas has never been described in other renal cell cancer histologies. Thus, initial studies of chromophobe cell carcinomas have identified both molecular and cytogenetic discriminators that will likely be useful diagnostically.

Oncocytoma

Oncocytomas are epithelial neoplasms composed of large cells that are typically eosinophilic because of the presence of abundant mitochondria. These neoplasms are regarded by most as benign, and are invariably cured after surgical resection. However, rare cases attain a large size (>10 cm), and many cases have substantial histologic overlap with "oncocytic" renal cell carcinomas. Such cases can be difficult to distinguish conclusively from renal cell carcinoma resulting in prognostic uncertainties. It is notable, therefore, that characteristic cytogenetic aberrations have been defined in some oncocytomas. In addition, oncocytomas lack several of the distinctive cytogenetic aberrations found in most renal cell carcinomas. Initial cytogenetic and molecular studies in a small number of oncocytomas did not reveal nonrandom chromosome aberrations, but were provocative nonetheless because most cases had altered mitochondrial DNA restriction patterns *(76,77,81)*. Mitochondrial DNA aberrations were not confirmed in a subsequent study of 10 oncocytomas *(76)*, but recent studies have established the presence of several nonrandom cytogenetic aberrations in these tumors. Concomitant loss of an entire chromosome 1 and a sex chromosome (either X or Y) was noted in 5 of 11 oncocytomas described in three reports *(82–84)*, and translocations involving chromosome band 11q13 have been described in four cases (Fig. 3) *(3,85,86)*. It is difficult to infer the actual frequency

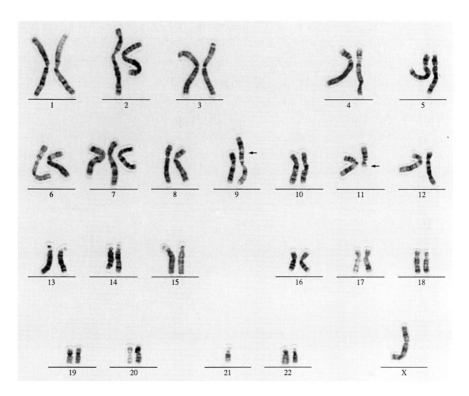

Fig. 3. Karyotype of an oncocytoma showing a balanced translocation t(9;11)(p24;q13) involving chromosome band 11q13. Arrows indicate translocation breakpoints.

of such nonrandom cytogenetic aberrations in oncocytomas because all reports to date involved either single oncocytomas or relatively small series of two to five cases. However, it is likely that no more than 50% of oncocytomas contain the aforementioned nonrandom chromosome aberrations. One extremely important conclusion can be drawn from these collective studies, however, which is that oncocytomas rarely if ever have the cytogenetic profiles typical of most clear cell/granular or chromophobe renal cell carcinomas.

Rhabdoid Tumor

Malignant rhabdoid tumors are highly malignant, histologically undifferentiated, tumors that arise in various primary sites including kidney, liver, soft tissues, and central nervous system. Rhabdoid tumors of the kidney are indistinguishable pathologically from those arising in other organs. Clonal chromosome aberrations have been reported for only one renal rhabdoid tumor after short-term tissue culture: that case had an unbalanced translocation t(8;22) resulting in deletion of the *BCR* region at 22q11 *(87)*. The 22q11 chromosomal region is also deleted nonrandomly in central nervous system rhabdoid tumors *(87)* thus, it is possible that rhabdoid tumors of the brain and kidney result from related genetic aberrations.

Wilms Tumor

Wilms tumors are by far the most common renal neoplasms diagnosed in children. They are typically composed of primitive blastemal cells resembling those in fetal kidney. These blastemal cells are felt to be the malignant progenitor in Wilms tumors, and in most cases some of the blastema differentiates into epithelial tubular and/or mesenchymal populations. The classic "triphasic" Wilms tumor contains an admixture of blastemal, epithelial, and mesenchymal components, and all three cell types in many such tumors contain the same clonal chromosome aberrations *(89)*. No single cytogenetic or molecular aberration has been identified in the majority of Wilms tumors, but several aberrations are individually found in at least 10% of cases. These aberrations include trisomies 6, 8, 12, and 18, and deletions of 11p13, 11p15, and 16q (Table 1, Fig. 4) *(9–13)*.

Deletion 11p13 is the best characterized aberration in Wilms tumors. This aberration became the focus of many studies after reports that individuals with the WAGR (Wilms tumor with aniridia, genitourinary malformations, and retardation) syndrome often had constitutional deletions at chromosome band 11p13. The Wilms tumor suppressor gene (*WT1*) deleted in WAGR syndrome has been cloned and characterized *(90)*, and this gene appears to play a critical role in urogenital development *(90–93)*. The WAGR phenotype results from deletions encompassing several genes: *WT1* gene deletion is responsible for the increased risk of Wilms tumors, whereas deletion of a neighboring gene, *PAX6*, results in aniridia *(94)*. A constitutional point mutation that inactivated *WT1*, but not

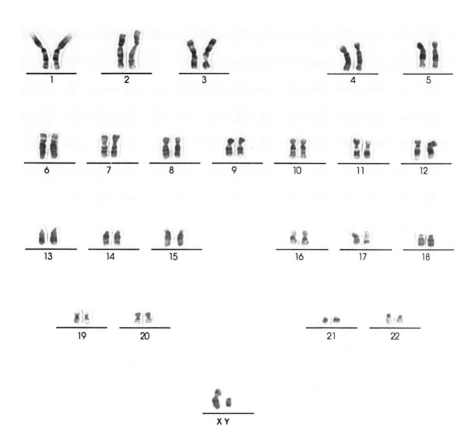

Fig. 4. Karyotype of Wilms tumor. Right hand member of the chromosome 11 pair has a short arm deletion encompassing bands 11p1?1-p15. WTI gene deletion was confirmed in this case by FISH.

neighboring genes, has been reported: this individual developed multiple Wilms tumors, but lacked the remaining features of WAGR syndrome *(95)*. Approximately 40% of kidneys involved by Wilms tumor also contain multifocal benign nephrogenic "rests" of blastema-like cells, and nephrogenic rests occasionally contain the same *WT1* point mutation found in an associated Wilms tumor *(96)*. Demonstration of *WT1* point mutations in nephrogenic rests proves that inactivation of this gene can be an early event in the genesis of certain Wilms tumors. The exact biologic mechanisms of *WT1* remain to be defined, but the protein encoded by *WT1* appears to have both transcription factor and mRNA splicing capabilities *(91)*.

Although most or all WAGR-associated Wilms tumors have complete inactivation of *WT1*, such inactivation is found in fewer than 20% of sporadic Wilms tumors.

A second 11p deletion region at chromosome band 11p15 has also been implicated in both constitutional deletions (Beckwith-Wiedemann syndrome) and in a minority of sporadic Wilms tumors. The gene targeted by this deletion has been named *WT2* but is yet to be cloned. A third deletion hotspot, within the 16q13-qter region *(98)*, is of particular clinical relevance because this deletion is associated with poor prognosis. Evaluation of 1p, 11p, and 16q LOH in 232 Wilms tumors demonstrated a 12-fold higher mortality rate among the 17% of patients with LOH at 16q. By contrast, LOH at 1p (12%) or 11p (33%) was not associated with poor prognosis *(13)*.

Several genetic aberrations are associated with anaplastic histologic features in Wilms tumor. Complex karyotypes with chromosome counts in the triploid-to-tetraploid range are generally found in tumors with either diffuse or focal anaplasia. Douglass et al. *(99)* reported chromosome aberrations in 21 Wilms tumors, and all cases ($N = 7$) with chromosome counts >70 contained anaplastic components. By contrast, all cases ($N = 14$) with chromosome counts <70 had favorable histology without anaplasia. Mutations of the *p53* tumor suppressor gene are infrequent in Wilms tumors, occurring in fewer than 10% of cases overall *(44,100)*. Those Wilms tumors with *p53* mutations generally have some degree of anaplasia *(44,101)*, and the *p53* mutations in those cases are often restricted to the anaplastic cells *(102)*. It is not yet known whether ploidy and *p53* evaluations provide independent prognostic information beyond that already apparent from the histologic examination.

Mesoblastic Nephroma

Mesoblastic nephromas are the most common renal tumors diagnosed in neonates, but are rarely encountered in children over the age of 1 yr. The original histologic description of mesoblastic nephroma was of a mesenchymal tumor composed of fascicles of bland, benign-appearing, spindle-cells: This histologic type is now referred to as "classic" *(103)*. Other mesoblastic nephromas are composed of much more cellular, undifferentiated mesenchyme and

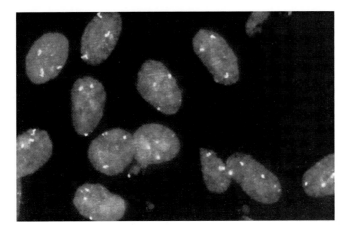

Fig. 5. FISH with a chromosome 11 centromere probe in cells disaggregated from 50 μ paraffin sections of a mesoblastic nephroma. Most cells are trisomic for chromosome 11.

often have worrisome histologic features such as frequent mitoses and abundant necrosis *(104,105)*. In addition, many mesoblastic neophromas have admixture of classic and cellular components, and in these cases it is presumed that the cellular populations arise from the more benign classic populations. Extra copy number of chromosome 11 was recognized as a consistent cytogenetic aberration in mesoblastic nephromas (Fig. 5) *(11,106,107)*, and recent FISH studies demonstrated that this aberration is restricted to mesoblastic nephromas containing cellular populations, *(14,15)*. Approximately 70% of cellular mesoblastic nephromas contain trisomy 11, and additional nonrandom aberrations found in 30–50% of cellular mesoblastic nephromas include trisomies for chromosomes 8 and 17 *(14)*. By contrast, clonal chromosome aberrations have not been identified in classic histology mesoblastic nephromas. These studies indicate that trisomy 11, with or without other clonal chromosome aberrations, is associated with progression from classic to cellular histology in mesoblastic nephroma. This observation is important clinically because differential diagnosis of mesoblastic nephroma includes Wilms tumor with predominantly mesenchymal differentiation. Trisomy 11, particularly as an isolated cytogenetic aberration, is uncommon in Wilms tumors *(9–12)*.

Bladder Tumors

Bladder cancers are among the most frequent adult cancers, and there is strong evidence that many bladder cancers arise following exposure to carcinogens. Bladder cancers are increasingly studied by cytogenetic and molecular methods, and such studies have a number of aims. One aim is to identify genetic aberrations present in the majority of cases and to elucidate the biologic consequences of these aberrations. Characterization of those aberrations might ultimately enable development of novel therapies that would be applicable to most patients with invasive cancer. Other aims are:

1. Identification of novel diagnostic and prognostic markers;
2. Implementation of noninvasive genetic approaches for monitoring bladder cancer recurrence through analysis of urine specimens; and
3. Evaluation of epidemiology and oncogenetic mechanisms in bladder cancer.

The latter aim might be accomplished by determining whether particular carcinogens are associated with specific genetic aberrations in bladder cancer *(108)*.

Approximately 90% of bladder cancers are transitional cell carcinomas and the remaining 10% are predominantly squamous cell or mixed squamous/transitional cell carcinomas. The uncommon histologies, including adenocarcinoma and sarcomas, are not discussed in this chapter. Most bladder cancers are superficial (noninvasive) at initial diagnosis, and many of these superficial lesions can be removed readily by transurethral resection or electrocautery. At least 50% of superficial carcinomas recur after conservative local excision or cautery, although it is not always clear whether an apparent local recurrence is a true recurrence or a second primary tumor. Many superficial bladder cancers arise following carcinogenic insult to the overall bladder mucosa, and it would seem likely that noncontiguous synchronous or metachronous tumors might represent independent primary tumors arising as a result of the carcinogen-associated epithelial "field-effect." However, preliminary studies indicate that multiple tumors are more likely to share an identical genetic fingerprint, suggesting that cells from one original primary tumor were able to migrate and take root in scattered regions of the bladder mucosa *(109)*. In any event, the strong likelihood of recurrence mandates careful monitoring of patients after therapy so that new cancer growth can be recognized and treated before becoming invasive. Such monitoring and early retreatment can spare patients the morbidity of cystectomy or radiotherapy.

The cytogenetic and molecular genetic aberrations implicated in bladder cancer are described comprehensively in a recent review by Sandberg and Berger *(17)*. The following sections focus on the most common cytogenetic and molecular aberrations in bladder cancer and also discuss novel diagnostic and prognostic approaches.

Nonrandom Chromosome Aberrations in Bladder Cancer

Virtually all of the published cytogenetic data in bladder cancer derives from studies of transitional cell carcinomas (Table 1). There is little cytogenetic or molecular data for squamous cell carcinomas of the bladder. Chromosome regions associated with cytogenetic deletion and/or loss of heterozygosity in at least 20% of transitional cell carcinomas include 1p, 3p, 4q, 6q, 9q, 9p, 11p, 13q, and 17p whereas chromosomes 7, 8, and 10 are often trisomic *(17)*. Genome-wide evaluations of transitional cell carcinoma somatic aberrations have been performed by karyotyping, allelotyping, and comparative genomic hybridization. Karyotyping and molecular cytogenetic (FISH) studies revealed several nonrandom aberrations including trisomy 1q, isochromosome 5p, trisomy 7, isochromosome 8q (resulting in monosomy 8p and trisomy 8q), monosomy 9, trisomy 10, and deletion 13q *(16,17,19,20,110)*. Allelotyping (loss of heterozygosity [LOH]) studies revealed allelic losses at 4p, 8p, 9q, 9p, 11p, 13q, 14q, and 17p *(21–28)*, and the overall frequency of these losses was greatest in higher grade tumors *(21–23,27)*. Comparative genomic hybridization studies revealed deletions at 3p, 8p, 9q, 9p, 11p, 14q, and 17p, but did not implicate any chromosome loci as consistent sites of high level amplification *(111,112)*. These genome-wide studies suggest, collectively, that inactivation of several tumor suppressor genes is a critical event in the genesis of most bladder cancers. The presence of a tumor suppressor locus at 3p13–p21.2 is supported by suppression of the tumorigenic phenotype in immortalized human uroepithelial cells after reintroduction of this chromosome region *(113)*. Several of the putative tumor suppressor loci have been localized further by LOH fine mapping. The 4p deletions appear to target two separate loci, one of which has been mapped to a critical 750-Kb interval *(26)*, likewise, the 14q deletions appear to target two separate critical loci at 14ql2 and 14q32 *(27)*. Chromosome 9 deletions have received special scrutiny because these aberrations are very common, even in early stage tumors, and are, therefore, candidates as initiating oncogenetic events in transitional cell carcinomas. One study combined karyotypic and FISH assessment of chromosome 9 copy number: monosomy 9 was found in 70% of superficial transitional cell carcinomas and in similar percentages of invasive carcinomas *(114)*. Another FISH study demonstrated monosomy 9 in 35% of superficial transitional cell carcinomas *(20)*. LOH studies have confirmed both 9p and 9q deletions, consistent with monosomy 9, in 50–75% of transitional cell carcinomas *(115–117)*. Because a majority of chromosome 9 deletions involve loss of the whole chromosome, it has been difficult to pinpoint the critical chromosome regions targeted by these events. However, large studies involving several hundred primary tumor specimens have revealed a handful of cases (5–25% of those with chromosome 9 deletion) with partial deletion of a chromosome 9 homolog. These informative cases had deletions of distinct regions on both 9p and 9q, suggesting the presence of at least two bladder cancer tumor suppressor loci on this chromosome. One locus maps to the short arm in or near band 9p21, whereas the other maps to the long arm in or near band 9q34 *(115,118,119)*. The probable existence of two independent tumor suppressor regions might explain the unusual frequency of monosomy 9 in bladder cancer, as loss of the entire chromosome accomplishes deletion of one allele at each tumor suppressor locus. One target of the 9p21 deletion is the *p16* CDK4-inhibitor tumor suppressor gene. Inactivating point mutations of *p16* were found in 3 of 33 primary bladder carcinomas *(120)*, and homozygous *p16* deletions were found in 18 of 31 bladder carcinomas with monosomy 9 and in each of 13 bladder carcinomas with partial chromosome 9 deletions including 9p21 *(121)*. A candidate gene in the chromosome 9 long arm deletion region has also been identified recently. This is the gelsolin gene, mapping to 9q33, which encodes a Ca^{2+}-binding and actin-regulatory protein. Gelsolin expression was undetectable or greatly reduced in 14 of 18 bladder cancers compared to expression in normal bladder epithelial cells, and transfection of gelsolin cDNA into a human bladder cancer cell line resulted in marked reduction in colony-forming ability and tumorigenicity in vivo *(122)*.

Cytogenetic and Molecular Aberrations Associated with Histologic Progression and Tumorigenic Properties

Allelic deletions at 13q typically involve the retinoblastoma (*RB*) gene, but these deletions are not always associated with inactivation of the remaining, nondeleted, RB allele *(28)*. Accordingly, it is possible that some 13q deletions target a second tumor suppressor gene in the *RB* region. Although *RB* inactivation is uncommon in low-grade superficial transitional carcinomas, *RB* mutations are found in at least 10% of high-grade transitional carcinomas *(28)*. A possible role for *RB* inactivation in carcinoma progression is supported by studies in which gene transfer of *RB* reversed tumorigenic properties (growth in nude mice and soft agar) of bladder carcinoma cell lines, but did little to slow their growth rate in monolayer cultures *(123–125)*. Preliminary clinical correlations suggest that patients with invasive bladder cancer and absent RB expression fare worse than those with invasive cancers that express RB normally *(30–33)*. The prognostic role of *RB* status in superficial bladder carcinomas has been difficult to evaluate because *RB* inactivation is an uncommon event in these lesions.

Several other genetic aberrations are associated with high histologic grade in transitional cell bladder carcinomas. Amplification of c-*erb*B-2 is uncommon in superficial transitional cell carcinomas, but is found in at least 20% of high-grade, invasive, transitional cell carcinomas *(126–128)*. Although c-*erb*B-2 amplification is clearly associated with higher histologic grade, clinical correlations indicate that c-*erb*B-2 status might have independent prognostic value. Patients with grade 3 tumors and concomitant c-*erb*B-2 amplification had the worst prognosis in one recent study *(126)*. Another genetic aberration associated with higher histologic grade is mutational inactivation of a *p53* tumor suppressor allele: such inactivating mutations are often accompanied by loss of the remaining allele (17p deletion) and overexpression of p53 protein. *p53* gene mutations are detected in fewer than 10% of superficial transitional cell carcinomas but are found in approx 50% of invasive carcinomas *(129,130)*. There is growing evidence that p53 overexpression and/or *p53* mutations identify a subset of invasive transitional cell carcinomas with particularly poor prognosis. Esrig et al. *(29)* evaluated p53 expression by immunohistochemical analysis of invasive transitional cell carcinomas from 243 patients treated by radical cystectomy. Five-year recurrence rates for patients with P1, P2, and P3a tumors were 7, 12, and 11%, respectively, when nuclear p53 staining was undetectable, but were 62, 56, and 80%, respectively, when p53 staining was evident *(29)*. In that study, p53 expression was the only independent predictor of recurrence and overall survival for patients with invasive carcinoma confined to the bladder.

Diagnosis and Surveillance of Well-Differentiated Transitional Carcinoma by FISH

A very exciting aspect of the evolving FISH technologies is that these methods can be employed to detect relatively low numbers of clonally aberrant cells. Diagnosis and monitoring of patients with superficial (low-stage) transitional bladder carcinomas is a promising application of FISH because the neoplastic cells from those carcinomas are shed freely into urine (Fig. 6). Although cytologic diagnosis of high-grade transitional cell carcinoma is straightforward, the neoplastic cells shed from low-grade (grade 1) lesions are often impossible to distinguish cytologically from nonneoplastic uroepithelial cells. Thus, FISH might be a useful adjunct to cytology that could spare patients the discomfort of invasive biopsy procedures. It should be emphasized that all patients treated for superficial transitional cell carcinomas are at high risk of local recurrence, particularly over the first few years after curative resection or electrocautery. The standard follow-up for these patients includes cystoscopic random biopsies, initially at 30-mo intervals. FISH evaluation of urine cytospins might be an effective alternate to cystoscopic biopsy in these patients.

The feasibility of molecular and FISH surveillance for neoplastic cells in urine specimens was first established in studies of *p53* point mutations and deletions *(131,132)*. As discussed previously, however, p53 aberrations are uncommon in superficial transi-

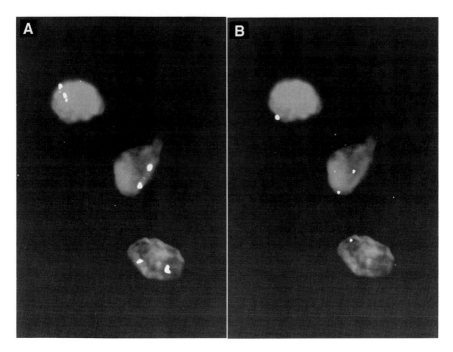

Fig. 6. FISH with chromosome 7 (**A**) and chromosome 10 (**B**) centromere probes in cells obtained from a urine specimen prior to transurethral biopsy. The urine cells were disomic for chromosome 7, but 60% of cells were monosomic for chromosome 10. Biopsy revealed a grade II/III noninvasive transitional cell carcinoma.

tional cell carcinomas, and are, therefore, poor markers of disease activity in patients with low-stage, low-grade, lesions. Other chromosome aberrations, including monosomy 9 and trisomy 7, are found in many low-grade transitional cell carcinomas, and these aberrations are appropriate targets for follow-up FISH studies in patients with a history of superficial bladder carcinoma. Meloni et al. *(133)* initially demonstrated the feasibility of FISH analyses in bladder cancer diagnosis and follow-up. These investigators evaluated copy number of chromosomes 7, 8, 9, 10, 11, X, and Y in urine specimens and bladder washings from 33 patients with active bladder cancer or with a history of bladder cancer. Comparison studies were also performed using urine and bladder washing specimens from 45 control patients. One or more clonal aberrations were detected in urine and/or bladder washings in seven of eight patients with transitional cell carcinoma at time of initial diagnosis and in five of seven patients at time of documented recurrence *(133)*. At least two other groups have confirmed the feasibility of FISH analyses in bladder washing specimens *(134,135)* Cajulis et al. *(134)* compared the diagnostic efficacy of conventional cytology, flow cytometry, and FISH evaluation of chromosomes 8 and 12 in bladder washes from 40 patients with suspected bladder cancer *(134)*. The bladder washes were obtained at time of initial biopsy, and the biopsies revealed transitional cell carcinoma in 26 patients, whereas the remaining 14 patients had nonneoplastic conditions. Cytology, flow cytometry, and FISH were concordant with the biopsy histology in 75, 74, and 83% of cases, respectively. The false-positive rates for cytology, flow cytometry, and FISH were 0, 20, and 0%, respectively, and the false-negative rates were 38.5, 28.5, and 27%, respectively. These findings support an adjunct diagnostic role for FISH, particularly if a urine or bladder washing specimen has inadequate cellularity for flow cytometric analysis *(134)*.

Potential diagnostic applications of FISH are not limited to follow-up of patients with superficial carcinomas. It is notable that several bladder cancer risk groups can be identified based on environmental and occupational exposures *(136,137)*. Known bladder carcinogens include cyclophosphamide, tobacco, and various chemicals used in synthesis of azo dyes and pigments *(136–139)*. Another risk group are those with chronic *Schistosoma haematobium* (bilharzial) infection of the bladder *(140)*. Patients with bilharzial bladder infection are at greatly increased risk for squamous cell carcinoma. Such infections are endemic in Egypt, and bilharzial bladder carcinoma is the most common malignant tumor diagnosed in Egypt, accounting for approx 20% of all cancers. FISH might a useful diagnostic adjunct in high-risk groups, particularly in patients with potential signs or symptoms, e.g., unexplained hematuria, of bladder cancer.

Acknowledgement

The author thanks Thomas Morgan for providing FISH images used in this chapter.

References

1. Kovacs G, Frisch S: Clonal chromosome abnormalities in tumor cells from patients with sporadic renal cell carcinomas. Cancer Res 49: 651–659, 1989.
2. Yamakawa K, Morita R, Takahashi E, Hori T, Ishikawa J, Nakamura Y: A detailed deletion mapping of the short arm of chromosome 3 in sporadic renal cell carcinoma. Cancer Res 51:4707–4711, 1991.
3. Presti Jr JC, Rao PH, Chen Q, Reuter VE, Li FP, Fair WR, Jhanwar SC: Histopathological, cytogenetic, and molecular characterization of renal cortical tumors. Cancer Res 51:1544–1552, 1991.
4. Dobin SM, Donner LR, Speights Jr VO: Mesenchymal chondrosarcoma. A cytogenetic, immunohistochemical and ultrastructural study. Cancer Genet Cytogenet 83:56–60, 1995.
5. Corless CL, Aburatani H, Fletcher JA, Housman DE, Amin MB, Weinberg DS: Papillary renal cell carcinoma: quantitation of chromosomes 7 and 17 by FISH, analysis of chromosome 3p for LOH, and DNA ploidy. Diagn Mol Pathol 5:53–64, 1996.
6. Kovacs G: Papillary renal cell carcinoma. A morphologic and cytogenetic study of 11 cases. Am J Pathol 134:27–34, 1989.
7. Henn W, Zwergel T, Wullich B, Thonnes M, Zang KD, Seitz G: Bilateral multicentric papillary renal tumors with heteroclonal origin based on tissue-specific karyotype instability. Cancer 72:1315–1318, 1993.
8. Kovacs G: The value of molecular genetic analysis in the diagnosis and prognosis of renal cell tumours. World J Urol 12:64–68, 1994.
9. Slater RM, Mannens MM: Cytogenetics and molecular genetics of Wilms' tumor of childhood. Cancer Genet Cytogenet 61:111–121, 1992.
10. Solis V, Pritchard J, Cowell JK: Cytogenetic changes in Wilms' tumors. Cancer Genet Cytogenet 34:223–234, 1988.
11. Kaneko Y, Homma C, Maseki N, Sakurai M, Hata J: Correlation of chromosome abnormalities with histological and clinical features in Wilms' and other childhood renal tumors. Cancer Res 51:5937–5942, 1991.
12. Wang-Wuu S, Soukup S, Bove K, Gotwals B, Lampkin B: Chromosome analysis of 31 Wilms' tumors. Cancer Res 50:2786–2793, 1990.
13. Grundy PE, Telzerow PE, Breslow N, Moksness J, Huff V, Paterson MC: Loss of heterozygosity for chromosomes 16q and 1p in Wilms' tumors predicts an adverse outcome. Cancer Res 54:2331–2333, 1994.
14. Schofield DE, Yunis EJ, Fletcher JA: Chromosome aberrations in mesoblastic nephroma. Am J Pathol 143:714–724, 1993.
15. Mascarello JT, Cajulis TR, Krous HF, Carpenter PM: Presence or absence of trisomy 11 is correlated with histologic subtype in congenital mesoblastic nephroma. Cancer Genet Cytogenet 77:50–54, 1994.
16. Gibas Z, Prout Jr GR, Connolly JG, Pontes JE, Sandberg AA: Nonrandom chromosomal changes in transitional cell carcinoma of the bladder. Cancer Res 44:1257–1264, 1984.

17. Sandberg AA, Berger CS: Review of chromosome studies in urological tumors. II. Cytogenetics and molecular genetics of bladder cancer. J Urol 151:545–560, 1994.

18. Hannon GJ, Beach D: p15INK4B is a potential effector of TGF-beta-induced cell cycle arrest. Nature 371:257–261, 1994.

19. Poddighe PJ, Ramaekers FC, Smeets AW, Vooijs GP, Hopman AH: Structural chromosome 1 aberrations in transitional cell carcinoma of the bladder: interphase cytogenetics combining a 22 centromeric, telomeric, and library DNA probe. Cancer Res 52:4929–4934, 1992.

20. Hopman AH, Moesker O, Smeets AW, Pauwels RP, Vooijs GP, Ramaekers FC: Numerical chromosome 1, 7, 9, and 11 aberrations in bladder cancer detected by in situ hybridization. Cancer Res 51:644–651, 1991.

21. Tsai YC, Nichols PW, Hiti AL, Williams Z. Skinner DG, Jones PA: Allelic losses of chromosomes 9, 11, and 17 in human bladder cancer. Cancer Res 50:44–47, 1990.

22. Knowles MA, Elder PA, Williamson M, Cairns JP, Shaw ME, Law MG: Allelotype of human bladder cancer. Cancer Res 54:531–538, 1994.

23. Olumi AF, Tsai YC, Nichols PW, Skinner DG, Cain DR, Bender LI, Jones PA: Allelic loss of chromosome 17p distinguishes high grade from low grade transitional cell carcinomas of the bladder. Cancer Res 50:7081–7083, 1990.

24. Fearon ER, Feinberg AP, Hamilton SH, Vogelstein B:: Loss of genes on the short arm of chromosome 11 in bladder cancer. Nature 318:377–380, 1985.

25. Shaw ME, Knowles MA: Deletion mapping of chromosome 11 in carcinoma of the bladder. Genes Chromosom Cancer 13:1–8, 1995.

26. Elder PA, Bell SM, Knowles MA: Deletion of two regions on chromosome 4 in bladder carcinoma: definition of a critical 750kB region at 4p16.3. Oncogene 9:3433–3436, 1994.

27. Chang WY, Cairns P, Schoenberg MP, Polascik TJ, Sidransky D: Novel suppressor loci on chromosome 14q in primary bladder cancer. Cancer Res 55:3246–3249, 1995.

28. Ishikawa J, Xu HJ, Hu SX, Yandell DW, Maeda S, Kamidono S, Benedict WF, Takahashi R: Inactivation of the retinoblastoma gene in human bladder and renal cell carcinomas. Cancer Res 51:5736–5743, 1991.

29. Esrig D, Elmajian D, Groshen S, Freeman JA, Stein JP, Chen SC, Nichols PW, Skinner DG, Jones PA, Cote RJ: Accumulation of nuclear p53 and tumor progression in bladder cancer. N Engl J Med 331:1259–1264, 1994.

30. Lipponen PK, Liukkonen TJ: Reduced expression of retinoblastoma (Rb) gene protein is related to cell proliferation and prognosis in transitional-cell bladder cancer. J Cancer Res Clin Oncol 121:44–50, 1995.

31. Cordon-Cardo C, Wartinger D, Petrylak D, Dalbagni G, Fair WR, Fuks Z, Reuter VE: Altered expression of the retinoblastoma gene product: prognostic indicator in bladder cancer. J Natl Cancer Inst 84:1251–1256, 1992.

32. Logothetis CJ, Xu HJ, Ro JY, Hu SX, Sahin A, Ordonez N, Benedict WF: Altered expression of retinoblastoma protein and known prognostic variables in locally advanced bladder cancer. J Natl Cancer Inst 84:1256–1261, 1992.

33. Vet JA, Debruyne FM, Schalken JA: Molecular prognostic factors in bladder cancer. World J Urol 12:84–88, 1994.

34. Fromowitz FB, Bard RH: Clinical implications of pathologic subtypes in renal cell carcinoma. Sem Urol 8:31–50, 1980.

35. Mancilla-Jimenez R, Stanley RJ, Blath RA: Papillary renal cell carcinoma: a clinical, radiologic, and pathologic study of 34 cases. Cancer 38: 2469–2480, 1976.

36. Mydlo JH, Bard RH: Analysis of papillary renal adenocarcinoma. Urology 30:529–534, 1987.

37. Dal Cin P, Gaeta J, Huben R, Li FP, Prout Jr GR, Sandberg AA: Renal cortical tumors. Cytogenetic characterization. Am J Clin Pathol 92:408–414, 1989.

38. Kovacs G, Fuzesi L, Emanual A, Kung HF: Cytogenetics of papillary renal cell tumors. Genes Chromosom Cancer 3:249–255, 1991.

39. Wolman SR, Camuto PM, Golimbu M, Schinella R: Cytogenetic, flow cytometric, and 24 ultrastructural studies of twenty-nine nonfamilial human renal carcinomas. Cancer Res 48:2890–2897, 1988.

40. Wolman SR, Waldman FM, Balazs M: Complementarity of interphase and metaphase chromosome analysis in human renal tumors. Genes Chromosom Cancer 6:17–23, 1993.

41. Teyssier JR, Ferre D: Chromosomal changes in renal cell carcinoma. No evidence for correlation with clinical stage. Cancer Genet Cytogenet 45:197–205, 1990.

42. de Jong B, Molenaar IM, Leeuw JA, Idenberg VJ, Oosterhuis JW: Cytogenetics of a renal adenocarcinoma in a 2-year-old child. Cancer Genet Cytogenet 21:165–169, 1986.

43. Ohjimi Y, Iwasaki H, Ishiguro M, Hara H, Ohgami A, Kikuchi M, Kaneko Y: Deletion (X)(p11): another case of renal adenocarcinoma with involvement of Xp11. Cancer Genet Cytogenet 70:77–78, 1993.

44. Tomlinson GE, Nisen PD, Timmons CF, Schneider NR: Cytogenetics of a renal cell carcinoma in a 17-month-old child. Evidence for Xp11.2 as a recurring breakpoint. Cancer Genet Cytogenet 57:11–17, 1991.

45. Tonk V, Wilson KS, Timmons CF, Schneider NR, Tomlinson GE: Renal cell carcinoma with translocation (X;1). Further evidence for a cytogenetically defined subtype. Cancer Genet Cytogenet 81:72–75, 1995.

46. Meloni AM, Dobbs RM, Pontes JE, Sandberg AA: Translocation (X;1) in papillary renal cell carcinoma. A new cytogenetic subtype. Cancer Genet Cytogenet 65:1–6, 1993.

47. Suijkerbuijk RF, Meloni AM, Sinke RJ, de Leeuw B, Wilbrink M, Janssen HA, Geraghty MT, Monaco AP, Sandberg AA, Geurts van Kessel A: Identification of a yeast artificial chromosome that spans the human papillary renal cell carcinoma-associated t(X;1) breakpoint in Xp11.2. Cancer Genet Cytogenet 71:164–169, 1993.

48. de Leeuw B, Suijkerbuijk RF, Olde Weghuis D, Meloni AM, Stenman G, Kindblom LG, Balemans M, van den Berg E, Molenaar WM, Sandberg AA, Geurts van Kessel A: Distinct Xp11.2 breakpoint regions in synovial sarcoma

revealed by metaphase and interphase FISH: relationship to histologic subtypes. Cancer Genet Cytogenet 73:89–94, 1994.

49. Clark J, Rocques PJ, Crew AJ, Gill S, Shipley J, Chan AM, Gusterson BA, Cooper CS: Identification of novel genes, SYT and SSX, involved in the t(X;18)(p11.2;q11.2) translocation found in human synovial sarcoma. Nat Genet 7:502–508, 1994.

50. Boldog F, Arheden K, Imreh S, Strombeck B, Szekely L, Erlandsson R, Marcsek Z, Sumegi J, Mitelman F, Klein G: Involvement of 3p deletions in sporadic and hereditary forms of renal cell carcinoma. Genes Chromosom Cancer 3:403–406, 1991.

51. Lubinski J, Hadaczek P, Podolski J, Toloczko A, Sikorski A, McCue P, Druck T, Huebner K: Common regions of deletion in chromosome regions 3p12 and 3p14.2 in primary clear cell renal carcinomas. Cancer Res 54:3710–3713, 1994.

52. Kovacs G, Erlandsson R, Boldog F, Ingvarsson S, Muller-Brechlin R, Klein G, Sumegi J: Consistent chromosome 3p deletion and loss of heterozygosity in renal cell carcinoma. Proc Natl Acad Sci USA 85:1571–1575, 1988.

53. Presti Jr JC, Reuter VE, Cordon-Cardo C, Mazumdar M, Fair WR, Jhanwar SC: Allelic deletions in renal tumors: histopathological correlations. Cancer Res 53:5780–5783, 1993.

54. Latif F, Tory K, Gnarra J, Yao M, Duh FM, Orcutt ML, Stackhouse T, Kuzmin I, Modi W, Geil L, Schmidt L, Zhou F, Li H, Wei MH, Chen F, Glenn G, Choyke P, Walther MM, Weng Y, Duan DSR, Dean M, Glavac D, Richards FM, Crossey PA, Ferguson-Smith MA, Paliser DL, Chumakov I, Cohen D, Chinault C, Maher E, Linehan WM, Zbar B, Lerman MI: Identification of the von Hippel-Lindau disease tumor suppressor gene. Science 260:1317–1320 26, 1993.

55. Kuzmin I, Stackhouse T, Latif F, Duh FM, Geil L, Gnarra J, Yao M, Orcutt ML, Li H, Tory K, Le Paslier D, Chumakof I, Cohen D, Chinault AC, Linehan WM, Lerman MI, Zbar B: One-megabase yeast artificial chromosome and 400-kilobase cosmid-phage contigs containing the von Hippel-Lindau tumor suppressor and Ca(2+)-transporting adenosine triphosphatase isoform 2 genes. Cancer Res 54:2486–2491, 1994.

56. Whaley JM, Naglich J, Gelbert L, Hsia YE, Lamiell JM, Green JS, Collins D, Neumann HP, Laidlaw J, Li FP, Klein-Szanto AJP, Seizinger BR, Kley N: Germ-line mutations in the von Hippel-Lindau tumor-suppressor gene are similar to somatic von Hippel-Lindau aberrations in sporadic renal cell carcinoma. Am J Hum Genet 55:1092–1102, 1994.

57. Shuin T, Kondo K, Torigoe S, Kishida T, Kubota Y, Hosaka M, Nagashima Y, Kitamura H, Latif F, Zbar B, Lerman MI, Yao M: Frequent somatic mutations and loss of heterozygosity of the von Hippel-Lindau tumor suppressor gene in primary human renal cell carcinomas. Cancer Res 54:2852–2855, 1994.

58. Gnarra JR, Tory K, Weng Y, Schmidt L, Wei MH, Li H, Latif F, Liu S, Chen F, Duh FM, Lubensky I, Duan DR, Florence C, Pozzatti R, Walther MM,

Bander NH, Grossman HB, Brauch H, Pomer S, Brooks JD, Isaacs WB, Lerman MI, Zbar B, Linehan WM: Mutations of the VHL tumour suppressor gene in renal carcinoma. Nat Genet 7:85–90, 1994.

59. Decker HJ, Klauck SM, Lawrence JB, McNeil J, Smith D, Gemmill RM, Sandberg AA, Neumann HH, Simon B, Green J, Seizinger BR: Cytogenetic and fluorescence in situ hybridization studies on sporadic and hereditary tumors associated with von Hippel-Lindau syndrome (VHL). Cancer Genet Cytogenet 77:1–13, 1994.

60. Tsuchiya E, Nakamura Y, Weng SY, Nakagawa K, Tsuchiya S, Sugano H, Kitagawa T: Allelotype of non-small cell lung carcinoma—comparison between loss of heterozygosity in squamous 27 cell carcinoma and adenocarcinoma. Cancer Res 52:2478–2481, 1992.

61. Brauch H, Tory K, Kotler F, Gazdar AF, Pettengill OS, Johnson B, Graziano S, Winton T, Buys CH, Sorenson GD, Poiesz BJ, Minna JD, Zbar B: Molecular mapping of deletion sites in the short arm of chromosome 3 in human lung cancer. Genes Chromosom Cancer 1:240–246, 1990.

62. Hibi K, Takahashi T, Yamakawa K, Ueda R, Sekido Y, Ariyoshi Y, Suyama M, Takagi H, Nakamura Y: Three distinct regions involved in 3p deletion in human lung cancer. Oncogene 7:445–449, 1992.

63. Yamakawa K, Takahashi T, Horio Y, Murata Y, Takahashi E, Hibi K, Yokoyama S, Ueda R, Nakamura Y: Frequent homozygous deletions in lung cancer cell lines detected by a DNA marker located at 3p21.3–p22. Oncogene 8:327–330, 1993.

64. LaForgia S, Lasota J, Latif F, Boghosian-Sell L, Kastury K, Ohta M, Druck T, Atchison L, Cannizzaro LA, Barnea G, Schlessinger J, Modi W, Kuzmin I, Tory K, Zbar B, Croce CM, Lerman M, Huebner K: Detailed genetic and physical map of the 3p chromosome region surrounding the familial renal cell carcinoma chromosome translocation, t(3;8)(p14.2;q24.1). Cancer Res 53:3118–3124, 1993.

65. Boldog FL, Gemmill RM, Wilke CM, Glover TW, Nilsson AS, Chandrasekharappa SC, Brown RS, Li FP, Drabkin HA: Positional cloning of the hereditary renal carcinoma 3;8 chromosome translocation breakpoint. Proc Natl Acad Sci USA 90:8509–8513, 1993.

66. Morita R, Ishikawa J, Tsutsumi M, Hikiji K, Tsukada Y, Kamidono S, Maeda S, Nakamura Y: Allelotype of renal cell carcinoma. Cancer Res 51:820–823, 1991.

67. Cairns P, Tokino K, Eby Y, Sidransky D: Localization of tumor suppressor loci on chromosome 9 in primary human renal cell carcinomas. Cancer Res 55:224–227, 1995.

68. Morita R, Saito S, Ishikawa J, Ogawa O, Yoshida O, Yamakawa K, Nakamura Y: Common regions of deletion on chromosomes 5q, 6q, and 10q in renal cell carcinoma. Cancer Res 51:5817–5820, 1991.

69. Limon J, Mrozek K, Heim S, Elfving P, Nedoszytko B, Babinska M, Mandahl N, Lundgren R, Mitelman F: On the significance of trisomy 7 and sex chromosome loss in renal cell carcinoma. Cancer Genet Cytogenet 49:259–263, 1990.

70. Elfving P, Cigudosa JC, Lundgren R, Limon J, Mandahl N, Kristoffersson U, Heim S, Mitelman F: Trisomy 7, trisomy 10, and loss of the Y chromosome in short-term cultures of normal kidney tissue. Cytogenet Cell Genet 53:123–125, 1990.

71. Emanuel A, Szucs S, Weier HU, Kovacs, G: Clonal aberrations of chromosomes X, Y, 7 and 10 in normal kidney tissue of patients with renal cell tumors. Genes Chromosom Cancer 4:75–77, 1992.

72. el-Naggar AK, van Dekken HD, Ensign LG, Pathak S: Interphase cytogenetics in paraffin-embedded sections from renal cortical neoplasms. Correlation with cytogenetic and flow cytometric DNA ploidy analyses. Cancer Genet Cytogenet 73:134–141, 1994.

73. Imai Y, Strohmeyer TG, Fleischhacker M, Slamon DJ, Koeffler HP: p53 mutations and MDM-2 amplification in renal cell cancers. Mod Pathol 7:766–770, 1994.

74. Oda H, Nakatsuru Y, Ishikawa T: Mutations of the p53 gene and p53 protein overexpression are associated with sarcomatoid transformation in renal cell carcinomas. Cancer Res 55:658–662, 1995.

75. Thoenes W, Storkel S, Rumpelt HJ, Moll R, Baum HP, Werner S: Chromophobe cell renal carcinoma and its variants—a report on 32 cases. J Pathol 155:277–287, 1988.

76. Kovacs A, Storkel S, Thoenes W, Kovacs G: Mitochondrial and chromosomal DNA alterations in human chromophobe renal cell carcinomas. J Pathol 167:273–277, 1992.

77. Kovacs G, Welter C, Wilkens L, Blin N, Deriese W: Renal oncocytoma. A phenotypic and genotypic entity of renal parenchymal tumors. Am J Pathol 134:967–971, 1989.

78. Welter C, Kovacs G, Seitz G, Blin N: Alteration of mitochondrial DNA in human oncocytomas. Genes Chromosom Cancer 1:79–82, 1989.

79. Kovacs A, Kovacs G: Low chromosome number in chromophobe renal cell carcinomas. Genes Chromosom Cancer 4:267, 268, 1992.

80. Speicher MR, Schoell B, du Manoir S, Schrock E, Ried T, Cremer T, Storkel S, Kovacs A, Kovacs G: Specific loss of chromosomes 1, 2, 6, 10, 13, 17, and 21 in chromophobe renal cell carcinomas revealed by comparative genomic hybridization. Am J Pathol 145:356–364, 1994.

81. Kovacs G, Szucs S, Eichner W, Maschek HJ, Wahnschaffe U, De Riese W: Renal oncocytoma. A cytogenetic and morphologic study. Cancer 59: 2071–2077, 1987.

82. Dobin SM, Harris CP, Reynolds JA, Coffield KS, Klugo RC, Peterson RF, Speights VO: Cytogenetic abnormalities in renal oncocytic neoplasms. Genes Chromosom Cancer 4:25–31, 1992.

83. Crotty TB, Lawrence KM, Moertel CA, Bartelt DH, Jr., Batts KP, Dewald GW, Farrow GM, Jenkins RB: Cytogenetic analysis of six renal oncocytomas and a chromophobe cell renal carcinoma. Evidence that-Y.-1 may be a characteristic anomaly in renal oncocytomas. Cancer Genet Cytogenet 61:61–66, 1992.

84. Meloni AM, Sandberg AA, White RD: -Y,-1 as recurrent anomaly in oncocytoma. Cancer Genet Cytogenet 61:108–109, 1992.

85. van den Berg E, Dijkhuizen T, Storkel S, de la Riviere GB, Dam A, Mensink HJ, Oosterhuis JW, de Jong B: Chromosomal changes in renal oncocytomas. Evidence that t(5;11)(q35;q13) may characterize a second subgroup of oncocytomas. Cancer Genet Cytogenet 79:164–168, 1995.

86. Fuzesi L, Gunawan B, Braun S, Boeckmann W: Renal oncocytoma with a translocation t(9;11)(p23;q13). J Urol 152:471, 472, 1994.

87. Shashi V, Lovell MA, von Kap-Herr C, Waldron P, Golden WL: Malignant rhabdoid tumor of the kidney: involvement of chromosome 22. Genes Chromosome Cancer 10:49–54, 1994.

88. Biegel JA, Rorke LB, Packer RJ, Emanuel BS: Monosomy 22 in rhabdoid or atypical tumors of the brain. J Neurosurg 73:710–714, 1990.

89. Weremowicz S, Kozakewich HP, Haber D, Park S, Morton CC, Fletcher JA: Identification of genetically aberrant cell lineages in Wilms' tumors. Genes Chromosome Cancer 10:40–48, 1994.

90. Haber DA, Buckler AJ, Glaser T, Call KM, Pelletier J, Sohn RL, Douglass EC, Housman DE: An internal deletion within an 11p13 zinc finger gene contributes to the development of Wilms' tumor. Cell 61:1257–1269, 1990.

91. Pelletier J, Bruening W, Li FP, Haber DA, Glaser T, Housman DE: WT1 mutations contribute to abnormal genital system development and hereditary Wilms' tumour. Nature 353:431–434, 1991.

92. Pelletier J, Bruening W, Kashtan CE, Mauer SM, Manivel JC, Striegel JE, Houghton DC, Junien C, Habib R, Fouser L, Fine RN, Silverman BL, Haber DA, Housman D: Germline mutations in the Wilms' tumor suppressor gene are associated with abnormal urogenital development in Denys-Drash syndrome. Cell 67:437–447, 1991.

93. Bruening W, Bardeesy N, Silverman BL, Cohn RA, Machin GA, Aronson AJ, Housman D, Pelletier J: Germline intronic and exonic mutations in the Wilms' tumour gene (WT1) affecting urogenital development. Nature Genet 1:144–148, 1992.

94. Ton CC, Hirvonen H, Miwa H, Weil MM, Monaghan P, Jordan T, van Heyningen V, Hastie ND, Meijers-Heijboer H, Drechsler M: Positional cloning and characterization of a paired box- and homeobox-containing gene from the aniridia region. Cell 67:1059–1074, 1991.

95. Huff V, Miwa H, Haber DA, Call KM, Housman D, Strong LC, Saunders GF: Evidence for WT1 as a Wilms tumor (WT) gene: intragenic germinal deletion in bilateral WT. Am J Hum Genet 48:997–1003, 1991.

96. Park S, Bernard A, Bove KE, Sens DA, Hazen-Martin DJ, Garvin AJ, Haber DA: Inactivation of WT1 in nephrogenic rests, genetic precursors to Wilms' tumour. Nat Genet 5:363–367, 1993.

97. Larsson SH, Charlieu JP, Miyagawa K, Engelkamp D, Rassoulzadegan M, Ross A, Cuzin F, van Heyningen V, Hastie ND: Subnuclear localization of WT1 in splicing or transcription factor domains is regulated by alternative splicing. Cell 81:391–401, 1995.

98. Maw MA, Grundy PE, Millow LJ, Eccles MR, Dunn RS, Smith PJ, Feinberg AP, Law DJ, Paterson MC, Telzerow PE, Callen DF, Thompson AD, Richards RI, Reeve AE: A third Wilms' tumor locus on chromosome 16q. Cancer Res 52:3094–3098, 1992.

99. Douglass EC, Look AT, Webber B, Parham D, Wilimas JA, Green AA, Roberson PK: Hyperdiploidy and chromosomal rearrangements define the anaplastic variant of Wilms' tumor. J Clin Oncol 4:975–981, 1986.

100. Waber PG, Chen J, Nisen PD: Infrequency of ras, p53, WT1, or RB gene alterations in Wilms tumors. Cancer 72:3732–3738, 1993.

101. Bardeesy N, Falkoff D, Petruzzi MJ, Nowak N, Zabel B, Adam M, Aguiar MC, Grundy P, Shows T, Pelletier J: Anaplastic Wilms' tumour, a subtype displaying poor prognosis, harbours p53 gene mutations. Nat Genet 7:91–97, 1994.

102. Bardeesy N, Beckwith JB, Pelletier J: Clonal expansion and attenuated apoptosis in Wilms' tumors are associated with p53 gene mutations. Cancer Res 55:215–219, 1995.

103. Bolande RP, Brough AJ, Izant RJ Jr: Congenital mesoblastic nephroma of infancy. A report of eight cases and the relationship to Wilms' tumor. Pediatrics 40:272–278, 1967.

104. Pettinato G, Manivel JC, Wick MR, Dehner LP: Classical and cellular (atypical) congenital mesoblastic nephroma: a clinicopathologic, ultrastructural, immunohistochemical, and flow cytometric study. Hum Pathol 20:682–690, 1989.

105. Beckwith JB, Weeks DA: Congenital mesoblastic nephroma. When should we worry? Arch Pathol Lab Med 110:98, 99, 1986.

106. Teyssier JR, Ferre D: Frequent clonal chromosomal changes in human non-malignant tumors. Int J Cancer 44:828–832, 1989.

107. Kovacs G, Szucs S, Maschek H: Two chromosomally different cell populations in a partly cellular congenital mesoblastic nephroma. Arch Pathol Lab Med 111:383–385, 1987.

108. Spruck CH 3rd, Rideout WM 3rd, Olumi AF, Ohneseit PF, Yang AS, Tsai YC, Nichols PW, Horn T, Hermann GG, Steven K, Ross RK, Yu MC, Jones PA: Distinct pattern of p53 mutations in bladder cancer: relationship to tobacco usage. Cancer Res 53:1162–1166, 1993.

109. Sidransky D, Frost P, Von Eschenbach A, Oyasu R, Preisinger AC, Vogelstein B: Clonal origin of bladder cancer. N Engl J Med 326:737–740, 1992.

110. Matsuyama H, Bergerheim US, Nilsson I, Pan Y, Skoog L, Tribukait B, Ekman P: Nonrandom numerical aberrations of chromosomes 7, 9, and 10 in DNA-diploid bladder cancer. Cancer Genet Cytogenet 77:118–124, 1994.

111. Kallioniemi A, Kallioniemi OP, Citro G, Sauter G, DeVries S, Kerschmann R, Caroll P, Waldman F: Identification of gains and losses of DNA sequences in primary bladder cancer by comparative genomic hybridization. Genes Chromosome Cancer 12:213–219, 1995.

112. Voorter C, Joos S, Bringuier PP, Vallinga M, Poddighe P, Schalken J, du Manoir S, Ramaekers F, Lichter P, Hopman A: Detection of chromosomal

imbalances in transitional cell carcinoma of the bladder by comparative genomic hybridization. Am J Pathol 146:1341–1354, 1995.

113. Klingelhutz AJ, Wu SQ, Huang J, Reznikoff CA: Loss of 3p13–p21.2 in tumorigenic reversion of a hybrid between isogeneic nontumorigenic and tumorigenic human uroepithelial cells. Cancer Res 52:1631–1634, 1992.

114. Smeets W, Schapers R, Hopman A, Pauwels R, Ramaekers F: Concordance between karyotyping and *in situ* hybridization procedures in the detection of monosomy 9 in bladder cancer. Cancer Genet Cytogenet 71:97–99, 1993.

115. Cairns P, Shaw ME, Knowles MA: Preliminary mapping of the deleted region of chromosome 9 in bladder cancer. Cancer Res 53:1230–1232, 1993.

116. Miyao N, Tsai YC, Lerner SP, Olumi AF, Spruck CH, 3d, Gonzalez-Zulueta M, Nichols PW, Skinner DG, Jones PA, Spruck CH: Role of chromosome 9 in human bladder cancer. Cancer Res 53:4066–4070, 1993.

117. Orlow I, Lianes P, Lacombe L, Dalbagni G, Reuter VE, Cordon-Cardo C: Chromosome 9 allelic losses and microsatellite alterations in human bladder tumors. Cancer Res 54:2848–2851, 1994.

118. Ruppert JM, Tokino K, Sidransky D: Evidence for two bladder cancer suppressor loci on human chromosome 9. Cancer Res 53:5093–5095, 1993.

119. Cairns P, Tokino K, Eby Y, Sidransky D: Homozygous deletions of 9p21 in primary human bladder tumors detected by comparative multiplex polymerase chain reaction. Cancer Res 54:1422–1424, 1994.

120. Gruis NA, Weaver-Feldhaus J, Liu Q, Frye C, Eeles R, Orlow I, Lacombe L, Ponce-Castaneda V, Lianes P, Latres E, Skolnick M, Cordon-Cardo C, Kamb A: Genetic evidence in melanoma and bladder cancers that p16 and p53 function in separate pathways of tumor suppression. Am J Pathol 146:1199–1206, 1995.

121. Williamson MP, Elder PA, Shaw ME, Devlin J, Knowles MA: *p16(CDKN2)* is a major deletion target at 9p21 in bladder cancer. Hum Mol Genet 4:1569–1577, 1995.

122. Tanaka M, Mullauer L, Ogiso Y, Fujita H, Moriya S, Furuuchi K, Harabayashi T, Shinohara N, Koyanagi T, Kuzumaki N: Gelsolin: a candidate for suppressor of human bladder cancer. Cancer Res 55: 3228–3232, 1995.

123. Goodrich DW, Chen Y, Scully P, Lee WH: Expression of the retinoblastoma gene product in bladder carcinoma cells associates with a low frequency of tumor formation. Cancer Res 52:1968–1973, 1992.

124. Zhou Y, Li J, Xu K, Hu SX, Benedict WF, Xu HJ: Further characterization of retinoblastoma gene-mediated cell growth and tumor suppression in human cancer cells. Proc Natl Acad Sci USA 91:4165–4169, 1994.

125. Takahashi R, Hashimoto T, Xu HJ, Hu SX, Matsui T, Miki T, Bigo-Marshall H, Aaronson SA, Benedict WF: The retinoblastoma gene functions as a growth and tumor suppressor in human bladder carcinoma cells. Proc Natl Acad Sci USA 88:5257–5261, 1991.

126. Lonn U, Lonn S, Friberg S, Nilsson B, Silfversward C, Stenkvist B: Prognostic value of amplification of c-*erb*-B2 in bladder carcinoma. Clin Can Res 1:1189–1194, 1995.

127. Sauter G, Moch H, Moore D, Carroll P, Kerschmann R, Chew K, Mihatsch MJ, Gudat F, Waldman F: Heterogeneity of erbB-2 gene amplification in bladder cancer. Cancer Res 53:2199–2203, 1993.

128. Underwood M, Bartlett J, Reeves J, Gardiner DS, Scott R, Cooke T: C-erbB-2 gene amplification: a molecular marker in recurrent bladder tumors? Cancer Res 55:2422–2430, 1995.

129. Fujimoto K, Yamada Y, Okajima E, Kakizoe T, Sasaki H, Sugimura T, Terada M: Frequent association of p53 gene mutation in invasive bladder cancer. Cancer Res 52:1393–1398, 1992.

130. Esrig D, Spruck CH, 3d, Nichols PW, Chaiwun B, Steven K, Groshen S, Chen SC, Skinner DG, Jones PA, Cote RJ, Spruck CH: p53 nuclear protein accumulation correlates with mutations in the p53 gene, tumor grade, and stage in bladder cancer. Am J Pathol 143:1389–1397, 1993.

131. Sidransky D, Von Eschenbach A, Tsai YC, Jones P, Summerhayes I, Marshall F, Paul M, Green P, Hamilton SR, Frost P, Vogelstein B: Identification of p53 gene mutations in bladder cancers and urine samples. Science 252:706–709, 1991.

132. Matsuyama H, Pan Y, Mahdy EA, Malmstrom PU, Hedrum A, Uhlen M, Busch C, Hirano T, Auer G, Tribukait B, Naito K, Lichter P, Ekman P, Bergerheim USR: p53 deletion as a genetic marker in urothelial tumor by fluorescence in situ hybridization. Cancer Res 54:6057–6060, 1994.

133. Meloni AM, Peier AM, Haddad FS, Powell IJ, Block AW, Huben RP, Todd I, Potter W, Sandberg AA: A new approach in the diagnosis and follow-up of bladder cancer. FISH analysis of urine, bladder washings, and tumors. Cancer Genet Cytogenet 71:105–118, 1993.

134. Cajulis RS, Haines GK, 3rd, Frias-Hidvegi D, McVary K, Haines GK, 3rd: Interphase cytogenetics as an adjunct in the cytodiagnosis of urinary bladder carcinoma. A comparative study of cytology, flow cytometry and interphase cytogenetics in bladder washes. Anal Quant Cytol Histol 16:1–10, 1994.

135. Wheeless LL, Reeder JE, Han R, O'Connell MJ, Frank IN, Cockett AT, Hopman AH: Bladder irrigation specimens assayed by fluorescence in situ hybridization to interphase nuclei. Cytometry 17:319–326, 1994.

136. Matanoski GM, Elliott EA: Bladder cancer epidemiology. Epidemiol Rev 3:203–229, 1981.

137. Anonymous: Occupational bladder cancer: a guide for clinicians. The BAUS Subcommittee on Industrial Bladder Cancer. Br J Urol 61:183–191, 1988.

138. Hartge P, Hoover R, Kantor A: Bladder cancer risk and pipes, cigars, and smokeless tobacco. Cancer 55:901–906, 1985.

139. Schulte PA, Ringen K, Hemstreet GP, Altekruse EB, Gullen WH, Tillett S, Allsbrook WC Jr, Crosby JH, Witherington R, Stringer W: Risk factors for bladder cancer in a cohort exposed to aromatic amines. Cancer 58:2156–2162, 1986.

140. El-Bolkainy MN, Mokhtar NM, Ghoneim MA, Hussein MH: The impact of schistosomiasis on the pathology of bladder carcinoma. Cancer 48:2643–2648, 1981.

Chapter 9

Cytogenetic Markers in Selected Gynecological Malignancies

Urvashi Surti and Lori Hoffner

Introduction

The gynecological tissues of a mature female, because of their reproductive function, contain examples of the most immature as well as mature cell types. Thus, representation of all three germ layers may be found in tumors originating from these tissues. Moreover, new tissue types appear in the course of pregnancy that may also develop aberrantly and give rise to neoplasms. Some of these tumors illustrate mechanisms of tumorigenesis that differ from those operating in other solid tumors and that appear uniquely related to early development.

Traditional cytogenetic and molecular analyses of gynecological malignancies have been well summarized in several recent reviews *(1–4)*. The predominant gynecologic malignancies are ovarian and uterine cervical cancers. Adenocarcinomas comprise 95% of all ovarian malignancies. As in many other epithelial neoplasms, ovarian adenocarcinoma is characterized by specific deletions, del(6)(q15–25)(29%), del(11)(p11–15)(26%), and del(1)(q21–44)(26%) *(3)*. Additional chromosomal abnormalities observed in about 200 cases of ovarian cancer include losses of

From: *Human Cytogenetic Cancer Markers*   Edited by S. R. Wolman and S. Sell
Humana Press Inc., Totowa, NJ

chromosomes X, 22, 17, 13, 14, and 8 in order of decreasing frequency, and a gain of chromosome 20. Numerous structural abnormalities involve chromosomes 1, 3, 11, 9, 7, 6, and 12. Molecular analysis has revealed amplification of *ERBB2* in 30% of cases, and loss of heterozygosity (LOH) at many loci including 3p, 4p, 8q, 11p, 12, 16, 17, and 19p. Analysis of about 30 benign tumors of the ovary has shown that trisomy 14 is common in granulosa cell tumor, and trisomy 12 in thecoma, fibroma, granulosa cell tumor, and adenoma.

Malignant germ cell tumors of the ovary have shown association with isochromosome 12p in a few of the reported cases. Benign germ cell tumors of the ovary have an apparently normal female karyotype in the majority of the more than 325 cases that have been analyzed, but the use of variable chromosomal heteromorphic regions indicates that the tumor karyotypes are *not* genetically identical to that of the normal somatic cells of the host. Although the observed genetic variations provide added insight into the origin of germ cell tumors, they are not usually addressed in discussion of chromosomal abnormalities of gynecological tumors *(1)*. The changes observed are unique to ovarian germ cell tumors and are discussed in detail in this chapter.

Tumors of the uterus may arise from the gland-forming epithelium lining the cavity or, rarely, from the stromal cells that surround and support them. Cytogenetic analysis of endometrial adenocarcinoma reveals a diploid mode with many cases containing a gain of the 1q21 to 1qter region by the formation of i(1)(q10) or unbalanced translocations. Rearrangement of 11q21–25 has been reported in 17% of cases having clonal changes and del(6)(q21–25) in 14% of cases *(4)*. In addition, frequent gains of chromosomes 10, 2, 7, and 12, and monosomy 22 have been reported. LOH for 22q, 3p, 9q, 10q, and 17p has also been observed. Eight cases of endometrial stromal tumor have revealed clonal abnormalities. The most frequent recurrent abnormalities are t(7;17)(p15–21;q11.2–21) (13%) and t(7;17), del(11)(q13–21q21–23) (25%) *(3)*. Analysis of eight benign endometrial polyps has shown rearrangement in the regions of 6p21 (62%) and 12q13–15 (38%). It has been suggested that rearrangements of these two breakpoints could define two cytogenetic subgroups *(5)*. Two cases with an identical translocation, t(6;20)(p21;q13), were reported.

Extensive cytogenetic analysis of uterine leiomyoma, the very common benign tumor originating from smooth muscle, indicates the presence of clonal chromosomal changes in 35–40% of cases. The most common abnormalities are 7q deletions, and translocation (12;14)(q13–15;q24), and other abnormalities involve chromosomes 12, 14, 6p, 3, 1, and 13. In contrast, very limited cytogenetic data have been reported on uterine leiomyosarcomas (LMS), which are rare malignant tumors of the smooth muscle. Abnormalities of 1p31, deletion 7q, and rearrangements of chromosomes 11, 10, 17, 12q13, and 14q24 have been observed. The similarities and differences of the changes observed in uterine leiomyomas and LMS provide a model for comparison of benign and malignant lesions from the same cell of origin, particularly interesting because of the high frequency of aberration in the benign lesions which do not progress to malignancy despite attaining large size.

Adenocarcinomas of the uterine cervix have revealed recurrent chromosomal abnormalities including isochromosomes for 4p and 5p (76%), rearrangements of 1p11–15 (31%) and rearrangements of 11p11–15(25%) *(3)*. In addition, del(10)(q24) is reported to be a nonrandom change along with frequent abnormalities of chromosomes 3, 17, 2, 6, and 9. Cytogenetic studies of carcinoma of the vulva and vagina describe abnormalities of chromosomes 3, 8, 22, 11, 10, 18, and 5.

Very few examples of choriocarcinoma and placental site tumors, rare malignant trophoblastic diseases, have been analyzed by cytogenetic or molecular techniques. Cytogenetic data from choriocarcinoma cell lines show frequent rearrangement of chromosomes 1, 3, 9, 13, 12, 7, and 21. Because of their probable gestational nature and association with hydatidiform molar pregnancies, these trophoblastic diseases constitute a model system for dissection of the developmental and malignant behavior of the first differentiating tissue of the conceptus, the trophoblast.

In this chapter, we address the molecular and cytogenetic analysis of three gynecological entities that have been examined in detail in our own laboratory over the last several years. These include:

1. Uterine leiomyomas and LMS;
2. Trophoblastic disease: including hydatidiform mole, choriocarcinoma, and placental site trophoblastic tumor; and
3. Ovarian germ cell tumors: focusing on benign ovarian teratomas and malignant ovarian germ cell tumors.

Leiomyoma and LMS

Uterine leiomyomas are benign smooth muscle cell tumors occurring in 20–30% of women over 30 yr of age. They are hormone-dependent tumors that grow during reproductive years and regress during menopause. The majority of patients present with multiple well-circumscribed leiomyomas and each leiomyoma is thought to be clonal, arising independently from a single initiated smooth muscle cell. The nature of this initial event is unknown. Histologically, the cells from a typical leiomyoma look identical to those from normal myometrium. Although leiomyomas are asymptomatic in many women, they are a frequent cause of abnormal uterine bleeding, pelvic pain, reduced fertility, fetal wastage, and they account for about 200,000 hysterectomies per year nationally. Treatment with a gonadotropin-releasing hormone analog to reduce endogenous estrogen reduces the size of the tumor, but enlargement to pretreatment size occurs after the therapy is stopped. Although these findings indicate an estrogen effect on the growth of these tumors in vivo, the addition of estrogen to leiomyoma cell cultures does not increase the growth rate, indicating that mechanism controlling the growth is affected indirectly by the hormones.

In the last few years, nonrandom, specific chromosomal abnormalities have been observed in several benign conditions such as leiomyoma, lipoma, and meningioma (6–9). These results indicate that specific chromosomal aberrations are not confined to malignant cells as previously thought. Identification of breakpoints provides an opportunity to pinpoint the areas of the genome that play an important role in pathogenesis of the benign conditions. More than 800 cases of leiomyoma have been karyotyped to date, and results of these investigations show that 35–40% of leiomyomas have an abnormal karyotype. Because the majority have normal karyotypes, it is clear that chromosomal abnormalities are not necessary for the formation of leiomyomas and do not represent the initial step; rather, chromosomal rearrangements arise later during the growth of leiomyomas. The most recurrent abnormalities are deletion of 7q, del(7)(q11.2–22q31–32), and the translocation t(12;14)(q13–15; q22–24), seen in about 35 and 20% of cytogenetically abnormal cases, respectively. Rearrangements involving 1p36 (9%) and 6p21(9%), monosomy 22 (6%), trisomy 12 (8%), and ring chromosomes (7%) have been observed in many cases *(3)*. Other abnormalities of chromosomes 1, 2, 3, 10, 12, 13, 14, and X have been reported as well. Recently an architectural factor gene, *HMGI-C*, located in the 12q13–15 region has been implicated in lipomas and uterine leiomyomas *(10,11)*. *HMGI-C* belongs to a family of high-mobility-group DNA-binding proteins with a role in transcriptional regulation. Null mutation of this gene results in development of a pygmy phenotype in the mouse. Its disruption in lipomas results in a chimeric transcript. The translocation breakpoint on chromosome arm 12q in uterine leiomyoma maps within 10–100 kb upstream of the *HMGI-C* locus, and higher expression of *HMGI-C* may play a role in the growth of leiomyoma cells *(10,11)*. In addition, the region 7q22 has been investigated for a possible tumor suppressor gene. LOH studies using dinucleotide repeat sequences have narrowed down the region of interest to 3cM *(12)*.

LMS are malignant neoplasms arising from smooth muscle, occurring most frequently in the female genital and gastrointestinal tracts. LMS behave very aggressively with frequent local recurrences and lung and liver metastases. Uterine LMS is an uncommon malignancy with an incidence of 0.67/100,000 in women over the age of 20. LMS represents 1.3% of all uterine malignancies and approx 25% of uterine sarcomas. The ratio of its incidence to that of the benign counterpart, uterine leiomyoma, is 1:800. Whereas over 800 leiomyomas have been cytogenetically analyzed, only 18 LMS have documented cytogenetic results *(13–20*; and unpublished data). Data were obtained from 8 primary tumors, 9 recurrent tumors, and 1 lung metastasis. Clonal chromosomal abnormalities were reported in 9 of these 18 cases. Modal chromosome numbers included hypodiploid, diploid, hypotriploid, and hypertriploid. Chromosomes 1, 7, 10, and 17 were most frequently altered. Chromosomes 1 and 7 were each altered in 6 of the 9 cytogenetically abnormal cases, and chromosomes 10 and 17 were each altered in 5 of the 9 cases. One LMS had a simple rearrangement, t(10;17)(q22;p13) *(15)*. Deletions of 7q were detected in 4 cases, del(7)(q11) *(15)*, del(7)(q22q32) *(19)*, and del(7)(q31) *(20)* in 2 cases. Alterations of 14q were observed in two cases, t(8;14)(q24;q24) *(16)*, and del(14)(q23) *(20)*. There was deletion of 12q in a single case, del(12)(q13q24) *(19)*. It is interesting to note these changes, as structural rearrangements of 7q, 12q13–15 and 14q22–24 have been found in many uterine leiomyomas. Five recurrent and four primary tumors all demonstrated a normal diploid karyotype. It is possible that this normal karyotype represents overgrowth of normal stromal cells or, alternatively, that the genetic changes in these tumors are not observable at the resolution level of traditional cytogenetics. Loss or rearrangement of chromosome 1, at bands 1p13–1pter, has been noted in many malignant tumors, including LMS. It is possible that the initiation or progression of all these tumors may be related to a tumor suppressor gene or genes in this region.

Trophoblastic Disease

Gestational choriocarcinoma is a rare malignancy of the trophoblast that is preceded by a hydatidiform molar pregnancy in more than 50% of cases. It can also follow a spontaneous abortion, ectopic pregnancy or, rarely, a normal term delivery. The incidence of choriocarcinoma varies geographically from 0.05–0.23/1000 live births. Choriocarcinoma is fatal if not treated in a timely manner, but can be treated successfully with chemotherapy in the majority of cases when diagnosed early. Malignant trophoblast metastasizes readily from the uterus to lung, liver, brain, and other organs. Placental site trophoblastic tumor consists of intermediate trophoblasts of the placental bed, whereas choriocarcinoma consists of cytotrophoblast as well as syncytiotrophoblast.

Hydatidiform mole is an abnormal pregnancy characterized by the early arrest of the embryonic development, swelling of all the placental villi, and trophoblastic hyperplasia. Molar pregnancy should be suspected when the pregnancy test is positive and the uterus is enlarged, but a fetal heartbeat is not detected. Unequivocal diagnosis is made by ultrasound, and the products of conception are either spontaneously aborted or evacuated by dilatation and curettage. All patients with a molar pregnancy are advised to use oral contraceptives and to participate in careful clinical follow-up programs because of the high risk (5–10%) of developing choriocarcinoma. The mechanism of increased susceptibility of the molar trophoblast for malignant transformation is not well understood.

Some nontraditional ways of analyzing chromosomes from molar pregnancies include analysis of Q- and C-banded chromosomal heteromorphic regions, located on the pericentromeric regions of chromosomes 1, 3, 4, 9, 13, 14, 15, 16, 21, and 22, and then comparing them to the heteromorphic regions of the corresponding normal tissues. The use of this technique revealed that complete hydatidiform moles contain only paternal chromosomes, while maternal chromosomes are absent *(21,22)*. Although the 46,XX karyotype of the hydatidiform mole seemed to be identical to that of the normal somatic cells of the patient in some 90% of cases, the comparison of the heteromorphisms established that the apparently normal karyotype is far from normal and is nullisomic for every maternal chromosome and disomic for every paternal chromosome. As more cases were karyotyped, our laboratory reported on the first case with a 46,XY karyotype, also of totally paternal origin *(23)*. About the same time, detailed morphologic and cytogenetic analysis of molar conceptions resulted in delineating two distinct syndromes of complete and partial hydatidiform moles *(24–26)*. The complete mole has a diploid androgenetic 46,XX or 46,XY karyotype, absence of an embryo or fetus in most cases, conspicuous trophoblastic hyperplasia, cistern formation, and necrobiosis of the connective tissue of the placental villi. A cistern is formed as hydropic swelling proceeds from edema to central fluid accumulation with decreasing cellularity. The partial mole has a triploid karyotype with 69 chromosomes and XXY, XXX, or XYY sex chromosomes, and is associated with the presence of a fetus with a partially molar placenta with trophoblastic inclusions and cistern formation. The extra haploid set of chromosomes in partial moles is usually derived from the father *(27–29)*. The risk of subsequent development of choriocarcinoma or persistent trophoblastic disease following a complete mole is substantial (5–10%) and the risk following a partial mole is less, with reports ranging from 0–4%. Additional studies done at many medical centers confirmed the above hypothesis *(30–36)*. These results have contributed insight into the developmental biology of hydatidiform moles and choriocarcinoma because they indicated, for the first time in humans, that the parental origin of the chromosomes (which determines genomic imprinting) is critical for normal development.

These early experiments relied on Q-banded chromosomal heteromorphic regions to determine the parental origin of the molar chromosomes. However, this method is limited in its ability to permit objective resolution of subtle variations in the length of heterochromatic segments, satellites, and satellite stalks on many of the chromosomes. With the availability of an increasing number of highly polymorphic DNA markers, the opportunity to explore the origin of various tumors in greater detail has become feasible. The use of DNA, HLA, and enzyme polymorphisms has confirmed the paternal origin of complete hydatidiform moles and established that more than 90% of complete moles arise by fertilization of an empty egg by a haploid 23,X sperm, with subsequent duplication of its genome. This results in a completely homozygous 46,XX karyotype. Eight to ten percent of complete moles arise by fertilization of an empty egg by two haploid sperm dispermy or one diploid sperm. This results in a 46,XX or 46,XY karyotype with some heterozygous and some homozygous loci. A 46,YY chromosomal complement is not viable. Interestingly, in complete moles the nuclear DNA is exclusively of paternal origin, while the mitochondrial DNA remains maternal *(37)*.

The cytogenetic analysis of choriocarcinoma reveals extensive chromosomal rearrangements, and a hyperdiploid to hypertriploid mode *(38–41)*. Direct analysis of one case of choriocarcinoma showed isochromosomes for 1q, 8q, and 12q with trisomies of 3, 10, and 12, along with a marker of unidentified origin *(42)*. Abnormalities identified in several choriocarcinoma cell lines involved chromosomes 1, 3, 6, 7, 9, 10, 12, 13, 15, 21, 22, and X *(38–41)*. The use of alpha satellite and paint probes for chromosome 12 demonstrated amplification of chromosome 12 DNA in a marker chromosome in one of the cell lines *(43)*.

The genetic origins of a few choriocarcinoma and placental site trophoblastic tumors have been determined, using the DNA polymorphisms from the patient, her partner, previous gestations, and the tumor *(44–46)*. Biparental, androgenetic, and parthenogenetic origins of gestational and nongestational choriocarcinomas have been reported. Biallelic expression of IGF2 and H19 loci has been reported in some choriocarcinoma tumors and cell lines, indicating a loss or relaxation of imprinting at these loci *(46)*. Surprisingly, in the cases of gestational choriocarcinoma, the pregnancy responsible for the malignant transformation of the trophoblast can be either the antecedent pregnancy or any previous molar or nonmolar pregnancy. Thus, choriocarcinoma arising from a complete mole represents a complete allograft with a tumor genotype foreign to the patient, whereas choriocarcinoma arising from a nonmolar conception is a partial allograft. Rejection of an allograft is thought to be one reason why choriocarcinoma following a complete mole is easier to cure. Additional cases of this rare tumor need to be studied to delineate the events responsible for genomic instability and malignant transformation of the molar trophoblast.

From the aforementioned observations, it is evident that paternally and maternally derived chromosomes behave differently even when present in the same nucleus. In order to gain insight into the biology of a particular tumor, the parental origin of the structurally abnormal chromosomes and of the chromosomes gained or lost should be investigated.

Ovarian Germ Cell Tumors (GCTs)

GCTs are thought to originate from pluripotent progenitor cells, such as primordial germ cells, or from embryonic and extraembryonic stem cells. Histologically, these tumors can contain mature and immature tissue from all three germ layers, giving rise to bone, hair, neural tissue, sebaceous material, skin, and teeth, as well as embryonal carcinoma, germinoma, choriocarcinoma, and yolk sac tumor. Benign cystic teratomas can range in size from <1 cm to >45 cm in diameter. Most adult GCTs occur in the gonads, whereas most pediatric GCTs originate in extra gonadal sites such as the sacroccygeum, mediastinum, retroperitoneum, and pineal gland *(47–49)*. In addition, the frequency of malignant gonadal GCTs varies widely between children and adults. Most pediatric testicular

GCTs are benign, but adolescent and adult testicular tumors are frequently malignant. Paradoxically, the opposite is true for ovarian tumors, as most adult GCTs are benign. Ninety-five percent of ovarian GCTs are benign mature cystic teratomas (dermoid cysts) *(47)*, that occur most frequently during childbearing years (median age of 31) *(48)*, but have been found in patients ranging in age from 2–88 yr.

Most benign human ovarian teratomas occur unilaterally, and have a 46,XX karyotype. However, approx 1–2% of ovarian teratomas undergo malignant degeneration *(50,51)*, 8–15% of cases occur bilaterally, and 4–7% of benign cases are chromosomally abnormal, with numerical and structural abnormalities *(48,52)*. Early cytogenetic analyses of mature ovarian teratomas revealed that even though these tumors were 46,XX, they frequently appeared to differ genetically from their host. For example, if the host was heterozygous for a particular centromeric heteromorphism, the teratoma was homozygous for that heteromorphism *(53,54)*. Further studies combined centromeric heteromorphic variations with distal enzyme, HLA, and DNA polymorphisms to determine the origin of mature teratomas *(54–58)*. These studies indicate that most ovarian teratomas originate via a defective meiotic process. Five mechanisms of origin have been postulated *(48)*:

1. Type I: Failure of meiosis I (M I) or fusion of the first polar body with the oöcyte.
2. Type II: Failure of M II or fusion of the second polar body with the oötid.
3. Type III: Duplication of the genome of a haploid ovum.
4. Type IV: Mitotic proliferation of a premeiotic germ cell.
5. Type V: Fusion of two haploid ova.

The precise nature of the meiotic error can be discerned in most cases by the use of chromosomal centromeric heteromorphism and distal polymorphic DNA markers. Type I teratomas would be expected to be heterozygous for all centromeric markers that were also heterozygous in the host. Distal markers could be heterozygous or homozygous depending on the occurrence and frequency of recombinational events. The absence of crossovers would result in heterozygous distal markers, a single crossover would result in 50% homozygosity at the distal marker and double crossovers would result

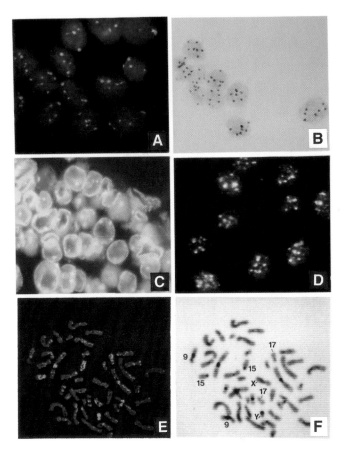

Plate 1 (Fig. 1; *see* **full caption on p. 48 and discussion in Chapter 3).**
Chromosome detection from a bladder tumor.

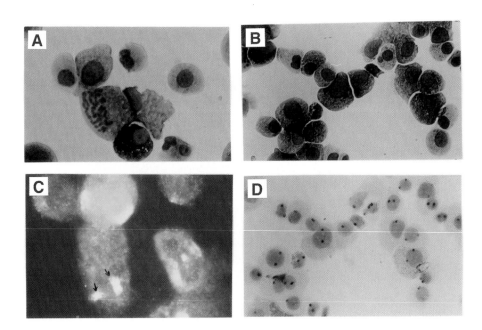

Plate 2 (Fig. 1; *see* full caption on p. 98 and discussion in Chapter 5). Cytospin preparation for bone marrow aspirate of a patient with myelo-dysplastic syndrome.

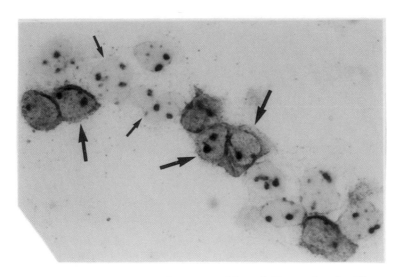

Plate 3 (Fig. 2; *see* full caption on p. 99 and discussion in Chapter 5).
Alkaline phosphatase antialkaline phosphatase (APAAP) staining followed by
in situ hybridization.

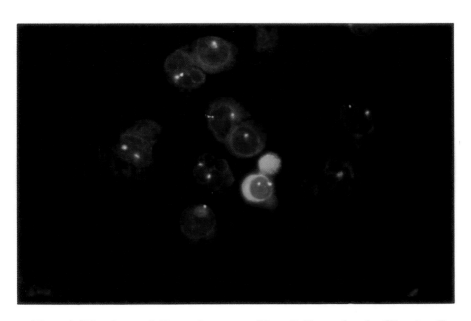

Plate 4 (Fig. 3; *see* full caption on p. 99 and discussion in Chapter 5).
Fluorescence (fluorescein isothiocyanate) immunostaining with glycophorin
A monoclonal antibody (erythroid cells).

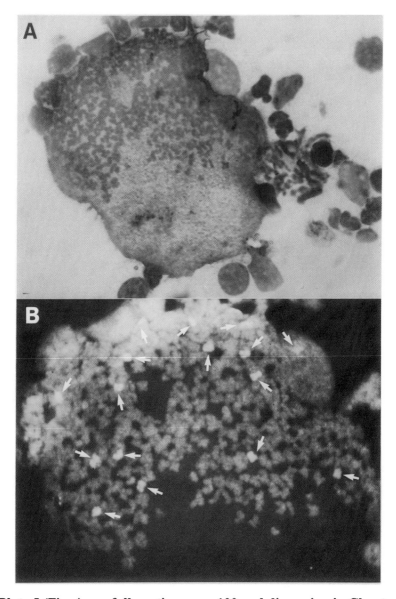

Plate 5 (Fig. 4; *see* full caption on p. 100 and discussion in Chapter 5).
Alkaline phosphatase antialkaline phosphatase immunostaining with CD61
megakaryocytic antibody.

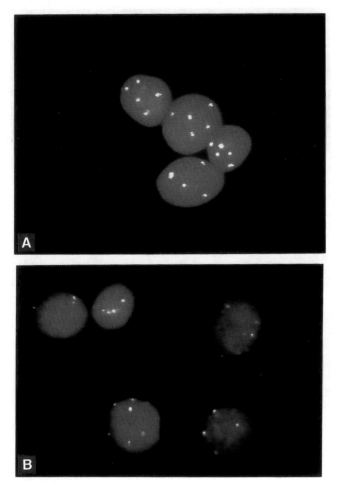

Plate 6 (Fig. 1; *see* full caption on p. 114 and discussion in Chapter 6).
Detection of numerical chromosomal aberrations in breast tumors by FISH.

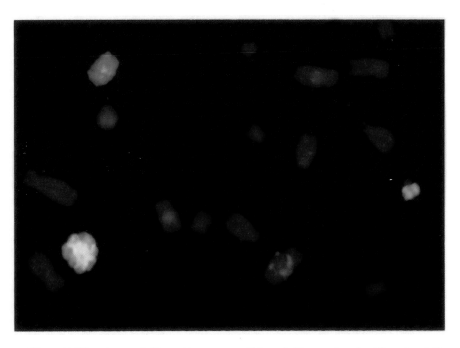

Plate 7 (Fig. 4; *see* full caption on p. 434 and discussion in Chapter 16).
Dual color FISH of a dermatofibrosarcoma protuberans metaphase cell with
digoxigenin-labeled chromosome 17 paint and biotin-labeled chromosome
22 paint.

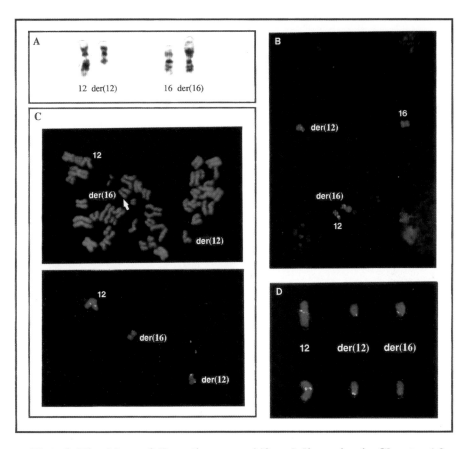

Plate 8 (Fig. 14; *see* full caption on p. 448 and discussion in Chapter 16).
FISH analysis of t(12;16) from a myxoid liposarcoma using the 100C4 YAC.

Table 1
Mechanisms of Origin of Ovarian Teratomas[a]

Type	Mechanism	Centromere	Distal marker
I	M I error	+	+, −
II	M II error	−	+, −
III	Endoreduplication	−	−
IV	No meiosis	+	+
V	Fusion of two ova	+, −	+, −

[a] +, Heterozygous; −, homozygous.

in 75% heterozygosity of distal markers. Type II teratomas would be homozygous for centromeric markers whereas the distal markers could be homozygous or heterozygous depending on crossover events. For type III teratomas, all markers, centromeric and distal, would be homozygous. Absence of meiosis in a primordial germ cell proliferating by mitosis would produce type IV. These tumors would be completely identical to the host at all centromeric and distal markers. Type V teratomas would have, on the average, an equal number of heterozygous and homozygous centromeric markers (*see* Table 1).

Our data indicate that 30% of benign ovarian teratomas are type I, 56% are type II, 11% are type III, and 3% are type IV *(59)*. Fusion of two ova (type V) has not yet been identified. The unique parthenogenetic origins of type I and II ovarian teratomas provide us with a useful tool to study recombination. Centromeric and distal markers can be used to define the heterozygosity or homozygosity of different segments of a chromosome, thus allowing detection of crossover events. Therefore, it has been recognized that type I and II teratomas are useful for gene-centromere mapping *(59,60)*.

Comparison of the recombination data from chromosome 1 in type I and II teratomas with chromosome 1 data from family studies suggests that the frequency of recombination in type II teratomas is normal or near normal, whereas the frequency of recombination in type I teratomas is abnormal *(59)*. The suppression of recombination on chromosomes that have undergone meiosis I nondisjunction in teratomas is similar to that reported in constitutional trisomies arising by maternal meiosis I nondisjunction *(61)*.

To date, over 325 cases of benign ovarian teratomas have been analyzed cytogenetically. The vast majority have shown a normal 46,XX karyotype. However, chromosomal abnormalities have been documented in 12 cases: 47,XX,+8 [4 cases]; 47,XX,+12; 47,XX,+14; 47,XX,+15; 47,XX,+16; 47,XX,–15,+21,+mar; 48,XX,+8,+8; 69, XXX; 92,XXXX/91,XXXX,–13 *(48,54–58,62)*. In contrast, in the approx 25 cases of malignant ovarian GCT with adequate cytogenetic data *(63–72)*, abnormalities are much more frequent; 80% of immature and malignant teratomas compared with 4% of benign teratomas. In these relatively few cases, nonrandom gains of chromosomes 3, 12, and 14 are apparent and have been observed in both near-diploid and polyploid malignant tumors. Most immature cases have simple numerical abnormalities, with one or two extra chromosomes, although a few cases have shown hypotriploid–hypertriploid modal numbers and structural abnormalities. Isochromosome 12p, which is a marker for over 80% of male germ cell tumors *(73)*, has also been observed in two ovarian dysgerminomas, one malignant mixed Mullerian carcinoma, and two malignant teratomas with yolk sac elements *(71,72,74,75)*. A near-diploid mature ovarian teratoma was reported to contain an i(12p), in addition to +der(6)t(1;6)(q11;q22),+8, and +12 *(76)*. This tumor was detected following initial diagnosis and prior surgical removal of an immature teratoma and a successful course of chemotherapy. The patient's previously elevated α-fetoprotein levels were normal and the mass was histologically diagnosed as mature teratoma.

Analysis of centromeric heteromorphisms and distal DNA markers indicate that immature malignant teratomas probably originate by similar mechanisms to those seen in benign cystic teratomas *(72,77)*. Increased copies of chromosome 12 in both benign and malignant ovarian GCT and the presence of i(12p) in both male and female GCT validate the need for additional investigation into the role of chromosome 12 in the development of germ cell tumors.

Both androgenetic trophoblastic disease and parthenogenetic ovarian germ cell tumors display an abnormal phenotype in the presence of a normal karyotype, illustrating the result of abnormal genomic imprinting. In recent years, a great deal of progress has been made in identifying imprinted genes and exploring the role of DNA methylation in genomic imprinting, as discussed in the following section.

Genomic Imprinting

Genomic imprinting is the germline-specific epigenetic modification that produces functional differences in the expression of genetic material depending on its parental origin. The evidence for genomic imprinting is derived from observations of specific human diseases and elegant mouse experiments. Nuclear transplantation experiments involving two male pronuclei (androgenesis) and two female pronuclei (gynogenesis) in the mouse demonstrated that it is essential to have one male and one female pronucleus in the zygote for normal development *(78)*. Androgenesis results in better development of the trophoblast but poor fetal development, whereas gynogenesis results in better development of the fetus but poor trophoblast. In humans, an interesting parallel is displayed in tumor development, in that hydatidiform moles are totally androgenetic and ovarian teratomas are parthenogenetic. Differential expression of the two parental alleles is found to be associated with differential maternal- and paternal-specific methylation imprinting *(79,80)*. In a normal embryo, there is a balance between the paternal and maternal effects, and current data suggest that the genes expressed from the paternal genome promote growth while the maternally expressed genes limit overgrowth. Several domains of imprinted genes have been identified in the mouse and human genomes.

The best understood examples of genomic imprinting in humans are Prader-Willi (PWS) and Angelman Syndromes (AS) on chromosome 15 and the Beckwith-Wiedemann Syndrome (BWS) on chromosome 11. Cytogenetic and molecular findings in PWS and AS indicate that PWS results either from the absence of the paternal copy of chromosome 15 (maternal uniparental disomy) or from molecular deletion of the paternal 15q11–q13 region. AS results from the absence of the maternal copy of the chromosome 15 (paternal uniparental disomy) or from molecular deletion of the maternal 15q11–q13 region in the majority of cases. These two syndromes have very different phenotypes that depend on the parental origin of the deleted region. Several imprinted genes with only paternal expression have been identified in this region including *SNRPN*, *ZNF127*, *PAR1*, *PAR5*, and *IPW*. *SNRPN* and *ZNF127* genes carry parental-specific methylation patterns. The putative maternally expressed gene for AS has not yet been identified. Paternal uni-parental disomy for chromosome 11 has been reported in BWS, a syndrome characterized by overgrowth and increased susceptibility for the development of Wilms' tumor and hepatoblastoma. In addition to the developmental abnormalities observed as a result of abnormal genomic imprinting, loss or relaxation of imprinting has been observed in several tumors such as Wilms' tumor, hepatoblastoma, rhabdomyosarcoma, and lung cancer *(81)*. In Wilms' tumor, 70% of cases show loss of imprinting resulting in expression of both the paternal and maternal copy of Igf2 located on chromosome 11.

In recent years, important advances have been made in our understanding of epigenetic modification of the mammalian genome in normal development. Thus far, at least 14 imprinted human genes have been identified *(82)*. Some of them are found to have biallelic expression in some tissues during normal development and certain disease processes. Although imprinted genes are generally expressed from one parental allele, they can switch from monoallelic to biallelic expression. Imprinted genes show replication asynchrony with earlier replication of the paternal allele. Future research will lead to additional identification and understanding of imprinted genes and domains that play a critical role in the phenotypic manifestations of androgenetic and parthenogenetic development in humans. The connections among genomic imprinting, abnormal development and cancer in trophoblastic disease, and the chromosomal determinants of some GCT add a new dimension to our understanding of relationships between normal and malignant growth and differentiation.

References

1. Heim S, Mitelman F: Cancer Cytogenetics, 2nd edition. New York: Wiley-Liss, 1995.
2. Taylor RR, Teneriello MG, Nash JD, Park RC, Birrer MJ: The molecular genetics of gynecologic malignancies. Oncology 8:63–70, 1994.
3. Sreekantaiah C, Chaganti RSK: Cytogenetic aberrations in solid tumors. In: Kaplan BJ, Dale KS (eds.), The Cytogenetic Symposia 1994. Burbank, CA: The Association of Cytogenetic Technologists, pp. 1–11, 1994.
4. Rodriquez E, Sreekantaiah C, Chaganti RSK: Genetic changes in epithelial solid neoplasia. Cancer Res 54:3398–3406, 1994.

5. Vanni R, Dal Cin P, Marras S, Moerman P, Andria M, Valdes E, Deprest J, Van Den Berghe H: Endometrial polyp: another benign tumor characterized by 12q13–q15 changes. Cancer Genet Cytogenet 68:32–33, 1993.

6. Heim S, Nibert M, Vanni R, Floderus U-M, Mandahl N, Liedgren S, Lecca U, Mitelman F: A specific translocation, t(12;14)(q14–15;q23–24), characterizes a subgroup of uterine leiomyomas. Cancer Genet Cytogenet 32:13–17, 1988.

7. Hu J, Surti U: Subgroups of uterine leiomyomas based on cytogenetic analysis. Hum Pathol 22:1009–1016, 1991.

8. Turc Carel C, Dal Cin P, Rao U, Karakousis C, Sandberg AA: Cytogenetic studies of adipose tissue tumors. I. A benign lipoma with reciprocal translocation t(3;12)(q28;q14). Cancer Genet Cytogenet 23:283–289, 1986.

9. Zang ZK: Cytological and cytogenetical study on human meningioma. Cancer Genet Cytogenet 6:249–274, 1982.

10. Ashar HR, Schoenberg Fejzo M, Tkachenko A, Zhou X, Fletcher JA, Weremowicz S, Morton CC, Chada K: Disruption of the architectural factor HMGI-C: DNA binding AT hook motifs fused in lipomas to distinct transcriptional regulatory domains. Cell 82:57–65, 1995.

11. Schoenberg Fejzo M, Ashar H, Tkachenko A, Fletcher JA, Weremowicz S, Yoong S-J, Krauter KS, Kucherlapati R, Chada K, Morton CC: HMGI-C: an architectural factor at 12q14–15 involved in frequent chromosomal rearrangement in benign tumors. Am J Hum Genet 57:A4, 1995.

12. Ishwad CS, Ferrell RE, Davare J, Meloni A, Sandberg AA, Surti U: Molecular and cytogenetic analysis of chromosome 7 in uterine leiomyomas. Genes Chromosom Cancer 14:51–55, 1995.

13. Bardi G, Johansson B, Pandis N, Heim S, Mandahl N, Bar-Jensen E, Frederiksen H, Sandberg AA, Mitelman F: Recurrent chromosome aberrations in abdominal smooth muscle tumors. Cancer Genet Cytogenet 62:43–46, 1992.

14. Fotiou SK, Tserkezoglou AJ, Mahera H, Konstandinidou AE, Agnantis NJ, Pandis N, Bardi G: Chromosome aberrations and expression of ras and myc oncogenes in leiomyomas and a leiomyosarcoma of uterus. Eur J Gynecol Oncol 13:340–345, 1992.

15. Fletcher JA, Morton CC, Pavelka K, Lage JM: Chromosome aberrations in uterine smooth muscle tumors: potential diagnostic relevance of cytogenetic instability. Cancer Res 50:4092–4097, 1990.

16. Nilbert M, Jin Y, Heim S, Mandahl N, Floderus UM, Willen H, Mitelman F: Chromosome rearrangements in two uterine sarcomas. Cancer Genet Cytogenet 44:27–35, 1990.

17. Boghosian L, Dal Cin P, Turc-Carel C, Rao U, Karakousis C, Sait SJ, Sandberg AA: Three possible cytogenetic subgroups of leiomyosarcoma. Cancer Genet Cytogenet 43:39–49, 1989.

18. Dal Cin P, Boghosian L, Sandberg AA: t(10;17) as the sole chromosome change in a uterine leiomyosarcoma. Cancer Genet Cytogenet 32:263–266, 1988.

19. Havel G, Dahlenfors R, Wedell B, Mark J: Similar chromosomal evolution in a uterine stromomyosarcoma and in one of two leiomyomas from the same patient. APMIS 94:143–146, 1989.

20. Laxman R, Currie JL, Kurman RJ, Dudzinski M, Griffin CA: Cytogenetic profile of uterine sarcomas. Cancer 71:1283–1288, 1993.
21. Kajii T, Ohama K: Androgenetic origins of hydatidiform mole. Nature 268:633,634, 1977.
22. Wake N, Takagi N, Sasaki M: Androgenesis as a cause of hydatidiform mole. J Natl Cancer Inst 60:51, 1978.
23. Surti U, Szulman AE, O'Brien S: Complete (classic) hydatidiform mole with 46,XY karyotype of paternal origin. Hum Genet 51:153–155, 1979.
24. Surti U, Szulman AE: Cytogenetics, morphology and clinical outcome of classical and partial hydatidiform moles. Am J Hum Genet 29:104A, 1977.
25. Szulman AE, Surti U: The syndromes of hydatidiform moles: I. Cytogenetic and morphologic correlations. Am J Obstet Gynecol 131:665–671, 1978.
26. Szulman AE, Surti U: The syndromes of hydatidiform moles: II. Morphologic evolution. Am J Obstet Gynecol 132:20–27, 1978.
27. Jacobs PA, Angell RR, Buchanan IM, Hassold TJ: The origin of human triploids. Ann Hum Genet 42:49–57, 1978.
28. Szulman, AE, Surti U: Clinico-pathological profile of partial hydatidiform mole. Obstet Gynecol 59:597–602, 1982.
29. Doshi N, Surti U, Szulman AE: Morphologic anomalies in triploid liveborn fetuses. Hum Pathol 14:716–723, 1983.
30. Jacobs PA, Wilson CM, Sprenkle JA, et al.: Mechanism of origin of complete hydatidiform moles. Nature 286:714–716, 1980.
31. Lawler SD, Povey S, Fisher RA, et al.: Genetic studies on hydatidiform moles II. The origin of complete moles. Ann Hum Genet 46:209, 1982.
32. Lawler SD, Fisher RA, Pickthall VJ, et al.: Genetic studies on hydatidiform moles I. The origin of partial moles. Cancer Genet Cytogenet 5:309–320, 1982.
33. Ohama K, Kajii T, Okamoto E, et al.: Dispermic origin of XY hydatidiform moles. Nature 292:551–552, 1981.
34. Surti U, Szulman AE, O'Brien S: Dispermic origin and clinical outcome of three complete hydatidiform moles with 46,XY karyotype. Am J Obstet Gynecol 144:84–87, 1982.
35. Surti U, Szulman AE, Wagner K, Leppert M, White R, O'Brien S: Two tetraploid partial hydatidiform moles with triple paternal contribution and 92,XXXY karyotype. Hum Genet 72:15–21, 1986.
36. Vejerslev LO, Fisher RA, Surti U, Wake N: Hydatidiform mole: cytogenetically unusual cases: implications for the present classification. Am J Obstet Gynecol 157:180–184, 1987.
37. Wallace DC, Surti U, Adams C, Szulman AE: Complete moles have paternal chromosomes but maternal mitochondrial DNA. Hum Genet 61:145–147, 1982.
38. Wake N, Tanaka K, Chapman V, Metsui S, Sandberg AA: Chromosomes and cellular origin of choriocarcinoma. Cancer Res 41:3137–3143, 1981.
39. Sheppard DM, Fisher RA, Lawler SD: Karyotypic analysis and chromosome polymorphisms in four choriocarcinoma cell lines. Cancer Genet Cytogenet 16:251–258, 1985.
40. Habibian R, Surti U: Cytogenetics of trophoblasts from complete hydatidiform moles. Cancer Genet Cytogenet 29:271–287, 1987.

41. Surti U, Habibian R: Chromosomal rearrangement in choriocarcinoma cell lines. Cancer Genet Cytogenet 38:229–240, 1989.
42. Bettio D, Giardino D, Rizzi N, Simoni G: Cytogenetic abnormalities detected by direct analysis in a case of choriocarcinoma. Cancer Genet Cytogenet 68:149–151, 1993.
43. Surti U, Juda S, Krishnan S, Alavizadeh S, Leger W: Characterization of chromosomes 7 and 12 abnormalities in gestational choriocarcinoma. Am J Hum Genet 51:4, 1992
44. Fisher RA, Paradinas FJ, Newland ES, Boxer GM: Genetic evidence that placental site trophoblastic tumours can originate from a hydatidiform mole or a normal conceptus. Br J Cancer 65:355–358, 1992.
45. Arima T, Imamura T, Amada S, Tsuneyoshi M, Wake N: Genetic origin of malignant trophoblastic neoplasms. Cancer Genet Cytogenet 73:95–102, 1994.
46. Hashimoto K, Azuma C, Koyama M, Ohashi K, Kamiura S, Nobunaga T, Kimura T, Tokugawa Y, Kanai T, Saji F: Loss of imprinting in choriocarcinoma. Nature Genetics 9:109,110, 1995.
47. Damjanov I: The pathology of human teratomas. In: Damjanov I, Knowles BB, Solter D (eds.), The Human Teratoma: Experimental and Clinical Biology. Clifton, NJ: Humana Press, pp. 23–54, 1983.
48. Surti U, Hoffner L, Chakravarti A, Ferrell R: Genetics of human ovarian teratomas: I. Cytogenetic analysis and mechanism of origin. Am J Human Genet 47:635–643, 1990.
49. Hoffner L, Deka R, Chakravarti A, Surti U: Cytogenetics and origin of pediatric germ cell tumors. Cancer Genet Cytogenet 74:54–58, 1994.
50. Climie ARW, Health LP: Malignant degeneration of benign cystic teratomas of the ovary. Review of the literature and report of a chondrosarcoma and carcinoid tumor. Cancer 22:824–832, 1968.
51. Tobon H, Surti U, Naus GJ, Hoffner L, Hemphill RW: Squamous cell carcinoma in situ arising in an ovarian mature cystic teratoma: report of one case with histopathologic, cytogenetic and flow cytometric DNA content analysis. Arch Pathol Lab Med 115:172–174, 1991.
52. Peterson WF, Prevost EC, Edmunds FT, Huntly JM, Morris FK: Benign cystic teratomas of the ovary: a clinicostatistical study of 1007 cases with a review of the literature. Am J Obstet Gynecol 70:368–382, 1995.
53. Linder D, Power J: Further evidence of post-meiotic origin of teratomas in the human female. Ann Hum Genet 34:21–30, 1970.
54. Patil S, Kaiser-McCaw B, Hecht F, Linder D, Lovrien E: Human benign ovarian teratomas: chromosomal and electrophoretic enzyme studies. Birth Defects Orig Article Ser 14:297–301, 1978.
55. Linder D, McCaw BK, Hecht F: Parthenogenic origin of benign ovarian teratomas. N Engl J Med 292:63–66, 1975.
56. Carritt B, Parrington JM, Welch HM, Povey S: Diverse origins of multiple ovarian teratomas in a single individual. Proc Natl Acad Sci USA 79:7400–7404, 1982.
57. Parrington J, West L, Povey S: The origin of ovarian teratomas. J Med Genet 21:4–12, 1984.

58. Ohama K: Androgenesis and parthenogenesis in humans. In: Vogel F, Springer K (eds.), Human Genetics. Berlin, Germany: Springer, pp. 245–249, 1987.

59. Deka R, Chakravarti A, Surti U, Hauselman E, Reefer J, Majumder PP, Ferrell RE: Genetics and biology of human ovarian teratomas: II. Molecular analysis of origin of non-disjunction and gene-centromere mapping of chromosome 1 markers. Am J Hum Genet 47:644–655, 1990.

60. Chakravarti A, Majumder PP, Slaugenhaupt SA, Deka R, Warren AC, Surti U, Ferrell RE, et al.: Gene-centromere mapping and the study of non-disjunction in autosomal trisomies and ovarian teratomas. In: Hassold TJ, Epstein CJ (eds.), Molecular and Cytogenetic Studies of Non-Disjunction. New York: Liss, pp. 45–79, 1989.

61. Warren AC, Chakravarti A, Wong C, Slaugenhaupt SA, Halloran SL, Watkins PC, Metaxotous C, Antonarakis SE: Evidence for reduced recombination on the nondisjoined chromosomes 21 in Down syndrome. Science 237:652–654, 1987.

62. Dahl N, Gustavson K-H, Rune C, Gustavsson I, Pettersson U: Benign ovarian teratomas—an analysis of their cellular origin. Cancer Genet Cytogenet 46:115–123, 1990.

63. Arias-Bernal L: Chromosomes of a malignant ovarian teratoma. Am J Obstet Gynecol 100:785–789, 1968.

64. Serr DM, Padeh B, Mashiach S, Shaki R: Chromosomal studies in tumors of embryonic origin. Obstet Gynecol 33:324–332, 1969.

65. Atkin NB, Baker MC, Robinson R, Gage SE: Chromosome studies in 14 near-diploid carcinomas of the ovary. Eur J Cancer 10:143–146, 1974.

66. Kusyk CJ, Terpening EL, Edwards CL, Wharton JT, Copeland LJ: Karyotype analysis of four solid gynecologic tumors. Gynecol Oncol 14:324–338, 1982.

67. Ihara T, Ohama K, Satoh M, Fujii T, Nomura K, Fujiwara A: A histologic grade and karyotype of immature teratoma of the ovary. Cancer 54:2944–2988, 1984.

68. Yang-Feng TL, Katz SN, Cacanjiu ML, Schwartz PE: Cytogenetic analysis of ependymoma and teratoma of the ovary. Cancer Genet Cytogenet 35:83–89, 1988.

69. King ME, DiGiovanni LM, Yung J-F, Clarke-Pearson DL: Immature teratoma of the ovary Grade 3 with karyotype analysis. Int J Gyn Pathol 9:178–184, 1990.

70. Gibas Z, Talerman A: Cytogenetic analysis of a metastatic immature teratoma of the ovary: Abstract No. B22. Fourth International Workshop on Chromosomes in Solid Tumors. Tucson, Arizona, 1991.

71. Jenkyn DJ, McCartney AJ: A chromosome study of three ovarian tumors. Cancer Genet Cytogenet 26:327–337, 1987.

72. Hoffner L, Shen-Schwarz S, Deka R, Chakravarti A, Surti U: Genetics and biology of human ovarian teratomas. III. Cytogenetics and origin of malignant ovarian germ cell tumors. Cancer Genet Cytogenet 62:58–65, 1992.

73. Oosterhuis JW, Looijenga LHJ, van Kessel AG, de Jong B: A cytogenetic classification of germ cell tumors and its biological relevance. Eur Urol 23:6–8, 1993.

74. Atkin NB, Baker MC: Abnormal chromosomes including small metacentric in 14 human ovarian cancers. Cancer Genet Cytogenet 26:355–361, 1987.

75. Speleman F, DePotter C, Dal Cin P, Mangelschots K, Ingelaere H, Laurey G, Benoit Y, Leroy J, Van den Berghe H: I(12p) in a malignant ovarian tumor. Cancer Genet Cytogenet 45:49–53, 1990.

76. Speleman F, Laureys G, Benoit Y, Cuvelier C, Suikerbuijk R, DeJong B: I(12p) in a near-diploid mature ovarian teratoma. Cancer Genet Cytogenet 60:216–218, 1992.

77. Ohama K, Normua K, Okamoto E, Fukuda Y, Ihara T, Fujiwara A: Origin of immature teratoma of the ovary. Am J Obstet Gynecol 152:869–890, 1985.

78. Barton SC, Surani MAH, Norris ML: Role of paternal and maternal genomes in mouse development. Nature 311:374–376, 1984.

79. Driscoll DJ, Waters MF, Williams CA, Zori RT, Glenn CC, Avidano KM, Nicholls RD: A DNA methylation imprint, determined by the sex of the parent, distinguishes the Angelman and Prader-Willi syndromes. Genomics 13:917–924, 1992.

80. Mowery-Rushton PA, Driscoll DJ, Nicholls RD, Locker J, Surti U: DNA methylation patterns in human tissues of uniparental origin using a zinc-finger gene (ZNF127) from the Angelman/Prader-Willi region. Am J Med Genet 61:140–146, 1996.

81. Feinberg AP, Rainier S, DeBaun MR: Genomic imprinting, DNA methylation, and cancer. J Natl Cancer Inst Monogr 17:21–26, 1995.

82. Wutz A, Smrzka OW, Barlow DP, Neumann B: Genomic imprinting: the parental connection. Appl Cytogenet 21:145–152, 1995.

Chapter 10

Prostate Cancer

Arthur R. Brothman and Briana J. Williams

Introduction

As the leading malignancy of males in Western countries, prostate cancer has become a major research focus, yet only recently have techniques become available for the accurate study of this complex tumor. Clinically, prostate tumors follow widely varying courses of progression, with a subset of tumors showing little or no advancement and rarely causing death, in contrast to aggressive tumors that metastasize to bone, lymph nodes or other sites and kill the patient. **There is currently no biological marker that can distinguish the indolent from the aggressive form of this disease.** Current methods for prostate cancer detection include digital rectal examination, ultrasonic analysis, and assay for serum levels of the prostatic specific antigen (PSA). Although PSA screening, combined with digital rectal examination is the most sensitive test to date, it fails to detect all tumors, gives false positive results, and cannot distinguish indolent from aggressive tumors. Treatment of early-stage prostate cancer in the United States often involves removal of the prostate gland, especially in otherwise healthy men, but the surgery is often complicated by significant side effects, including incontinence and impotence which negatively affect the quality of postsurgical life. An understanding of the molecular

From: *Human Cytogenetic Cancer Markers*   Edited by S. R. Wolman and S. Sell
Humana Press Inc., Totowa, NJ

pathogenesis of prostate cancer may allow for improved patient management, especially if markers can be identified to differentiate aggressive from nonlife threatening tumors.

As is apparent from the previous chapters, cytogenetics often can serve as a powerful tool to identify chromosomal regions involved in specific cancers. In combination with molecular biological techniques, it permits a broad genomic analysis from the complete karyotype down to submicroscopic regions that can lead to identification of functional genes affecting tumor growth. The present heightened interest in prostate cancer research is at least in part the result of recent advances in genetic methodologies. For example, the initial work done in cell culturing and classical cytogenetics of prostate tumors set the stage for many of the subsequent studies. Our intent is to review the literature of many of these related studies of prostate cancer, and show how the concerted interaction of multiple scientific disciplines has led to an improved understanding of this disease. Much work is still needed to further understand mechanisms and prognostic implications of genetic abnormalities in prostate cancer, and although some candidate genes have been identified, others most surely exist that are responsible for different stages of the carcinogenic pathway.

We have separated our discussions into three main categories: classical cytogenetics, molecular analyses, and molecular cytogenetic studies of prostate cancer. Each has offered significant information, but it must be emphasized that each broad technique has strengths and weaknesses. Classical cytogenetics, which requires living, dividing cells, shows the entire genome at a glance, albeit with the limited sensitivity of the light microscope. If banding resolution in a cytogenetic study is approx 550 bands/haploid karyotype, each karyotype can provide information at a resolution of approx 10–20 Mb throughout the entire genome. Molecular analyses provide such a focused assessment of genetic rearrangement that they can detect single base changes, whereas major genetic alterations elsewhere in the genome go undetected. Molecular cytogenetics, including techniques such as fluorescence *in situ* hybridization (FISH) and comparative genomic hybridization (CGH) combines strengths and weaknesses of the previous two technologies, and has proven to be one of the most powerful tools in the study of prostate cancer. A major advantage of molecular cytogenetics is that it confers the ability to examine nondividing nuclei. FISH using most conventional DNA probes allows for detailed analysis on single cells, but again is limited to the specific regions being evaluated. CGH, alternatively, offers a genome-wide screening, but will not detect near-balanced rearrangements and to date has approximately the same resolution limits as conventional cytogenetics. When the three methods are used in a complementary fashion, however, information can be obtained that is likely to yield insights into some of the genetic mechanisms of prostate cancer. The conclusion of this chapter deals with functional aspects of the disease, with examples from an experimental system of microcell-mediated chromosome transfer into living prostate cells; finally, data accumulated are discussed in relationship to clinical outcome and potential prognostic implications.

Classical Cytogenetics

Since the prostate gland is anatomically difficult to access, tumor tissue has not been widely available for study. The cellular heterogeneity of the gland, including the presence of normal, nontumor cells, such as differentiated epithelial secretory cells and a large fibroblastic stromal component further complicates analysis. Furthermore, prostate tumors are usually very slow growing in vivo, apparently based on low mitotic index. Because so few mitotic cells are present in a tumor specimen, the initial cytogenetic studies of prostate cancers were limited, and provided only a glimpse of the chromosomal abnormalities associated with the disease. Over 70% of primary prostate tumors studied by classical cytogenetics had normal male karyotypes, with only 106 of the 319 reported cases showing abnormalities *(1–18)*. The most common structural abnormalities involved chromosomal regions on 1p, 1q, 2p, 2q, 7q, and 10q, as well as numerical changes such as +7 and –Y *(see* Table 1).

The preponderance of normal results suggests that the standard method for culturing prostate tumor cells may actually select against cytogenetically abnormal clones and may not accurately reflect the cellular composition of the tumor. Studies by Konig's group and our group *(10,19)* have indicated that there is selective loss of abnormal

Table 1
Classical Cytogenetic Studies of Prostate Cancer

Refs.	Clonal abnormalities	No. tumors	No. abnormal
3	+7	4	1
11	dmin	2	2
8	−1, −2, −3, t(8;12), t(1;21)	1	1
12	−7q, −10q	1	1
17	iso(17q)	1	1
2	del (10q), del (17q), −7p, der (1), −Y	5	5
5	+4, +7, +14, +20, +22, rearranged 2p, 7q, 10q, dmin	30	9
6	−Y, +Y, dmin, tetraploid	20	5
55	−Y, −14, −19, t(Y;22), +7,+8,+12,+18, 9p+	14	
13	−Y, clonal structural abnormality of 1, 7, and 10; dmin	57	15
1	−Y, del(10q24), +7	32	16 clonal

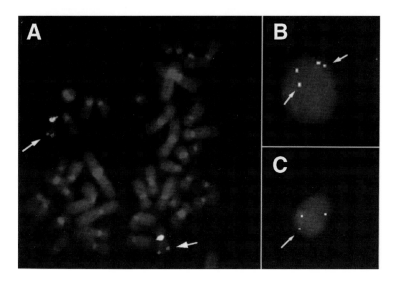

Fig. 1. Gray scale image illustrating the localization of a P1 phage probe for MXI1 at 10q25 and its use in deletion detection in uncultured prostate tumor cells. (**A**) Illustration of biotinylated MXI1 signals (arrows) hybridized with a digoxigenin-labeled chromosome 10 pericentromeric α-satellite probe (Oncor) on a normal male metaphase. (**B**) Uncultured prostate tumor cell with dual-color FISH with no deletion (two copies) of the biotinylated MXI1 P1 (arrows) and two copies of the digoxigenin-labeled chromosome 10 pericentromeric probe (Oncor). (**C**) Similar dual-color FISH illustrating loss of one copy of the biotinylated MXI1 P1 signal suggesting partial deletion of one chromosome 10.

cells in vitro, indicating that efforts to improve cell culturing systems are needed.

It is interesting to note, however, that at least one of the cytogenetic abnormalities observed in some prostate tumors (deletion on the long arm of chromosome 10) has resulted in the identification of a putative prostate-specific tumor suppressor gene, MXI1, at 10q25, illustrated in Fig. 1 *(20)*. Thus, although classical cytogenetic studies have not yielded a definitive and consistent abnormality such as the diagnostic changes seen in the leukemias and some other solid tumors, chromosome aberrations once again are likely to shed light on potential mechanisms involved in the development of this disease.

Molecular Analyses

Molecular studies, such as loss of heterozygosity (LOH) or allelic imbalance (AI), may provide a more detailed view of genetic abnormalities than cytogenetic techniques *(15,21–45)*. It is impractical to screen the entire genome with this technique, but it is powerful when used at specific loci to look for genomic imbalance. As is the case with all of the techniques described in this chapter, molecular studies are not without their limitations. LOH and AI studies require highly polymorphic markers, most of which are not intragenic, as well as high levels of constitutional genetic heterozygosity in the patients. Since these are DNA-based evaluations, they are very sensitive to the normal cell contamination inherent in prostate tumors. For those regions, however, where fine mapping of deletions is desirable, and the other problems can be adequately overcome, Southern blot or polymerase chain reaction (PCR)-based LOH or AI studies have proven to be informative (*see* Table 2).

Loss of 8p loci have probably been more extensively studied by more laboratories than any other chromosomal sites in prostate cancer; it appears from these studies that there are at least three distinct regions of loss associated with the disease. Regions of loss have been reported which are centered around the LPL and MSR loci at 8p22, and at two other regions, one centered around the NEFL locus at 8p21 and the other more proximal including the ANK locus at 8p11–21 *(15,22,30,35,42,44)*.

In addition to loss from 8p, LOH or AI studies also indicate frequent loss on 7q, 10q, 13q, 16q, 17p and q, and 18q in a significant number of tumors. Many of these regions of LOH or AI were not specific for any particular gene in the region of loss, and may be the sites of novel prostate-specific suppressor genes, but in some cases LOH or AI of a known tumor or metastasis suppressor locus was detected. For example, imbalances at DCC (18q21.3), BRCA1 (17q21), APC (5q21), TP53 (17p13), RB (13q14), and the metastasis suppressor locus, nm23-H1 (17q21.3) have been detected in varying numbers and stages/grades of tumors *(23,24,31,32,34,39)*. Abnormal expression of known genes with putative suppressor functions from these regions has also been observed in prostate cancers, such as e-cadherin (16q22), her2/neu (17q21), p53 (17p13),

Table 2
Molecular Studies of Prostate Cancer[a]

Refs.	LOH/AI or molecular abnormality detected	No. tumors	No. abnormal
33	8p, 10, 16q, 18q	18	11/18
26	10q, 16q	24 + 4 mets	13/24 tumors, 4/4 mets
21	8p, 10, 16q	10 + 8 mets	
36	17p	23	1/23
31	18q (DCC)	14	5/11 LOH, 12/14, ↓expression
28[b]	17p (p53)	10 + 2 mets	1/10 tumors, 1/2 mets
22	8p, +8q (myc)	52	32/51
39	5q (APC), 10, 13q (RB), 16q	21	
23	5q (APC), 17p (p53), 18q	30	
35	8p	63	29/63
34	7q, 8p, 10q, 18q	20	
32	17q	21	11/21
45	7q	16	12/16
24	13q (RB)	41	11/41
25	17q	23	5/23
44	8p	38 + 6 mets	26/44
41	8p, 10q, 16q	19	

[a]Abbreviations: AI, allelic imbalance; APC, adenomatous polyposis coli; LOH, loss of heterozygosity; mets, metastases; RB, retinoblastoma; DCC, deleted in colon cancer.
[b]This study used single-strand conformational polymorphism and sequencing of TP53 only. Most of these studies examined a limited number of sites.

and DCC (18q21.3) *(27,29,31,38,40)*. There may be novel prostate-specific suppressor genes at these same locations, as well as in the others where a genetic imbalance has not yet been linked to particular gene. The most exciting recent discoveries in prostate cancer genetic research have undoubtedly been the characterizations of prostate-specific tumor suppressor genes, such as mxi-1 at 10q25 and the newly cloned metastasis suppressor, KAI-1 at 11p11.2, as well as the amplification of the androgen receptor gene at Xq12 from regions previously defined by genetic imbalance studies *(20,27,46)*. These may well be the first gene-based biomarkers useful in the detection or clinical monitoring of prostate cancer.

Molecular Cytogenetics

FISH

The advent of molecular cytogenetic techniques has had a major impact on the field of cytogenetics. One of the most pronounced advantages of FISH techniques over classical cytogenetics is the ability to examine nondividing cells by FISH, allowing for the study of uncultured tissue. FISH, using either locus- or chromosome-specific DNA probes, is highly sensitive and allows for the rapid detection and enumeration of defined DNA sequences in both metaphase and interphase nuclei. Both types of FISH studies have contributed to a significant understanding of clonal abnormalities in prostate tumors, but an advantage of locus-specific probes over chromosome-specific, centromere enumeration probes is that specific genetic loss or gain can be evaluated directly. With the enumeration probes, loss and gain of whole chromosomes is extrapolated from the number of fluorescent signals, which are specific to the pericentromeric region alone.

In contrast with classical cytogenetic results, clonal abnormalities have been detected in nearly 70% of the tumors studied by FISH *(47–61)*. Although a number of centromere-based FISH studies of prostate cancer have been performed, relatively few abnormalities are common to the majority of the studies (*see* Table 3). Losses of 8p, 10q, 16q, 17, 18q, and Y have been observed in significant numbers of cases from multiple studies, as has gain of chromosomes 7, 8, and the X chromosome, illustrated in Fig. 2A. There

Table 3
Molecular Cytogenetic Studies of Prostate Cancer with Combined Methodologies[a]

Refs.	Clonal abnormalities	No. tumors	No. abnormal
50	−7, −8, −10, −16, −17, −18, +7, +8, +10, +16, +17, +18	10	9
37	8p, 10q (LOH), −10, −Y (FISH), +4, +7, +8, +10 (FISH)	13	10/12 (FISH)
4[b]	−Y, t(1;10), tetraploid	26, 5 FISH	15 cyto, 2/5 FISH
19[b]	+1 and/or tetraploid	14	5/14
16	−10, −Y (FISH), +7 (cyto), +8 (FISH)	7	5/7
15[c]	−8p, −8q, −8cen (FISH), 8p (LOH), +8q (FISH)	9	7/9
57[b,d]	TET, +7 and +8 (FISH)	50	24/50
51	−12, −17, +X	20	17/20
52	−8, −9, −12, −17, −18, +7, +8, +10, +11, +18, +Y	40	16/40
60[e]	−Y (cyto) and −7 (FISH), +7 (cyto) and +7 (FISH)	53	5/41 cyto, 41/53 FISH
58[b]	−7, −10, −16, +1, +7, +8, +10, +17, +X, and +Y	23 tumors	17/23
9	+7, +10, +17, +X, and +Y	31	23/31 FISH
48	+7	15 + 16 mets	29/31
49	−1, −1p(tel), −7, −8, −10, −18, and −Y, +7, +8, +X, and +Y	35	34/35
54[c]	−8p	42 tumors	30/34
10	−17 (FISH), +7, tetraploid (FISH)	20 + 2 mets	5/20
47[b]	−8, −10, −15, −Y, +7, +8	25 tumors	13/25
53[c]	−16q24	30	15/30
61[c]	−17q21-22	23	16/23

(continued)

Table 3 (continued)

Refs.	Clonal abnormalities	No. tumors	No. abnormal
62	−8p, +8q, +13q, +16, +17, +20q, +Y	17	13/17
63	−6q, −8p, −9p, −13q, −16q, −18q, −22q, +7, +19p, +X	40	30/40
46	+Xq11–13	23	7/23

[a]Many of these studies examined a limited number of chromosomes or regions. cyto, classical cytogenetics.
[b]Also included flow cytometry results.
[c]Used single-copy probes.
[d]Used needle biopsies.
[e]Used touch preparations and paraffin-embedded tissues.

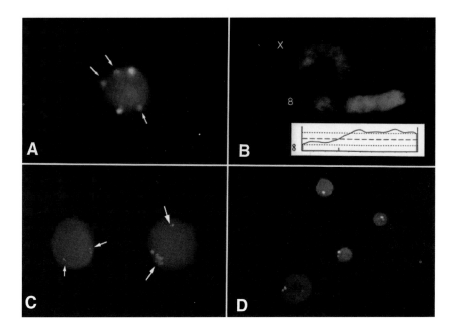

Fig. 2. Gray scale images illustrating various molecular cytogenetic analyses. (**A**) Dual-color FISH of an uncultured prostate tumor cell using a biotinylated chromosome 17 pericentromeric probe (Oncor) and at the arrows, a digoxigenin-labeled probe for the X chromosome (Oncor). (**B**) CGH image, courtesy of Wiley-Liss, reprinted with permission from ref. *63*, of chromosomes X and 8 illustrating the overall decreased signal intensity of the X chromosome and the p arm of chromosome 8, as well as the increased signal intensity of 8q. The CGH profile of chromosome 8 indicates the color intensity ratios at all points along the chromosome. (**C**) Dual-color FISH with two copies of the X chromosome centromere and the copy number of androgen receptor-specific P1 signals (arrows), reproduced courtesy of Nature Publishing, reprinted with permission from ref. *47*. The cell on the left shows two copies of each probe, whereas the cell on the right illustrates the use of FISH to detect the increased copy number of androgen-receptor signals. (**D**) Single-color FISH of several prostate cancer cells hybridized with a chromosome 17 pericentromeric probe (Oncor) illustrating the close association of the signals in three cells and apparent monosomy in the top cell.

have been comparatively few FISH studies of prostate cancer using single-copy probes, but they have been useful in localizing small regions deleted from chromosome arms such as 8p, 16q, and 17q, presumably where important genes are located. A single-copy probe for the androgen receptor was shown to be useful in evaluating gene amplification in recurrent prostate cancer, as illustrated in Fig. 2C.

While a recent study indicated that homologous chromosomes associate at opposite poles in the prometaphase nucleus *(75)*, evidence by FISH now suggests that some chromosomes may actually pair in the interphase prostate nucleus. In studies from both our laboratory and from the Mayo clinic, association of homologous centromeres of chromosomes 9 and 17 have been observed *(52,59)*. The centromeric association, as illustrated in Fig. 2D, creates a problem in the interpretation of FISH results, since signals lie so close together that they are often mis-scored as single signals, resulting in overestimation of chromosomal loss in some cases. The biological consequence of this unexplained phenomenon may be an increase in the potential for exchange of genetic material near the centromere, increasing the likelihood of expression of a mutant or rare allele or the disruption of a functional gene.

CGH

CGH was introduced in 1992 for the detection of deletions and amplifications in solid tumors, and the technique is without rival as a one-step genome-wide screening for such numerical abnormalities. The technique, however, is appropriate only for the detection of numerical imbalances, and cannot detect polyploidy, balanced translocations, inversions, or point mutations. The deletion detection limit of CGH is approx 20–30 Mb in primary tumors; approximately the size of an average chromosomal band. Although this provides CGH with essentially the sensitivity of traditional cytogenetic evaluation, it is not limited by the low mitotic index of most prostate tumors. One of the most serious limitations of both CGH and AI studies of prostate cancer is that they are based on DNA extracted from tissue which may have a high degree of cellular contamination by normal prostate epithelial and/or stromal cells; a limitation as noted in the Classical Cytogenetics section to the establishment of primary prostate tumor cell cultures as well. The use of paraffin-embedded tissues (PET) for CGH analysis (and for LOH/AI studies) may overcome some of the limitations of cellular heterogeneity since a tumor sample can be carefully microdissected after histological and pathological evaluation. Use of PET will also make possible large retrospective studies of prostate cancer genetics with clinical correlations.

There have been three CGH studies to date reporting evaluation of prostate tumors *(46,62,63)*. The changes observed most frequently were loss of 8p; gain of 8q; and loss of 13q, 16q, 17q, 18q, and the proximal Y chromosome. Novel deletions on 6q, 9p, 22q, as well as gain of chromosome 19 and Xq11–13, previously undetected by karyotyping, FISH or LOH, were also observed in these studies. With the exception of the androgen receptor gene on Xq, the specific genes on these chromosomes important to the initiation or progression of prostate tumors have not yet been identified, but the CGH results have given investigators new regions to analyze. In fact, gain or loss of every chromosome except chromosome 21 has been reported in at least one prostate tumor using CGH. Some false positive results are to be expected from a screening technique, but this result may reflect a formidable hurdle in genetic studies of prostate cancer, i.e., gross genetic heterogeneity. CGH results have also been compared with molecular LOH or AI results in prostate cancer, with concordance in at least 76% of the cases studied *(62,63)*.

In addition to the novel, although anonymous, regions, CGH has led to the identification of a particular genetic abnormality in prostate cancer. The localized gain of genetic material in the proximal Xq region detected by CGH has been associated with the amplification of the androgen receptor gene in hormone-refractory disease *(see* Fig. 2C) *(46)*. Use of multiple molecular and cytogenetic techniques confirmed that the androgen receptor, located at Xq12, is overexpressed in nearly one-third of cases of recurrent, hormone-refractory disease, but not in the primary prostate tumors from those patients. The clinical significance of this discovery is discussed in the Clinical Correlations section of this chapter.

The technique has also provided evidence for interesting, but unexplained, genomic imbalances such as the loss of genetic material on 8p and the concommitant gain of genetic material on 8q illustrated in Fig. 2B. This particular imbalance has been observed in CGH studies of other solid tumors, such as uveal melanoma and small cell lung carcinoma, as well as gains of 8q reported in acute myeloid leukemia *(64–67)*. In prostate tumors, the imbalance has been suggested to reflect the formation of an isochromosome, but no examples of an 8q isochromosome have been seen in classical cytogenetic studies of prostate tumors. A study by Macoska and colleagues *(15)* used cosmids specific for 8p and 8q loci and a chromosome 8 centromere-specific probe to address the imbalance on chromosome 8, but found only 2/8 cases with 8p loss and concurrent gain of the centromere and 8q signals. Although the existence of an isochromosome is still is question, the imbalance of chromosome 8 in such a wide variety of tumor types makes the "8p loss/8q gain conundrum" an interesting mechanistic question which CGH may help to resolve.

It is necessary to keep in perspective that any single technique plays a role in genetic analysis, but many coordinated techniques may be necessary to determine the complete genetic makeup of a particular tumor or to draw conclusions about mechanisms of progression. Regardless of its limitations, CGH is one of the most interesting and promising techniques recently introduced to play a role in the genetic analysis of prostate cancer.

Microcell-Mediated Chromosome Transfer (MMCT)

The specific aim of many genetic studies of prostate cancer is to identify oncogenes or tumor suppressor genes involved in the natural history of the disease. Once genetic regions of interest are identified, testing of candidate chromosomes or chromosomal regions for their tumor inducing or suppressing abilities can proceed. One technique useful for such evaluation is MMCT. In MMCT, the goal is to introduce a single human chromosome, or chromosomal region, into recipient tumor cells of interest and to look for morphological changes presumably caused by the expression of genes on the introduced chromosome or chromosomal fragment. Once stable clones containing the transferred human chromosome or fragment are made, experiments may be done to test the altered phenotype conferred by the newly introduced chromosome, such as in vitro growth/morphology changes, in vivo tumorigenicity, soft agar colony formation, and so on.

In MMCT studies of prostate cancer, fragments of chromosomes 3, 11, 12, and 17 have been introduced into the highly metastatic rat AT6.1 cell line, a subline of the Dunning R3327H rat prostate cell line, as well as into the tumorigenic human PPC-1 or DU145 cell lines *(68–71)*. For example, Berube and colleagues *(68)* demonstrated that introduction of chromosome 3 into DU145 cells had no effect, however addition of a region of chromosome 12 (12pter-12q13) completely suppressed tumor growth in nude mice. Loss of a small fragment from this region resulted in re-expression of the malignant phenotype, strongly suggesting the presence of a tumor suppressor at 12q13.

In the study by Murakami et. al. *(70)*, one of the tumor-suppressing clones contained an approx 28-cM fragment of chromosome 17, that included the hereditary breast/ovarian cancer susceptibility gene, BRCA1, at 17q21. Several studies, both epidemiologic and genetic, have suggested the involvement of a tumor suppressor gene on proximal 17q in prostate cancer, and have speculated whether it might be BRCA1 itself *(72–74)*. It is interesting to note that the same 28-cM fragment when transferred into two breast cancer cell lines suppressed tumorigenicity at a significantly higher level than it did in PPC-1, suggesting either that BRCA1 suppresses tumors strongly in breast tissues and more weakly in prostate, or that multiple tumor suppressor genes may be located in the 28-cM region of 17q surrounding BRCA1 whose direct involvement in prostate cancer remains to be determined.

Studies of MMCT in prostate tumors have also been useful in the actual localization of a putative prostate-specific metastasis suppressor gene. Ichikawa and colleagues *(69)* first reported the localization of a prostate-specific metastasis suppressor gene to the 11p11.2–13 region of chromosome 11, excluding the Wilms tumor locus. This region of 11p was sufficient to suppress metastasis of the highly metastatic AT6.1 prostate cancer subline, but did not suppress proliferation, suggesting it was an authentic metastasis suppressor gene. In subsequent studies from this group, the same region of 11p has been unable to suppress metastases in the breast cancer cell line, R1564, thereby demonstrating its tissue specificity, and KAI1, a prostate-specific metastasis suppressor gene at 11p11.2 has recently been cloned *(27,71)*. The KAI1 cDNA was able to suppress the number of lung metastases of AT6.1 cells in nude mice, but not the growth rate of the primary tumor, demonstrating that this gene product is able to produce the phenotype seen in the earlier studies. In addition, KAI1 was also shown to have reduced expression in cell lines, such as PC-3, DU 145, LNCap, and TSUPr1, derived from metastatic human prostate tumors.

Clinical Correlations

Clinical correlations with genetic abnormalities in prostate cancer have been limited. There have been several studies looking at mutations in the TP53 gene which appears to be overexpressed in a subset of late stage prostate tumors; it is thus unlikely to be involved in early carcinogenesis. There are correlations between both Gleason grade (histological grading system for prostate cancer) and length of survival after diagnosis with the appearance of abnormal karyotypes in prostate tumors. The studies and chromosomal changes that have been associated at some frequency with prostate tumors create a puzzling dilemma: What do these changes mean regarding prognosis of the disease? Unfortunately, only a few studies to date have been reported that show clinical correlations.

DNA ploidy changes detected by flow cytometry (FCM) have been associated with poor prognosis, whereas tumors that are diploid show no correlation with outcome. FISH studies using centromeric probes correlate well with the detection of abnormal populations by FCM, and have been able to detect copy number changes in tumors diploid by FCM. Using pericentromeric probes for only chromosomes 8 and 12, Person's study indicated that FISH and flow data from touch preparations were concordant in 82% of cases, but FISH was able to identify aneusomic tumors not detected by FCM *(57)*. In addition to the correlation of FISH/flow cytometry studies, this group has also shown that archival prostate tumors are valuable resources for FISH data collection, and that retrospective analyses enable correlations between genetic abnormalities and clinical outcome.

Several cytogenetic studies cited in this chapter, including those from our laboratory, have indicated that tumors with any clonal chromosomal changes are associated with a higher overall cancer grade, suggesting a more aggressive disease. This is helpful and can be informative, but only after the cumbersome methods involved in culturing primary tissue. FISH studies appear to be more promising in that regard, since nondividing cells from many sources can be used for molecular cytogenetic analysis. Diagnostic abnormalities could be identified from specimens obtained from biopsy prior to radical prostatectomy, or from samples obtained at the time of surgery. Although biopsy specimens have been analyzed in FISH studies, e.g., in the study by Takahashi et. al. *(57)*, biopsies are small, and not routinely available for research in many institutions. Once a diagnostic or predictive marker is available, however, evaluation of biopsy material may become useful in screening.

For example, intriguing evidence using FISH suggests that gains of chromosomes 7 and 8 are relatively common abnormalities in prostate tumors, and that gain of chromosome 7 is a marker for prostate cancer progression. Overall, there was an increase in LOH or AI with advanced tumor stage and grade, and imbalance at multiple loci within a tumor was generally correlated with a poor prognosis. A number of LOH studies showing loss from 8p generally support the notion that the frequency of 8p deletions increases with histopathologic grade of the tumor. The deletions are observed in resultant metastases, yet studies such as those of Emmert-Buck and colleagues *(30)* also had reported significant loss of 8p12 in both prostatic intra-epithelial neoplasia and primary tumors, suggesting the alternative view that loss of this region may be an early event in prostate tumor progression.

Certain genes may be markers for initiation or progression of prostate cancer. For example, our group has shown that a subset of prostate tumors have lost *MXI1* sequences at 10q25, and the identification of point mutations within this gene in some of the tumors reported by Eagle et al. *(20)* is intriguing. The map location and usefulness of a FISH probe specific for the *MXI1* gene in deletion detection in prostate tumor cells is illustrated in Fig. 1. The mxi1 gene product may function as a tumor suppressor by forming protein heterodimers with max, a myc-binding protein, which competes with myc–max heterodimers for myc DNA binding sites. The mxi1–max heterodimer lacks the transcriptional activation function of the myc–max heterodimer and thus its proliferative effect. Studies of deletions/mutations within this gene could elucidate a primary mechanism of prostate cancer initiation. Basic genetic studies such as these have only just begun, but are necessary to determine if the function of a gene of interest is necessary in the pathway in prostate cancer development.

CGH as well has defined several new chromosomal sites that appear to be involved in prostate cancer and that may serve as markers of disease progression. Of particular interest is the amplification of genetic sequences at Xq11–13, and subsequent identification of over-representation of the androgen receptor (AR) gene at this site in patients with hormone-refractory disease (*see* Fig. 2C). Amplification of this genetic sequence makes biological sense as androgen deprivation is a common treatment for advanced prostate tumors. Cell growth is presumably facilitated by amplification of AR in individuals with low circulating androgen concentrations or because changes in the ligand specificity allow a wider range of hormones to potentiate cell growth through the AR. Screening for AR copy number could be helpful as a means of early identification of tumors that will have metastasized.

Likewise, the work which was derived from MMCT experiments ultimately led to the identification of the KAI1 gene at 11p11.2. As a member of a membrane glycoprotein family presumably involved in cell–cell interactions, KAI1 may be a marker for the progression of prostate tumors.

Summary and Conclusions

Prostate cancer is clearly a complex and heterogeneous disease. The first cytogenetic analysis of a prostate tumor cell was done in 1975, and the accumulation of virtually all the data discussed in this chapter has occurred in the past 20 yr. Moreover, the majority of the work reviewed, especially the molecular and molecular cytogenetic studies, has been reported since 1990. As the field of biological sciences advances and new technologies become available, we are almost certain to experience quantum gains in our knowledge of the basic mechanisms of cancer and their relevance to human health.

The interaction of clinical and basic scientists, and technically complementary approaches to the study of diseases such as prostate cancer are imperative for thorough and timely answers to the specific questions asked in this review. This exciting time of scientific progress is unfortunately coupled with an increased incidence and mortality of prostate cancer. Future studies using the methods described herein, and other techniques not yet discovered will be key to helping the many men who suffer from this often aggressive and untreatable disease.

References

1. Arps S, Rodewald A, Schmalenberger B, Carl P, Bressel M, Kastendieck H: Cytogenetic survey of 32 cancers of the prostate. Cancer Genet Cytogenet 66:93–99, 1993.
2. Atkin NB, Baker MC: Chromosome study of five cancers of the prostate. Hum Genet 70:359–364, 1985.
3. Babu VR, Miles BJ, Cerny JC, Weiss L, Van Dyke DL: Cytogenetic study of four cancers of the prostate. Cancer Genet Cytogenet 48:83–87, 1990.
4. Breitkreuz T, Romanakis K, Lutz S, Seitz G, Bonkhoff H, Unteregger G, Zwergel T, Zang KD, Wullich B: Genotypic characterization of prostatic carcinomas: a combined cytogenetic, flow cytometry, and *in situ* DNA hybridization study. Cancer Res 53:4035–4040, 1993.
5. Brothman AR, Peehl DM, Patel AM, McNeal JE: Frequency and pattern of karyotypic abnormalities in human prostate cancer. Cancer Res 50: 3795–3803, 1990.
6. Brothman AR, Peehl DM, Patel AM, MacDonald GR, McNeal JE, Ladaga LE, Schellhammer PF: Cytogenetic evaluation of 20 cultured primary prostatic tumors. Cancer Genet Cytogenet 55:79–84, 1991.
7. Debruyne FMJ, Collins VP, van Dekken H, Jenkins RB, Klocker H, Schalken JA, Sesterhenn IA: Cytogenetics of prostate cancer. Scand J Urol Nephrol Suppl 162:65–71, 1994.
8. Gibas Z, Pontes JE, Sandberg AA: Chromosome rearrangements in a metastatic adenocarcinoma of the prostate. Cancer Genet Cytogenet 16:301–304, 1985.
9. Henke R-P, Kruger E, Ayhan N, Hubner D, Hammerer P: Frequency and distribution of numerical chromosomal aberrations in prostatic cancer. Hum Pathol 25(5):476–484, 1994.
10. Jones E, Zhu XL, Rohr LR, Stephenson RA, Brothman AR: Aneusomy of chromosomes 7 and 17 detected by FISH in prostate cancer and the effects of selection in vitro. Genes Chromosome Cancer 11:163–170, 1994.
11. Limon J, Lundgren R, Elfving P, Heim S, Kristoffersson U, Mandahl N, Mitelman F: Double minutes in two primary adenocarcinomas of the prostate. Cancer Genet Cytogenet 39:191–194, 1989.
12. Lundgren R, Kristoffersson U, Heim S, Mandahl N, Mitelman F: Multiple structural chromosome rearrangements, including del(7q) and del(10q), in an adenocarcinoma of the prostate. Cancer Genet Cytogenet 35:103–108, 1988.
13. Lundgren R, Mandahl N, Heim S, Limon J, Henrikson H, Mitelman F: Cytogenetic analysis of 57 primary prostatic adenocarcinomas. Genes Chromosome Cancer 4:16–24, 1992.

14. Lundgren R, Heim S, Mandahl N, Anderson H, Mitelman F: Chromosome abnormalities are associated with unfavorable outcome in prostatic cancer patients. J Urol 147:784–788, 1992.

15. Macoska JA, Trybus TM, Sakr WA, Wolf MC, Benson PD, Powell IJ, Pontes JE: Fluorescence in situ hybridization analysis of 8p allelic loss and chromosome 8 instability in human prostate cancer. Cancer Res 54:3824–3830, 1994.

16. Micale MA, Sanford JS, Powell IJ, Sakr WA, Wolman SR: Defining the extent and nature of cytogenetic events in prostatic adenocarcinoma: paraffin FISH vs. metaphase analysis. Cancer Genet Cytogenet 69:7–12, 1993.

17. Oshimura M, Sandberg AA: Isochromosome 17 in prostatic cancer. J Urol 114:249,250, 1975.

18. Sandberg AA: Chromosomal abnormalities and related events in prostate cancer. Hum Pathol 23(4):368–380, 1992.

19. Konig JJ, Teubel W, van Dongen JW, Hagemeijer A, Romijn RC, Schroder FH: Tissue culture loss of aneuploid cells from carcinomas of the prostate. Genes Chromosome Cancer 8:22–27, 1993.

20. Eagle LR, Yin X, Brothman AR, Williams BJ, Atkin NB, Prochownik EV: Mutation of the MXI1 gene in prostate cancer. Nat Genet 9:249–255, 1995.

21. Bergerheim USR, Kunimi K, Collins VP, Ekman P: Deletion mapping of chromosomes 8, 10, and 16 in human prostatic carcinoma. Genes Chromosome Cancer 3:215–220, 1991.

22. Bova GS, Carter BS, Bussemakers MJG, Emi M, Fujiwara Y, Kyprianou N, Jacobs SC, Robinson JC, Epstein JI, Walsh PC, Isaacs WB: Homozygous deletion and frequent allelic loss of chromosome 8p22 loci in human prostate cancer. Cancer Res 53:3869–3873, 1993.

23. Brewster SF, Browne S, Brown KW: Somatic allelic loss at the DCC, APC, nm23-H1 and p53 tumor suppressor gene loci in human prostatic carcinoma. J Urol 151:1073–1077, 1994.

24. Brooks JD, Bova GS, Isaacs WB: Allelic loss of the retinoblastoma gene in primary human prostatic adenocarcinomas. Prostate 26:35–39, 1995.

25. Brothman AR, Steele MR, Williams BJ, Jones E, Odelberg S, Albertsen HM, Jorde JB, Rohr LR, Stephenson RA: Loss of chromosome 17 loci in prostate cancer detected by polymerase chain reaction quantitation of allelic markers. Genes Chromosome Cancer 13:278–284, 1995.

26. Carter BS, Ewing CM, Ward WS, Treiger BF, Aalders TW, Schalken JA, Epstein JI, Isaacs WB: Allelic loss of chromosomes 16q and 10q in human prostate cancer. Proc Natl Acad Sci USA 87:8751–8755, 1990.

27. Dong J-T, Lamb PW, Rinker-Schaeffer CW, Vukanovic J, Ichikawa T, Isaacs JT, Barrett JC: KAI1, a metastasis suppressor gene for prostate cancer on human chromosome 11p11.2. Science 268:884–886, 1995.

28. Effert PJ, Neubauer A, Walther PJ, Liu ET: Alterations of the p53 gene are associated with the progression of a human prostate carcinoma. J Urol 147:789–793, 1992.

29. Effert PJ, McCoy RH, Walther PJ, Liu ET: p53 gene alterations in human prostate carcinoma. J Urol 150:257–261, 1993.

30. Emmert-Buck MR, Vocke CD, Pozzatti RO, Duray PH, Jennings SB, Florence CD, Zhuang Z, Bostwick DG, Liotta LS, Linehan WM: Allelic loss on chromosome 8p12–21 in microdissected prostatic intraepithelial neoplasia. Cancer Res 55:2959–2962, 1995.

31. Gao X, Honn KV, Grignon D, Sakr W, Chen YQ: Frequent loss of expression and loss of heterozygosity of the putative tumor suppressor gene DCC in prostatic carcinomas. Cancer Res 53:2723–2727, 1993.

32. Gao X, Zacharek A, Salkowski A, Grignon DJ, Sakr W, Porter AT, Honn KV: Loss of heterozygosity of the BRCA1 and other loci on chromosome 17q in human prostate cancer. Cancer Res 55:1002–1005, 1995.

33. Kunimi K, Bergerheim USR, Larsson I-L, Ekman P, Collins VP: Allelotyping of human prostatic adenocarcinoma. Genomics 11:530–536, 1990.

34. Latil A, Baron J-C, Cussenot O, Fourier G, Soussi T, Boccon-Gibod L, Le Duc A, Rouesse J, Lidereau R: Genetic alterations in localized prostate cancer: identification of a common region of deletion on chromosome arm 18q. Genes Chromosome Cancer 11:119–125, 1994.

35. MacGrogan D, Levy A, Bostwick D, Wagner M, Wells D, Bookstein R: Loss of chromosome arm 8p loci in prostate cancer: mapping by quantitative allelic imbalance. Genes Chromosome Cancer 10:151–159, 1994.

36. Macoska JA, Powell IJ, Sakr W, Lane M-A: Loss of the 17p chromosomal region in a metastatic carcinoma of the prostate. J Urol 147:1142–1146, 1992.

37. Macoska JA, Micale MA, Sakr WA, Benson PD, Wolman SR: Extensive genetic alterations in prostate cancer revealed by dual PCR and FISH analysis. Genes Chromosome Cancer 8:88–97, 1993.

38. Morton RA, Ewing CM, Nagafuchi A, Tsukita S, Isaacs WB: Reduction of E-cadherin levels and deletion of the α-catenin gene in human prostate cancer cells. Cancer Res 53:3585–3590, 1993.

39. Phillips SMA, Morton DG, Lee SJ, Wallace DMA, Neoptolemos JP: Loss of heterozygosity of the retinoblastoma and adenomatous polyposis susceptibility gene loci and in chromosomes 10p, 10q, and 16q in human prostate cancer. Br J Urol 73:390–395, 1994.

40. Sadasivan R, Morgan R, Jennings S, Austenfeld M, Van-Veldhuizen P, Stephens R, Noble M: Overexpression of her-2/neu may be an indicator of poor prognosis in prostate cancer. J Urol 150(1):126–131, 1993.

41. Sakr WA, Macoska JA, Benson P, Grignon DJ, Wolman SR, Pontes JE, Crissman JD: Allelic loss in locally metastatic, multisampled prostate cancer. Cancer Res 54:3273–3277, 1994.

42. Suzuki H, Emi M, Komiya A, Fujiwara Y, Yatani R, Nakamura Y, Shimazaki J: Localization of a tumor suppressor gene associated with progression of human prostate cancer within a 1.2 Mb region of 8p22–p21.3. Genes Chromosome Cancer 13:168–174, 1995.

43. Taplin M-E, Bubley GJ, Shuster TD, Frantz ME, Spooner AE, Ogata GK, Keer HN, Balk SP: Mutation of the androgen-receptor gene in metastatic androgen-dependent prostate cancer. NEJM 332(21):1393–1398, 1995.

44. Trapman J, Sleddens HFBM, van der Weiden MM, Dinjens WNM, Konig JJ, Schroder FH, Faber PW, Bosman FT: Loss of heterozygosity of chromosome

8 microsatellite loci implicates a candidate tumor suppressor gene between the loci D8S87 and D8S133 in human prostate cancer. Cancer Res 54: 6061–6064, 1994.

45. Zenklusen JC, Thompson JC, Troncoso P, Kagan J, Conti CJ: Loss of heterozygosity in human primary prostate carcinomas: a possible tumor suppressor gene at 7q31.1. Cancer Res 54:6370–6376, 1995.

46. Visakorpi T, Hyytinen E, Koivisto P, Tanner M, Keinanen R, Palmberg C, Palotie A, Isola J, Kallioniemi O-P: In vivo amplification of the androgen receptor gene and progression of human prostate cancer. Nat Genet 9: 401–406, 1995.

47. Alers JC, Krijtenburg PJ, Vissers KJ, Bosman FT, van der Kwast TH, van Dekken H: Interphase cytogenetics of prostatic adenocarcinoma and precursor lesions: analysis of 25 radical prostatectomies and 17 adjacent prostatic intraepithelial neoplasias. Genes Chromosome Cancer 12:241–250, 1995.

48. Bandyk MG, Zhao L, Troncoso P, Pisters LL, Palmer JL, von Eschenbach AC, Chung LWK, Liang JC: Trisomy 7: a potential cytogenetic marker of human prostate cancer progression. Genes Chromosome Cancer 9:19–27, 1994.

49. Baretton GB, Valina C, Vogt T, Schneiderbanger K, Diebold J, Lohrs U: Interphase cytogenetic analysis of prostatic carcinomas by use of nonisotopic in situ hybridization. Cancer Res 554:4472–4480, 1994.

50. Brothman AR, Patel AM, Peehl DM, Schellhammer PF: Analysis of prostatic tumor cultures using fluorescence in-situ hybridization (FISH). Cancer Genet Cytogenet 62:180–185, 1992.

51. Brothman AR, Watson MJ, Zhu XL, Williams BJ, Rohr LR: Evaluation of 20 archival prostate tumor specimens by fluorescence in situ hybridization (FISH). Cancer Genet Cytogenet 75:40–47, 1994.

52. Brown JA, Alcaraz A, Takahashi S, Persons DL, Lieber MM, Jenkins RB: Chromosomal aneusomies detected by fluorescent in situ hybridization analysis in clinically localized prostate carcinoma. J Urol 152:1157–1162, 1994.

53. Cher ML, Ito T, Weidner N, Carroll PR, Jensen RH: Mapping of regions of physical deletion on chromosome 16q in prostate cancer cells by fluorescence in situ hybridization (FISH). J Urol 153:249–254, 1995.

54. Matsuyama H, Pan Y, Skoog L, Tribukait B, Naito K, Ekman P, Lichter P, Bergerheim USR: Deletion mapping of 8p in prostate cancer by fluorescence in situ hybridization. Oncogene 9(10):3071–3076, 1994.

55. Micale MA, Mohamed A, Sakr W, Powell IJ, Wolman SR: Cytogenetics of primary prostate adenocarcinoma: clonality and chromosome instability. Cancer Genet Cytogenet 61:165–173, 1992.

56. Persons DL, Gibney DJ, Katzmann JA, Lieber MM, Farrow GM, Jenkins RB: Use of fluorescent in situ hybridization for deoxyribonucleic acid ploidy analysis of prostatic adenocarcinoma. J Urol 150:120–125, 1993.

57. Takahashi S, Qian J, Brown JA, Alcaraz A, Bostwick DG, Lieber MM, Jenkins RB: Potential markers of prostate cancer aggressiveness detected by fluorescence in situ hybridization in needle biopsies. Cancer Res 54:3574–3579, 1994.

58. Visakorpi T, Hyytinen E, Kallioniemi A, Isola J, Kallioniemi O-P: Sensitive detection of chromosome copy number aberrations in prostate cancer by fluorescence in situ hybridization. Am J Pathol 145(3):624–630, 1994.

59. Williams BJ, Jones E, Brothman AR: Homologous centromere association of chromosomes 9 and 17 in prostate cancer. Cancer Genet Cytogenet, 85: 143–152, 1995.

60. Zitzelberger H, Szucs S, Weier H-U, Lehmann L, Braselmann H, Enders S, Schilling A, Bruel J, Hofler H, Bauchinger M: Numerical abnormalities of chromosome 7 in human prostate cancer detected by fluorescence in situ hybridization (FISH) on paraffin-embedded tissue with centromere-specific DNA probes. J Pathol 172:325–335, 1994.

61. Williams BJ, Jones E, Zhu XL, Steele MR, Stephenson RA, Rohr LR, Brothman AR: Evidence for a tumor suppressor gene distal to BRCA1 in prostate cancer. J Urol 155:720–725, 1996.

62. Cher ML, MacGrogan D, Bookstein R, Brown JA, Jenkins RB, Jensen RH: Comparative genomic hybridization, allelic imbalance, and fluorescence in situ hybridization on chromosome 8 in prostate cancer. Genes Chromosome Cancer 11:153–162, 1994.

63. Visakorpi T, Kallioniemi AH, Syvanen A-C, Hyytinen ER, Karhu R, Tammela T, Isola JJ, Kallioniemi O-P: Genetic changes in primary and recurrent prostate cancer by comparative genomic hybridization. Cancer Res 55:342–347, 1995.

64. Gordon KB, Thompson CT, Char DH, O'Brien JM, Kroll S, Ghazvini S, Gray JW: Comparative genomic hybridization in the detection of DNA copy number abnormalities in uveal melanoma. Cancer Res 54(17):4764–4768, 1994.

65. Levin NA, Brzoska P, Gupta N, Minna JD, Gray JW, Christman MF: Identification of frequent novel genetic alterations in small cell lung carcinoma. Cancer Res 54:5086–5091, 1994.

66. Nacheva E, Grace C, Holloway TL, Green AR: Comparative genomic hybridization in acute myeloid leukemia. Cancer Genet Cytogenet 82: 9–16, 1995.

67. Ried T, Petersen I, Holtgreve-Greve H, Speicher MR, Schrock E, duManoir S, Cremer T: Mapping of multiple DNA gains and losses in primary small cell lung carcinomas by comparative genomic hybridization. Cancer Res 54:1801–1806, 1994.

68. Berube NG, Speevak MD, Chevrette M: Suppression of tumorigenicity of human prostate cancer cells by introduction of human chromosome del (12) (q13). Cancer Res 54:3077–3081, 1994.

69. Ichikawa T, Ichikawa Y, Dong J, Hawkins AL, Griffin CA, Isaacs WB, Oshimura M, Barrett JC, Isaacs JT: Localization of metastasis suppressor gene(s) for prostatic cancer to the short arm of human chromosome 11. Cancer Res 52:3486–3490, 1992.

70. Murakami Y, Brothman AR, Leach RJ, White RL: Suppression of malignant phenotype in a human prostate cancer cell line by fragments of normal chromosomal region 17q. Cancer Res 55:3389–3394, 1995.

71. Rinker-Schaeffer CW, Hawkins AL, Ru N, Dong J, Stoica G, Griffin CA, Ichikawa T, Barrett JC, Isaacs JT: Differential suppression of mammary and prostate cancer metastasis by human chromosomes 17 and 11. Cancer Res 54:6249–6256, 1994.
72. Arason A, Barkadottir TB, Egilsson V: Linkage analysis of chromosome 17q markers and breast–ovarian cancer in Icelandic families, and possible relationship to prostatic cancer. Am J Hum Genet 52:711–716, 1993.
73. Tulinius H, Egilsson V, Olafsdottir GH, Sigvaldson H: Risk of prostate, ovarian, and endometrial cancer among relatives of women with breast cancer. Br Med J 305:855–860, 1992.
74. Ford D, Easton DF, Bishop DT, Narod SA, Goldgar DE: Risks of cancer in BRCA1 mutation carriers. Lancet 343:692–695, 1994.
75. Nagele R, Freeman T, McMorrow L, Lee H: Precise spatial positioning of chromosomes during prometaphase: evidence of chromosomal order. Science 270:1831–1835, 1995.

Chapter 11

Chromosomes in Lung Cancer

Daphne W. Bell and Joseph R. Testa

Introduction

Lung carcinomas are now the leading cause of neoplastic deaths among both men and women in the United States *(1)*. With the increasing incidence of lung cancer, it is apparent that new diagnostic and staging techniques are needed. Because of the inadequacies of current therapeutic protocols, < 10% of all patients will achieve long-term survival and potential cures *(2,3)*. Most therapeutic modalities currently available are specific to the histopathological type, i.e., small cell lung carcinoma (SCLC) versus nonsmall cell lung carcinoma (NSCLC). Our understanding of the biology of lung cancer indicates shared features among several histological variants *(4)*. Identification of cytogenetic markers could allow for a better comprehension of this relationship that should, in turn, expand our knowledge of the overall disease process and offer the possibility of new treatment options. However, despite the high incidence of lung cancer, the cytogenetic data available are rather limited in this neoplasm compared to that for the hematological malignancies *(5)*. The reasons for this are several-fold:

1. Low rate of cell growth in these tumors;
2. Presence of cells in various stages of differentiation, many of which will not enter mitosis;

From: *Human Cytogenetic Cancer Markers*   Edited by S. R. Wolman and S. Sell
Humana Press Inc., Totowa, NJ

3. Areas of necrosis and hypoxia where cell division does not occur; and
4. Difficulty in adapting these tumor cells to in vitro culture and to induce the malignant stem cell population to divide (*6*).

Moreover, the karyotypes can be extremely complex with many additional chromosomes, complicating efforts to identify consistent changes.

Thus far, reports describing detailed karyotypes of primary SCLC specimens have been limited to only a few cases (*7–9*). Whang-Peng et al. (*10*) described a nonrandom clonal abnormality, deletion of 3p, in tumor cells from SCLC patients. Other recurrent deletions have also been described in SCLC (*9,11*), and are summarized in this chapter. In addition, double minutes (dmins) and homogeneously staining regions (hsrs), two cytogenetic manifestations of gene amplification, have been reported in SCLC, particularly in cell lines derived from these tumors (*9,12,13*). Karyotypic analysis of SCLC specimens has often been performed on cell lines originating from tumor cells found in bone marrow, effusions, or metastatic lesions. Two recent series, including one from this laboratory, have described successful karyotypic analyses of short-term cultures of fresh SCLC specimens, eight of which were from primary lung tumors (*8,9*). It should be noted, however, that it is sometimes not possible to obtain adequate numbers of analyzable metaphase spreads from SCLC specimens until the cells have been cultured for weeks or even months.

To examine karyotypes of primary or low passage NSCLC cultures, considerable attention must be focused on the mitotic index in the cultures. Since the growth rate of NSCLC is low (>200-d doubling times in vivo are not uncommon (*1*)), the number of mitotic events is relatively small. Moreover, despite multiple harvests, many tumors from NSCLC patients fail to yield adequate numbers of metaphase cells for detailed karyotypic analysis. Consequently, until 1994 detailed reports of karyotypes of primary NSCLC were limited to several small series, usually of fewer than 10 cases (*14–18*), or several selected cases or case reports (*19–24*). Other descriptions of cytogenetic changes in NSCLC had been published (*25–34*), but these either did not provide complete karyotypes or reported on metastatic tumors, effusions, or established cell lines that had been cultured for many passages. More recently, there have been two cytogenetic reports of relatively large series of primary NSCLCs. We *(35)* reported detailed cytogenetic findings in 63 NSCLCs, and Johansson et al. *(36)* described abnormal karyotypes of 20 bronchial large cell carcinomas (LCCs). We discuss the findings of Johansson et al. separately, because this selected series was restricted to a subtype of NSCLC which comprises a minority (10–20%) of all NSCLCs *(37)*. Even though karyotypes in NSCLC are generally very complex, recurrent cytogenetic changes have been identified. For example, Lukeis et al. *(16)* described a nonrandom chromosomal abnormality, deletion of the short arm of 9, in 9 of 10 NSCLC they examined, and frequent numerical loss of chromosome 9 has also been reported *(15,35,38)*. Other recurrent alterations have also been described and are reviewed here.

This chapter presents a summary of known cytogenetic alterations in lung cancer determined by conventional karyotyping and the newer molecular cytogenetic techniques of interphase fluorescence *in situ* hybridization (FISH) and comparative genomic hybridization (CGH) that can overcome some of the limitations inherent in karyotypic analysis. The biological implications and specificity of chromosome changes is discussed. The translational roles of conventional and newer cytogenetic techniques in relation to molecular genetic changes and DNA ploidy are also reviewed.

Conventional Karyotypic Analysis

SCLC

In SCLC, karyotypic changes are usually quite extensive, even in newly diagnosed primary tumors. Thus far, this laboratory has carried out cytogenetic analyses on fresh specimens and low passage cell lines from 17 SCLCs *(9,39)*. In many cases, most or all of the recurrent chromosome abnormalities described in this section occurred in combination. The total number of such changes ranged from 11 to more than 60 per tumor. In our series, 10 fresh specimens were examined, including 7 lung primaries, and each case displayed multiple numerical and structural changes. DeFusco et al. *(8)* examined 11 fresh SCLC specimens (including four primary tumors) and also found numerous chromosomal alterations in every case. The ploidy level of SCLC tumors may be distributed over a wide range. In our SCLC series, the modal chromosome number was hypodiploid in 3 cases, near-diploid in 1 case, hyperdiploid in 2 cases, near-triploid in 10 cases, and near-tetraploid in 1 case.

In SCLC, certain chromosomes frequently participate in structural rearrangements, prominent among them being chromosomes 1, 3, 5, and 17 *(7–9,11)*. Among our 17 SCLC, breakpoints clustered at 3p (15 cases, including those with isochromosomes of 3q that result in loss of the entire short arm), 5q (11 cases), 1p (9 cases), and 17p (8 cases). A description of common changes seen in SCLCs follows.

Loss of 3p

In 1982, Whang-Peng et al. *(10)* reported deletions of 3p in each of 20 SCLC cell lines and fresh tumor specimens derived from bone marrow. A deletion of 3p in SCLC has been consistently identified in several other studies as well *(7,9,12,40–44)*. However, in other reports only a minority of SCLC cell lines exhibited a 3p deletion *(11,13,25)*. Furthermore, DeFusco et al. *(8)* examined fresh SCLC tumors grown in short-term culture and found alterations of 3p in only 5 of 11 cases. However, loss of heterozygosity (LOH) analysis of 3p markers in SCLC confirms an almost universal loss of genetic material in this region *(45–47)*.

Of the 17 SCLC tumors and cell lines that we examined, cytogenetic evidence for loss of 3p was found in 16 cases *(9,39)*. Fifteen of these cases exhibited structural changes of 3p. Among these, 3 had terminal or interstitial deletions, 6 had one or more unbalanced derivative chromosomes involving partial loss of 3p, 3 had an i(3q), 2 had both a deletion and either a der(3) or an i(3q), and 1 near-tetraploid tumor had an i(3q), a der(3), and a numerical loss of 3. Another specimen had an unbalanced translocation derivative in which breakage occurred in the long arm of chromosome 3, resulting in loss of 3pter→q21. The shortest region of overlap (SRO) of losses of 3p is located at 3p21–p25. LOH analysis was carried out on 5 tumor specimens that exhibited cytogenetic alterations of 3p, and allelic losses of 3p were identified in each case *(41)*. Only 1 of our 17 SCLC specimens did not have a visible structural alteration of chromosome 3, but molecular analysis of this tumor indicated that LOH had occurred at both the DNF15S2 (chromosome band

3p21) and *RAF1* proto-oncogene (3p25) loci, when compared to DNA from normal lymphoblastoid cells from this patient *(9)*. Thus, taken collectively, the cytogenetic and LOH findings indicate that every one of these 17 SCLC cases had losses involving 3p.

Some of the interlaboratory differences concerning the frequency of cytogenetic deletions of 3p may be attributed to difficulties in precisely assigning breakpoints in some cases, particularly when the quality of the chromosome preparation is suboptimal *(41)*. Clearly, interstitial or terminal deletions of 3p are not seen uniformly in SCLC, but losses of 3p by mechanisms such as unbalanced translocations or isochromosome formation have a comparable net result *(48)*. In our series, only 5 cases had intrachromosomal deletions of 3p, and 11 others showed losses of 3p caused by other types of unbalanced rearrangements. The remaining case had (allelic) losses of 3p that were not detected karyotypically. The SRO of 3p losses among our cases was found to be at 3p21–p25. In other reports, the SRO was placed at 3p14–p23 *(10)*, 3p21–p22 *(47)*, or 3p23–p24 *(49)*. In contrast to these reports, our interpretation of the minimal 3p deletion extends more distally to 3p25 and is in agreement with molecular analyses demonstrating consistent LOH at the *RAF1* locus at band 3p25 in SCLC *(41,50,51)*. In addition, other reports of LOH have demonstrated that almost all SCLC tumors lose heterozygosity within the chromosomal region 3p14–p21, as well *(45–47)*. Therefore, the deleted segment in SCLC usually is very large. This consistent allelic loss at 3p strongly supports the hypothesis that one or more tumor suppressor genes important in the pathogenesis of SCLC reside within this chromosomal region. The search for such a gene(s) may be facilitated by the recent identification of 3p DNA markers that are homozygously deleted in some SCLC cell lines *(52,53)*. Yamakawa et al. *(53)* detected homozygous deletions in 4 of 26 SCLC cell lines and 1 of 10 NSCLC cell lines with a DNA marker located at 3p21.3–p22 *(53)*. The region of homozygous loss has been estimated to consist of <1 Mb of DNA and may contain at least 1 of the tumor suppressor genes associated with lung carcinogenesis. A different homozygous deletion of 3p was identified in the DNA of the SCLC cell line U2020. This deletion removed an approx 5-Mb chromosomal segment within 3p13–p14, including the locus D3S3 *(52,54,55)*.

Loss of 5q

We previously reported that alterations of 5q are frequently involved in SCLC *(9)*. In addition, our review of karyotypic data presented in two earlier reports revealed losses of 5q in approx one-half of all SCLC specimens examined *(8,11)*. Among the 17 SCLC cases that we have analyzed, 12 showed either a numerical loss of chromosome 5, an i(5p) resulting in loss of the entire long arm of chromosome 5, a derivative chromosome resulting in loss of part of 5q, or an interstitial deletion of 5q. The SRO of deleted segments on 5q resides at 5q13–q21. The recurrent loss of 5q13–q21 suggests that this region also may contain a tumor suppressor gene important in the pathogenesis of SCLC. Several cell regulatory genes are located at band 5q13, including the gene encoding phosphatidylinositol-3 kinase associated protein, p85α, which has been shown to modulate interactions between certain activated receptors and the phosphatidylinositol-3 kinase *(56,57)*, and the *RASA* locus that encodes the GTPase activating protein involved in signal transduction *(58)*. In addition, the putative tumor suppressor genes *APC* and *MCC*, which have been shown to be somatically altered in some colorectal tumors, are located at 5q21 *(59)*. A study of polymorphic sites within the *APC* and *MCC* loci revealed frequent LOH in SCLC *(60)*. Among 23 SCLC samples examined in the latter study, 21 were informative for one or more polymorphic sites within these loci, and allelic losses were found in 17 (81%) cases. However, no mutations or homozygous deletions of these genes have been documented in SCLCs. It is also noteworthy that Wieland et al. *(61)* used a genomic subtraction hybridization procedure to isolate three different DNA sequences deleted in the SCLC cell line SK-LC-17, one of which has been mapped on chromosome 5. Probes for these sequences specifically hybridized with normal human DNA, but not with tumor DNA from SK-LC-17 cells, suggesting that the identified clones are derived from independent genetic loci encoding candidate tumor suppressor genes *(61)*.

Loss of 13q

Loss of chromosome 13 has been described in some cytogenetic studies of SCLC *(9,11)*. Numerical losses of chromosome 13 in the absence of structural change were observed in 10 of the 17

SCLC cases we examined. Another 3 cases had structural alterations with breakpoints at 13q14, site of the *RB1* tumor suppressor gene *(62,63)*. Thus, 13 of our 17 (76%) SCLC cases had changes that affected 13q14. Interestingly, a similar proportion (nearly 80%) of SCLC tumors exhibit absent or very low levels of expression of *RB1* *(64)* suggesting that in many SCLCs cytogenetic changes could unveil an inactivated *RB1* allele on the remaining, karyotypically normal chromosome 13 homolog.

Loss of 17p

Morstyn et al. *(11)* identified abnormalities of chromosome 17 in 8 of 10 SCLC cell lines they examined, although the specific types of alterations and breakpoints were not described. In another report, rearrangements of chromosome 17 were described in 4 of 11 SCLC specimens, including 3 cases with breakpoints at 17p11–p13 resulting in losses of part of 17p *(8)*. Loss of part or all of 17p was observed in 14 of our 17 SCLCs. In 4 of these cases, the only alteration of chromosome 17 was a numerical loss. Ten others had structural alterations that were interpreted as unbalanced rearrangements resulting in loss of part or all of band 17p13; 9 of these specimens had partial deletions or various derivative chromosomes with breakpoints in 17p or proximal 17q, and 1 tumor had both a dicentric (15p;17p) and a der(17).

Yokota et al. *(65)* reported LOH at 17p in each of five SCLCs they examined. The *TP53* tumor suppressor gene is located at band 17p13.1, and *TP53* has been shown to be a frequent target for molecular alteration in lung cancer *(66,67)*. The finding of frequent cytogenetic losses of 17p appears to be consistent with this molecular evidence, because a mutated *TP53* allele may exist on the remaining copy of 17p.

Dmins and hsrs

The novel cytogenetic alterations, dmins and hsrs, have been reported in a number of cases of SCLC, particularly in cell lines derived from these tumors. Dmins or hsrs were reported in 3 of 16 (19%) SCLC cell lines studied by Whang-Peng et al. *(12)* and in 4 of 17 (24%) cases examined by our laboratory *(39)*. However, in an investigation of SCLC specimens from late-stage, heavily pretreated patients with extensive distant metastases, Wurster-Hill et al.

(13) found dmins or hsrs in 11 of 15 cases; 7 of the 15 specimens were obtained at autopsy. In our series, variable numbers of dmins were observed in four SCLC cell lines, three of which were derived from patients who had received prior cytotoxic therapy. In one of these SCLC lines, there were two cell populations: one with numerous dmins, and another with a large hsr instead of dmins. The karyotype of these two cell populations was otherwise nearly identical. In another case, dmins were identified in only a few cells, but a marker chromosome containing an hsr was present in nearly all cells examined.

Dmins and hsrs are associated with amplification of oncogenes or genes involved in drug resistance *(68,69)*. Southern blot analysis revealed amplification of specific oncogenes in each of our four cell lines displaying dmins. Two of these cases exhibited a 5- to 10-fold level of amplification of either *MYC* or *MYCN* oncogenes. In each of the latter two cell lines, dmins were observed in a minority of the cells examined cytogenetically. The level of amplification of *MYC* or *MYCN* was approx 60-fold in the other two cell lines. In each of the latter cases, all of the metaphase spreads examined contained a large hsr or multiple dmins, including a few mitoses with more than 100 dmins. FISH of a nonisotopically labeled *MYCN* probe to metaphase cells of the SCLC tumor having approx 60-fold amplification of this gene demonstrated that the amplified sequences reside within the dmins and hsr.

Amplification of various members of the *MYC* family of oncogenes is relatively common in SCLC cell lines *(70–72)*. However, such amplification appears to be less common in primary tumors. In one study of SCLC primaries, amplification of *MYC* or *MYCN* was reported in only 5 of 45 (11%) SCLC specimens *(73)*. Cytogenetic evidence for gene amplification was found in 3 of our 7 established cell lines, but in only 1 of 10 fresh specimens. Among the 4 patients whose tumor cells contained dmins and hsrs, 3 received prior cytotoxic therapy. Overall, dmins/hsrs were observed in 3 of 5 specimens from previously treated patients vs only 1 of 12 (8%) from untreated patients. Similarly, Brennan et al. *(74)* detected amplification of one of the *MYC* family genes in 28% of tumor specimens from previously treated SCLC patients, compared to only 8% of specimens from untreated patients. This evidence and the relatively low incidence of *MYC* family gene amplification in primary tumors *(73)* implies that such amplification is unlikely to represent an initial, transformation-related event in SCLC.

NSCLC

Most NSCLCs have many numerical and structural changes. We recently reported karyotypic findings in 63 NSCLCs, only 3 of which had <10 clonal chromosomal changes *(35)*. Some of these tumors showed as many as 60–70 different structural and numerical changes. The number of cytogenetic changes per tumor was similar among different histological subgroups. Other studies have also documented numerous chromosomal alterations in most primary NSCLCs *(15–18,20)*. In the 20 cytogenetically abnormal cases of NSCLC described by Johansson et al. *(36)* simple karyotypes were observed in 3 cases whereas the remaining 17 displayed complex chromosomal changes.

There have been several reported cases of NSCLC displaying only a single numerical change (i.e., gain of chromosomes 7 or 12) *(14,19,23,36)*. Cell populations carrying an extra chromosome 7 as the sole karyotypic change have been described in cultures from several malignant disorders, such as bladder, brain, colon, and kidney as well as in cultured cells from nonneoplastic tissue obtained from the lung, brain, kidney, placenta, Dupuytren's contracture, and Peyronie's disease *(75)*. In some series, approx 10% of cultured cells from all nonneoplastic kidney samples examined displayed trisomy 7 *(75,76)* and trisomy 7 and trisomy 10 have been shown to characterize subpopulations of tumor-infiltrating lymphocytes in kidney tumors and in the surrounding kidney tissue *(77)*. Moreover, in ovarian cancer, trisomy 12 has been found to represent a recurrent chromosome aberration in benign ovarian tumors, particularly in fibromas, rather than in tumors of epithelial origin *(78)*. Thus, in NSCLC it is unclear whether clones exhibiting simple karyotypes with gains of either chromosome 7 or chromosome 12 actually reflect changes in the malignant cell population. Johansson et al. *(23)* described two tumors bearing sole karyotypic abnormalities of a t(1;6) and loss of the Y chromosome, respectively. They attributed these aberrations to changes in the stromal cells rather than changes in the cells that were part of the tumor parenchyma. A third tumor was described that contained a supernumerary ring chromosome as the only cytogenetic alteration. This structure is generally rare in epithelial tumors, but has been described repeatedly in mesenchymal tumors. In an earlier study by this same group, pseudodiploid karyotypes with one or a few clonal structural rearrangements were reported in two adenosquamous carcinomas, leading them to conclude that this relatively rare histological subtype differs from other lung cancers by having simple pseudodiploid, or near-diploid, instead of massively aneuploid tumor cells *(23)*. Only one other short-term cultured adenosquamous carcinoma with an abnormal karyotype has been reported, and that tumor had trisomy 12 as the sole abnormality *(19)*. Pejovic et al. *(22)* reported a well-differentiated adenocarcinoma of the lung with a relatively simple mosaic karyotype: 49,XX,+5,+5,+7,+7,–17/50,XX,+5,+5,+7,+7,–17,+r. Their findings and other literature data indicate that exclusively numerical changes are much more common in highly differentiated epithelial tumors than in moderately or poorly differentiated carcinomas, and they proposed that numerical changes may reflect early-onset genomic instability that may precede the emergence of complex structural changes and more aggressive phenotypic features.

Tumor Ploidy and Numerical Changes

In our series of 63 NSCLCs, the modal chromosome number was near-diploid in 16 cases (25%), near-triploid in 35 cases (56%), and near-tetraploid to near-hexaploid in 12 cases (19%) *(35)*. Near-triploidy was the most common ploidy in each of the histological categories (46% of adenocarcinomas, 61% of squamous cell carcinomas, and 80% of other NSCLCs). Among the 20 karyotypically abnormal cases of LCC reported by Johansson et al. *(36)* the modal chromosome number was near-diploid in 6 cases (30%), near-triploid in 8 cases (40%), near-tetraploid in 2 cases (10%), and near-hexaploid in 1 case (5%). Additionally, 2 tumors (10%) contained cell populations with chromosome numbers ranging from diploid to tetraploid and 1 case (5%) from triploid to hexaploid.

These findings demonstrate that karyotypes in NSCLC generally are very complicated, even in newly diagnosed primary tumors. This complex cytogenetic pattern appears to be part of the natural course of NSCLC, because the two largest studies of primary NSCLCs have focused on samples obtained prior to initiating cytotoxic therapy *(35,36)*. Moreover, it is unlikely that this genomic complexity can be attributed to in vitro karyotypic evolution, as most of the analyses are from relatively short-term (1–10 d) cultures of tumor cells. In addition, in a separate study of 12 NSCLCs, we observed complete agreement between the modal chromosome number of cultured tumor cells and the DNA index of the corresponding tumor tissue, indicating that the cells that proliferate in culture are representative of the major aneuploid or near-diploid component of the solid tumor *(79)*.

In NSCLC, all chromosomes contribute to numerical changes. In our series, losses of chromosomes 9 (41 of 63 cases, 65%) and 13 (45 cases, 71%) were the two most frequent numerical changes. Loss of the Y was observed in 25 of 43 (58%) tumors from male patients. Gain of chromosome 7 was also a frequent finding (26 of 63 cases, 41%). Gains of chromosomes 5 and 12 were common as well, each occurring in approx 20% of cases. Polysomy for all or part of chromosome 7 in NSCLC has been reported by a number of investigators *(14–17,20,26–29,34,36,38,80)*. Trisomy 7 has been proposed as an early change in NSCLC that can be found in premalignant lung tissue in a subset of patients *(14)*. Frequent numerical loss of chromosome 9 has been described in several other studies of NSCLC *(15,38)* and Lukeis et al. *(16)* reported loss of material from 9p in 9 of 10 NSCLCs *(16)*. Losses of chromosomes 13 and Y have also been observed in other studies of primary NSCLC *(15,16)*. In LCC, recurrent numerical changes appeared to be less frequent than in NSCLC generally, and the spectrum of chromosomes involved was somewhat different *(36)*. The most frequent numerical change was loss of the X chromosome (4 of 5 female cases). Loss of the Y chromosome was also frequent, being observed in 6 of 15 (40%) tumors from males. With regard to the autosomes, losses of 14 and 18 were the most frequent numerical changes with each being lost from 3 of 20 (15%) cases with clonal chromosome abnormalities *(36)*. Losses of 4, 9, 10, 13, 15, and 21 were each seen in 2 cases.

Structural Changes

We summarized the structural changes seen in short-term cultures of 97 primary NSCLCs for which complete karyotypic details have been published *(14–24,35)*. The most common sites of chromosomal breakage seen in NSCLC were at or near the hete-rochromatic centromere regions of chromosomes 1, 3, 5, 6, 7, 8, 9, 11, 13, 14, 15, and 17. Other regions of chromosomes 1, 3, 6, 7, 9p, 11, and 19 were also prone to rearrangement. In LCC, the chromosomes most frequently involved in structural rearrangements were 1, 2, 3, 5, 6, 7, 8, 10, 11, 13, 14, and 17 *(36)*. Many rearrangements in LCCs also occurred near centromeres.

Balanced translocations appear to be relatively rare in NSCLC. In contrast, losses as a result of missing chromosomes or apparently unbalanced rearrangements (deletions and derivative chromosomes) are frequently observed. Losses of chromosomal material because of combined numerical and structural alterations are a prominent feature in NSCLC. In our series of 63 NSCLCs, all chromosome arms except 7p and 7q exhibited partial or complete losses in at least 25% of tumors *(35)*. The chromosome arm most frequently contributing to losses was 9p (52 of 63 tumors, 83%). Other chromosome arms lost in at least 60% of cases included 3p, 6q, 8p, 9q, 13q, 17p, 18q, 19p, 21q, 22q, and the short arms of each of the acrocentric chromosomes. Losses of 3p, 8p, 9, 13, 14, 15, and Y were each observed in two smaller series of primary NSCLCs *(15,16)*. Nonrandom losses of 6q, 17p, 18, and 19 were also described in one report *(16)*.

Gains of chromosomal material because of either numerical or structural changes are also common in NSCLC. In our series, the chromosome arms most frequently involved in gains were 7p and 7q *(35)*. Among the entire 63 tumors, gains of part or all of 7p and 7q were observed in 60 and 59% of cases, respectively. Extra copies of chromosome arms 1p, 1q, 3q, 5p, 11q, and 12q were also common.

We compared our cytogenetic findings in 35 adenocarcinomas with those in 18 squamous cell carcinomas and found only a few statistically significant differences between these two groups *(35)*. The percentage of cases with loss of 3p was significantly higher in squamous cell carcinomas (94%) than in adenocarcinomas (60%, *p* value of difference <0.01). Similarly, allelotype studies have revealed LOH from 3p in 81–100% of informative cases of squamous cell carcinoma, but in a significantly lower percentage of adenocarcinomas *(81,82)*. In addition, our investigation revealed a statistically significant increase in the proportion of cases with gains of 1q, 7p, and 11q in adenocarcinomas as compared to squamous cell carcinomas.

Loss of 3p

Loss of all or part of 3p was observed in approx 75% of the NSCLC cases we examined. LOH for alleles on 3p has been reported in 25–100% of NSCLC cases in different series *(46,47,65,83–85)*. The SRO of chromosome losses appears to be at 3p21. Allelic loss at 3p21 has been reported in all major types of lung cancer *(46,47)*. The frequency of loss of 3p material in LCC is comparable to the frequency seen in other NSCLCs *(36)*. Whereas deletion of 3p14–p23 was initially reported as a specific chromosome aberration in SCLC *(10)* subsequent analyses revealed frequent deletions of 3p in a number of other malignancies including renal cell carcinoma, mesothelioma, ovarian cancer, and breast cancer *(5)*. Thus, loss of 3p could represent an important generalized tumorigenic event common to variety of solid neoplasms.

Loss of 9p

Deletion of 9p has been proposed as a critical change in NSCLC *(16)*. Even though only a minority of our cases had either an interstitial deletion or terminal deletion of 9p, many others had either a numerical loss of 9 or an apparently unbalanced rearrangement resulting in a net loss of 9p. However, loss of 9p does not appear to be a frequent observation in LCC *(36)*. Homozygous losses of DNA sequences from 9p21–p22 have been reported in some NSCLCs *(86)*. The putative tumor suppressor gene, *p16/MTS1/CDKN2* located in 9p21–p22, has recently been cloned and shown to be altered in cell lines from multiple tumor types *(87,88)*. Homozygous deletion of this gene has been demonstrated in 6 of 20 (30%) NSCLC cell lines, but not in any of the 20 SCLC cell lines analyzed *(89)*. The presence of these deletions in the corresponding tumor tissue was confirmed, thus excluding the possibility that the deletions were in vitro artifacts. Similarly an analysis of *p16* at the protein level showed that in primary resection specimens p16 was undetectable in 18 of 27 (66%) NSCLC specimens, but was abundant in four of five SCLC specimens *(90)*.

Loss of 17p

Alterations of 17p are a frequent observation in NSCLC, including LCC. The structural changes of 17p include partial deletions and various derivative chromosomes. DNA analyses have demonstrated that loss of alleles from 17p is a common occurrence in NSCLC *(83)*. Our data suggest that visible cytogenetic changes may be the cause of the allelic loss detected by molecular methods, at least in some cases. As in SCLC, the cytogenetic and molecular evidence suggests that loss of 17p containing a normal *TP53* allele could unmask a mutant allele on the remaining, karyotypically normal, homologue.

i(5p), i(8q), and Other Isochromosomes

Even though nonrandom balanced reciprocal translocations have not been reported in NSCLC, several recurrent isochromosomes have been identified. In our studies, the most frequent isochromosome was i(5p), which was observed in 9 of 63 (14%) tumors, 8 of which had adenomatous features *(35)*. An i(8q) was identified in 6 of our cases, including 5 adenocarcinomas and 1 large cell lung carcinoma. Several other groups have also reported isochromosomes of 5p and 8q in NSCLC *(15,16,20,28,29,31,32)*. Other common isochromosomes found in our NSCLC series include i(1q), i(3q), i(6p), i(7p), and i(14q), each seen in 4 to 5 cases *(35)*. An association between i(8q) and adenocarcinoma of the lung has been reported by several investigators *(20,91)*. However, i(8q) and i(5p) are not specific for this tumor type. An i(8q) has been reported in various types of leukemia and in several different solid tumors; likewise, i(5p) has been observed in several different types of solid neoplasms and appears to be particularly frequent in tumors of the uterus and bladder *(5)*. Moreover, among the 17 SCLC cases we analyzed, one had an i(5p) and another had an i(8q) *(9)*. Isochromosomes involving 5 and 8 were not observed in the cases of LCC analyzed by Johansson et al. *(36)*. They did, however, report the presence of an i(7)(p10), in three tumors.

Dmins and hsrs

Dmins were observed in 6 of our 63 (9.5%) specimens *(35)*. Two cases had an hsr, including 1 of the 6 cases having dmins. Tumor material was available for Southern blot analysis in 5 of our

7 NSCLC cases that exhibited dmins and/or an hsr. The DNA studies revealed amplification of *MYC* in 2 cases and *EGFR* in 1 case. Eight different oncogene probes were tested in the other 2 cases, but an amplified sequence was not identified. In two other series of NSCLC specimens examined by Southern blot analysis, amplification of the *MYC* oncogene was documented in 3 of 36 (8%) and 4 of 25 (16%) cases *(92,93)*. Amplification of *KRAS2* has also been reported in a case of NSCLC that had dmins *(94)*.

Metastatic NSCLC

Two recent reports focused on chromosome changes in metastatic tumors from NSCLC patients *(32,34)*. In one study of NSCLC cell lines mostly derived from metastatic lesions, statistical analysis revealed that the structural alterations were distributed nonrandomly among the chromosomes *(32)*. A statistically significant number of clonal breakpoints was observed at chromosome regions 1q1, 1q3, 3p1, 3p2, 3q1, 3q2, 7q1, 13p1, 14p1, 15p1, and 17q1. Most of these regions undergo frequent rearrangement in primary tumors as well, although breakage at 1q3 does not appear to be a prominent change in primary tumors. Furthermore, breakage at 5cen, 6p1→6q1, 8cen→8p1, 9p2, 11p1→11q1, 17p1, and 19p1 appeared to be much less frequent in these metastatic tumors than in primary tumors. Whether these discrepancies are because of karyotypic evolution during tumor progression, evolution occurring during prolonged growth in vitro, or differences in the interpretation of karyotypes is presently unclear.

In the second report, pleural effusions containing metastatic or invasive tumor cells were analyzed *(34)*. Recurrent breakpoint regions included 1p1, 3p10–p21, 3q11–q25, 6p11–p25, 6q13–q23, 7q11–q36, 9q32–q34, 11p1, 11q13–q24, 13p, 14p, 15p, 17p, and 19p. Most of these regions are also frequently involved in primary tumors, although breakage at 3q11–q25 and 6p11–p25 have not been reported to be nonrandomly involved in primary tumors. Lukeis et al. *(34)* noted a lower frequency of 9p loss in pleural effusions compared to primary tumors, whereas breakpoints at 9q32–q34 were observed almost exclusively in effusions (4 of 11 cases) and, therefore, could represent a change associated with tumor progression. Four other metastatic tumors from NSCLC

patients have been reported to have a breakpoint at this region
(31,32). Lukeis et al. *(16,34)* also observed that loss of chromosome
8 or 8p, loss of Y, and rearrangement of 5q are less common in effusions than in primary tumors, whereas extra or rearranged chromosome 7, extra 20, loss of 22, and dmins occur at a higher frequency
in effusions than in primary tumors.

Molecular Cytogenetic Analysis

Although recent technical advances in cell culture and cytogenetics have improved the overall success rate and quality of chromosome studies in lung cancer, it has not been possible to examine
karyotypes of the malignant cells in every specimen for reasons outlined in the introduction to this chapter. In addition, karyotypic
analysis is very time consuming, and it is not feasible to routinely
cut out karyotypes of large numbers of metaphase spreads.
Furthermore, in vitro culturing of tumor cells may result in selective
outgrowth of cells that may not be representative of the whole tumor
cell population. As a result, it is uncertain whether the high incidence of certain chromosome changes (e.g., polysomy 7) described
in conventional karyotypic studies of NSCLC is indicative of their
frequency in this malignancy generally. Moreover, lung cancer
karyotypes are often very complicated and may display numerous
unidentified marker chromosomes, hindering efforts to identify
chromosome segments that are consistently lost or gained.

Two techniques have emerged that circumvent some of the
problems inherent in conventional karyotypic analysis, namely
interphase FISH *(95–107)* and CGH *(108,109)*. These techniques
utilize interphase nuclei and genomic DNA, respectively, and thus
are not limited by restraints such as cell growth rate, mitotic index,
and in vitro cell culture. Interphase FISH provides information with
respect to specific chromosome copy number. CGH accounts for all
chromosome segments in the tumor cell genome, including those
present in hsrs, dmins, and marker chromosomes whose origin cannot be determined by conventional banding analysis. Therefore,
CGH is invaluable for the analysis of tumors displaying complex
karyotypes, permitting the identification of net gains and losses of
chromosome material that might escape detection by routine cyto-

genetic approaches. However, CGH yields no information regarding balanced translocations or actual chromosome copy number.

Interphase FISH

Interphase FISH permits investigators to directly examine interphase cells from tissue sections or cell suspensions of tumor specimens and has been used successfully to analyze many types of solid tumors including neuroectodermal *(95)*, gastric *(96)*, breast *(97)*, bladder *(98,99)*, brain *(100)*, prostate *(101)*, ovarian *(102)*, endometrial *(103)*, renal *(104,105)*, male germ cell *(106)*, and lung tumors *(107)*. Because of the relative ease of scoring FISH preparations, it is possible to rapidly count the number of target sites in a large number of tumor cells. Besides enhancing karyologic investigations of tumor specimens, interphase cytogenetics may represent a useful approach to assess "noninvolved" bronchial tissues and premalignant lesions for the presence of cells with early (primary) chromosome changes.

Initial studies suggest that interphase FISH is a useful tool for the analysis of lung cancers. Kim et al. *(107)* performed such a study on paraffin-embedded tissue sections from 30 cases of NSCLC using pericentromeric probes for chromosomes 3, 7, 9, 11, and 17. Polysomy for a set of probes was detected in all except 4 cases that showed monosomy for only chromosome 3 or 7 in 2 cases and disomy for only chromosome 3 or 11 in 2 cases. Among the set of chromosomes examined, the frequency of polysomy was significantly higher for chromosomes 9 and 17 than for others. No significant difference was detected between centromere copy number and histology or clinical stages of tumors.

We applied interphase FISH to the analysis of processed cell suspensions obtained from 17 disaggregated primary NSCLCs using a panel of centromeric DNA probes specific for chromosomes 6, 7, 8, 9, 12, 17, and 18 (T. Taguchi et al., unpublished observations). FISH evidence for aneuploidy was observed in every specimen, with most tumors displaying extra copies of multiple chromosomes. Gain of part or all of chromosome 7 was a particularly prominent change, occurring in a large population of cells in each of 14 tumors (82%). Extra copies of chromosomes 6, 12, and 17 were also common, being observed in 9–11 cases each. Gain of chromosome 9 was infrequent (3 of 19 tumors). In 2 cases, most of the nuclei had only a single chromosome 9 signal. In addition to the FISH analyses with autosomal probes, tumor specimens from 26 males with NSCLC were assayed with a Y-specific centromeric sequence. Loss of the Y was observed in 13 cases (50%).

Karyotypic data were available on 6 of the 17 cases examined with autosomal probes. Generally, for each chromosome-specific probe tested, the modal number of fluorescent signals per nucleus was consistent with the results of karyotyping, although several differences were observed. Combined interphase and karyotypic data indicate that the overall centromeric copy number of chromosome 7 may be higher in the subset of specimens that are successfully cultured and karyotyped, suggesting that gain of chromosome 7 could provide a proliferative advantage in vitro. As noted earlier, polysomy of all or part of chromosome 7 is a common finding in karyotypic studies of NSCLCs *(14–17,20,26–29,34,36,38)*, and has been suggested to be an early change in this malignancy *(14)*.

These investigations demonstrate the feasibility of interphase FISH for the detection of numerical chromosome changes in a high percentage of NSCLCs, even in the absence of adequate numbers of dividing cells required for karyotypic analysis. Such interphase studies complement karyotypic analysis and can provide evidence of aneuploidy even in small or nonsterile specimens.

Comparative Genomic Hybridization

This method has been used in the analysis of various solid tumors to identify gains or losses of whole chromosomes or chromosome segments as well as to map amplified genes *(108–118)*. Tumor types analyzed so far include prostate cancer *(111,112)*, SCLC *(110,113)*, renal cell carcinoma *(114)*, bladder cancer *(115)*, and breast cancer *(116)*. Interestingly, a recent CGH analysis of prostate carcinomas identified increased DNA-sequence copy number at Xq11–q13 *(112)*. Subsequent analysis at the molecular level revealed amplification of the androgen receptor gene, located within this chromosomal region, in 30% of recurrent prostate tumors *(117)*.

CGH analysis of 13 primary SCLC specimens demonstrated frequent chromosome losses expected in this tumor type (i.e., 3p-, 13q-, and 17p-), as well as several recurrent abnormalities that had not been recognized in previous karyotypic studies of SCLC: 4q-, 10q-, and amplification of 19q13 *(110)*. The detection of decreases in copy number of 3p, 13q, and 17p using CGH were confirmed in a second study of 18 SCLC cell lines *(113)*. This group also identified over-representation of the chromosomal sites 1p22–p32, 2p24–p25, and 8q24, sites of the genes *MYCL*, *MYCN*, and *MYC*, respectively, which are frequently amplified in SCLC cell lines *(70–72)*. In addition, novel copy number increases were detected at 5p, 1q24, and Xq26 whereas novel decreases involved 22q12.1–q13.1, 10q26, and 16p11.2. Two types of SCLC cell lines were analyzed by Levin et al. *(113)*. These were classified as "classic" or "variant" depending on their cellular morphology, growth phenotypes, enzymatic activity, and response to ionizing radiation. The variant cell lines were radioresistant whereas the classic cell lines were radiosensitive. Based on the CGH results several differences were found between the two classes of cell lines. A statistically significant increase in the copy number of 1p22–p32 and loss of 18p were preferentially associated with the variant cell lines. Over-representation of 18q21 and loss of 10p were preferentially seen in cell lines of the classic phenotype.

Recently, we have performed CGH analyses on nine established NSCLC cell lines (Sonoda et al., unpublished observations). Gains of part or all of 1q, 3q, 5p, 7p, 8q, 15q, 17q, and 20p and losses of 13q were prominent changes, each occurring in at least three different cell lines. The most frequent change was a gain of 7p, observed in 7 of 9 cell lines. Karyotypic data available on some of these NSCLC cell lines indicate that the specific imbalances identified by CGH analysis are consistent with those observed by karyotypic analysis. DNA amplification was detected in three of the nine NSCLC cell lines. Two of these lines had two different sites of amplification. The amplified sequences were located at 3q25–q26, 8q24 (two cases), 11q13–q21, and 20q13. An obvious candidate target gene in 8q24 is the *MYC* oncogene, which has previously been shown to be amplified in some NSCLCs *(35,92,93)*.

Cytogenetics in Relation to DNA Content and Molecular Alterations

The poor prognosis of lung cancer patients may be attributed to the high incidence of unresectable tumors at diagnosis *(3)*. Although patients with resectable disease have improved survival, recurrent disease will develop in >50% of cases within the first 5 yr postoperatively. There is a strong association between patient outcome and tumor size, presence of nodal metastases, distant spread and, to a lesser extent, cell type (119,120). The American Joint Committee on Cancer (AJCC) tumor staging was reported to be the most accurate predictor of survival in patients with NSCLC (121). Despite the value of tumor staging, an estimated 37% of patients with AJCC stage I adenocarcinoma and 40–50% with stage I squamous cell carcinoma will die of their disease within 5 yr (122). Therefore, it is important from a therapeutic standpoint to identify patients at high risk within these favorable subgroups. A major challenge then is to identify better prognostic indicators that can be used to accurately predict patient outcome.

Chromosomal alterations are thought to play a fundamental role in tumorigenesis. Some of these structural or numerical changes, or a combination of them, may be specific for a particular histological subtype or may correlate with tumor behavior. For example, as we noted earlier, there are differences in the pattern of karyotypic alterations seen in SCLC and NSCLC. Furthermore, certain cytogenetic losses appear to be more frequent in squamous cell carcinomas than in adenocarcinomas (35). At the molecular level, allelotyping has shown both quantitative and qualitative differences in the losses observed in different NSCLC subtypes, i.e., most chromosomal arms showed a higher frequency of LOH in squamous cell carcinomas than in adenocarcinomas (82). With respect to tumor grade, LOH for chromosome arms 2q, 3p, and 17p was more frequent in moderately and poorly differentiated adenocarcinomas than in well-differentiated carcinomas (81). In addition, in adenocarcinomas the frequency of allelic loss on 3p was significantly higher in stage II and stage III tumors considered together than in stage I tumors. Therefore, either specific karyotypic or molecular alterations or overall genetic imbalances may prove to be useful prognostic markers. The DNA content of a tumor cell population can be measured accurately by flow cytometry, whereas the overall genetic imbalances in a tumor cell genome can be determined by CGH. As discussed below, research aimed at identifying such markers in lung cancer has, in many instances, yielded contradictory results. Much of this research has employed flow cytometry to measure the total DNA content of tumor cell populations. In future investigations it will be of interest to compare the results of CGH analyses with clinical characteristics of patients to determine the influence of overall genetic imbalances on tumor progression and patient prognosis.

DNA Content

As noted earlier in our review of karyotypic analyses, most lung tumors appear to be near-triploid to near-tetraploid. Flow cytometry studies have also demonstrated a high frequency of abnormal cellular DNA content, or aneuploidy, in lung carcinomas. Aneuploidy has been shown to have prognostic value in a number of solid tumor types including breast, ovarian, bladder, and colon cancers *(123–126)*. With respect to lung cancer, however, the prognostic value of DNA content is, at present, unclear. Several studies reported a correlation between DNA content and prognosis *(127–135)*, whereas others have failed to detect such a relationship *(121,136–141)*. Flow cytometric measurements on fresh tumor specimens of mixed stage and histology have shown a significant correlation between ploidy and prognosis. Volm et al. *(127)* used flow cytometry to measure the DNA content and estimate the cell cycle phase of 240 surgical specimens of mixed stage and histology from patients with NSCLC. A correlation between DNA content and prognosis was reported. Patients with aneuploid tumors (83% of cases) and those with tumors comprised of multiple stem lines (20% of cases) had a significantly shorter survival rate than those with diploid tumors or only one stemline. In addition, patients whose tumors showed a low G0/G1-cell proportion or a high proliferation pool (S and G2/M-proportion) had a poor prognosis. In a similar analysis of fresh NSCLC and SCLC cases, again of mixed stage and histology, at least one aneuploid subpopulation of cells was present in 91% and 50% of cases, respectively *(131)*. Considering all the malignant tumors together, a statistically significant correlation between diploidy and increased survival was observed.

Analysis of archival material has yielded results similar to those just described for fresh specimens. Zimmerman et al. *(129)* successfully analyzed archival paraffin blocks from 100 cases of NSCLC of mixed stage and histology, 45% of which were aneuploid. Patients with aneuploid tumors had a significantly shorter overall survival than those with diploid tumors. There was no apparent relationship between ploidy and the clinical and pathological characteristics examined. In another retrospective study of mixed types of NSCLC, 70% of 136 cases examined were found to be aneuploid and had a statistically significant shorter survival time *(132)*. Again aneuploidy was found to be independent of tumor size, histology, grade of differentiation, regional lymph node involvement, age, and sex. In a retrospective study of 74 patients with lung cancer, Ogawa et al. *(135)* reported that those cases (48%) with aneuploid tumors had higher frequencies of lymphatic invasion and metastasis to the mediastinal lymph nodes and shorter survival times than cases with diploid tumors.

Several groups reported that DNA content is a useful prognostic indicator but only for certain tumor subsets. For example, in one flow cytometric study, ploidy level could distinguish two subgroups of identically staged patients with different prognoses *(128)*. In another investigation of stage I tumors, DNA content of well-differentiated and smaller (T1) tumors was correlated with tumor recurrence *(130)*. There is also evidence indicating that the clinical value of DNA content differs between squamous cell carcinoma and adenocarcinoma *(133)*. Investigations have demonstrated that DNA content is a significant independent prognostic factor in patients presenting with squamous cell carcinoma but not in nonsquamous cell carcinoma *(133,134)*.

Despite this body of evidence supporting a role for DNA content as a prognostic indicator for at least certain forms of lung cancer, several other groups were unable to confirm this association even though aneuploidy was detected in 56–85% of cases *(121,136–141)*. These studies analyzed both fresh clinical samples *(121,136,139)* and archival paraffin-embedded tissue samples *(137,138,140,141)*. Although none of these studies demonstrated a significant association between the prognosis and DNA content, one did reveal a significant correlation between the percentage of aneuploid tumor cells and survival *(139)*.

Several reasons have been postulated to account for these conflicting data. It has been suggested that a fundamental problem is that some studies have been based on the analysis of tumor series that include carcinomas of all TNM categories and histologic types, making it problematic to conclude that aneuploidy precedes either tumor size or metastases *(141)*. Studies limited to an analysis of stage I squamous cell carcinoma *(139)*, stage I adenocarcinoma *(138)*, or T1N0 NSCLC *(141)* did not find survival differences between patients with diploid and aneuploid tumors. It has also been proposed that the variability of interlaboratory results could reflect differences in the source of tumor material and the method of specimen preparation *(121)*. In particular, fresh tumor specimens have been shown to be superior to paraffin-embedded tumor material for flow cytometric analyses *(142)*. The latter source may give variable results because of differential tissue fixation, dehydration temperature, embedding variables, and the presence of cell fragments. However, the reports cited above that show a positive association between DNA ploidy and prognosis appear to be independent of whether or not the specimens were paraffin-embedded tissue or fresh tumor; five were retrospective studies *(129,130,132–134)* and four were performed on fresh specimens *(127,128,131,135)*. Of the reports that failed to find an association, four were retrospective *(137,138,140,141)* and three analyzed fresh tumor material *(121,136,139)*. Large intergroup studies, which take into account tumor stage and histological subtype, are needed to verify whether DNA ploidy can be used as a reliable prognostic indicator in lung carcinomas.

Molecular Alterations

Gene alterations may represent molecular manifestations of visible chromosomal changes. It is now well-recognized that tumorigenesis is a multistep process. In colorectal cancer the sequential nature of gene changes has been defined *(143,144)*. Currently there is little known about the sequence of such events in lung cancer. If the order of genetic alterations in lung cancer can be delineated, perhaps it will be feasible to distinguish between early and late changes and to determine the prognostic importance of any such changes. Activation of the oncogenes *MYC (145)*, *KRAS (146,147)*, *ERBB2 (148)* and *BCL2 (149,150)* have been described in certain subsets of SCLC and/or NSCLC. Known tumor suppressor genes such as *TP53 (66,67)*, *RB1 (62–64)*, and *p16/MTS1/CDKN2 (89,90)* are also altered in lung cancer. In addition, loss or inactivation of putative, as yet unidentified, tumor suppressor genes located on chromosomes 3p *(46,47)* and 5q *(151)* have been implicated in lung cancer. Several groups have now reported correlations between specific gene changes and prognosis of lung cancer patients, thus paving the way towards the identification of potentially improved prognostic indicators in lung cancer. These correlations are discussed below.

TP53

As we noted previously in this chapter, karyotypic losses involving chromosome 17p are frequent observations in both SCLC and NSCLC. Molecular alterations of the *TP53* tumor suppressor gene, located at 17p13.1, are often detected in lung cancer *(66,67)*. Thus, the cytogenetic and molecular evidence suggests that loss of 17p containing a normal *TP53* allele could unveil a mutant allele on the remaining, cytogenetically normal homolog. Evidence for such a mechanism comes from combined cytogenetic and molecular genetic studies of a case of NSCLC *(35)*. This tumor had an unbalanced translocation resulting in loss of part of one 17p; the remaining *TP53* allele had a nonsense mutation and no detectable TP53 mRNA or protein *(152)*.

In SCLC, the frequency of *TP53* mutation is very high (~90% of cases *(153)*), so that it is unlikely to be of value as a prognostic indicator *(154)*. In NSCLC, mutation of *TP53* occurs in approx 45% of cases *(155,156)*. There is evidence to suggest that *TP53* mutation may be of value as a prognostic indicator of NSCLC, although data from reports addressing this issue are contradictory. Immunohistochemical analysis of stage I and II adenocarcinomas and squamous cell carcinomas initially indicated a correlation between TP53 protein accumulation and decreased survival *(157)*. This association was confirmed molecularly in that patients whose tumors had *TP53* mutations survived for a shorter time interval than patients for whom no mutation was identified *(158,159)*. This association held for the subset of patients with stage I or II disease, which generally have a favorable response to treatment. In contrast, others investigators have reported the presence of *TP53* mutations to be a negative prognostic indicator for patients with advanced forms of the disease (stages III and IV), but not for those with early stage disease *(160)*.

The results of one group, however, contradict these findings of a correlation between TP53 protein staining and reduced survival times. Using immunohistochemistry to detect TP53, an association between TP53 staining and an increased rate of disease-free survival, especially in patients with early stage disease was reported *(161)*. Both investigations employing immunohistochemistry used the monoclonal antibody PAb1801 that recognizes both the wild-type and mutant forms of the protein *(157,161)*. It has been suggested that there might not be a simple relationship between TP53 protein expression and prognosis, as both the detection of wild-type TP53 and different oncogenic potential by different mutant TP53 proteins may greatly impact on tumor behavior *(162)*. In a study that investigated the utility of *TP53* gene mutation and immunostaining as prognostic factors for the same cohort of patients, mutations in the gene were not found to be adverse prognostic factors for survival whereas immunostaining was associated weakly with poor survival, but was not an independent prognostic indicator *(154)*. Future standardized investigations are required to resolve this issue.

KRAS

There is evidence to suggest that *KRAS* gene mutation may identify lung cancer patients with poor prognosis. Activated *ras* genes *(KRAS, HRAS* and *NRAS)* have been reported in approx 20% of NSCLC specimens *(146,147)*, with the majority of mutations occurring in adenocarcinomas largely in the 12th codon of these genes *(146,163)*. *KRAS* mutations have been reported to be a negative prognostic indicator in NSCLC *(164,165)*. In a retrospective study of adenocarcinomas (stages I–IIIa) that were completely resectable, tumors positive for *KRAS* point mutations tended to be smaller and less differentiated than those without such mutations *(164)*. Mutations in codon 12 of this gene were detected in 27% (29 of 69) of cases. A point mutation in codon 12 was a strong, independent, negative prognostic indicator as evidenced by both the duration of disease-free survival and overall survival. Analysis of a broader set of patients in terms of both disease extent and treatment confirmed the correlation between *KRAS* mutation and shortened survival *(165)*. Of interest is the association of *KRAS* mutation and smoking history *(166)*. *KRAS* mutations were found in 30% of adenocarcinoma samples from smokers or exsmokers, but in only 5% of tumors from patients who had never smoked. *KRAS* mutations, therefore, currently hold promise as a negative prognostic indicator in NSCLC.

ERBB2

Amplification of the *ERBB2* oncogene, located at 17q11.2–q12, correlates with patient relapse and survival in breast cancer *(167,168)*. It has been shown that amplification of this gene corre- lates with immunohistochemical staining for the corresponding 185 kDa protein *(169)*. In NSCLC, there are preliminary data that indi- cate that overexpression of *ERBB2* may be of prognostic value. Immunohistochemistry has shown that *ERBB2* protein overexpres- sion is greater in adenocarcinomas than in squamous cell carcinomas of the lung *(148)*. Positive staining was observed in 28% of cases of adenocarcinoma compared to 2% of squamous cell carcinomas. There was a statistically significant difference between the 5-yr sur- vival of positive patients in comparison to ERBB2 negative patients, suggesting that overexpression of the *ERBB2* gene may be of some prognostic importance in NSCLC. Similarly, Kern et al. *(170)* reported a significant correlation between ERBB2 overexpression and survival in adenocarcinomas, but not in squamous cell carcino- mas. A subsequent study by this same group revealed that ERBB2 expression was associated with a poor survival outlook but *KRAS* mutation was not. However, the influence of both factors on survival, collectively, was additive and highly significant *(171)*.

BCL2

The *BCL2* gene, located at chromosome band 18q21, is involved in the t(14;18) translocation found in many non-Hodgkin's B-cell lymphomas *(172)*. This translocation juxtaposes *BCL2* with the immunoglobulin heavy chain locus at 14q32 resulting in tran- scriptional deregulation leading to abnormally high levels of the *BCL2* protein *(173)*. In our interphase FISH analysis described ear- lier, we noted increased copy number of chromosome 18 in 4 of 17 (23%) cases. Overexpression of *BCL2* has been demonstrated in several types of solid tumors, including lung cancer *(149,150)*. Moreover, there is preliminary evidence that *BCL2* expression may serve as a useful prognostic indicator in lung cancer. In a study of 101 cases of primary resectable NSCLC, immunostaining for both BCL2 and TP53 protein expression was performed *(150)*. No relationship was observed between BCL2 protein expression and other clinicopathological or biological parameters such as tumor histology, grade, tumor status, nodal metastasis, or proliferative activity *(150)*. However, the mean BCL2 expression was significantly lower in patients who developed metastases during follow-up or who died of metastatic disease. Furthermore, survival probability was higher for those patients whose tumors expressed the BCL2 protein. In contrast, TP53 protein expression was observed in tumors with metastatic nodal involvement or in patients who developed metastasis at a later date. There was an inverse correlation between BCL-2 and TP53 expression in this series.

LOH from 5q

Our karyotypic analyses of 63 NSCLCs revealed that i(5p) is the most frequent isochromosome in this tumor type *(35)*. Formation of i(5p) would lead to overall loss of 5q sequences reflected in molecular loss of the *APC/MCC* gene cluster. A recent investigation showed that deletions of the *APC/MCC* gene cluster at chromosome 5q21 occur in about 30% of NSCLCs *(151)*. LOH involving this gene cluster correlated significantly with a worse survival and also with involvement of the medastinal and/or hilar nodes. Thus, 5q21 deletion may prove to be a valuable negative prognostic indicator for lung cancer.

MYC

As we noted earlier, amplification of *MYC* genes, although rarely reported in NSCLC, is a frequent observation in cell lines derived from SCLCs *(70–72)* and involves all members of this gene family, namely *MYC*, *MYCL*, and *MYCN (174)*. The frequency of amplification has been found to be higher in tumors and tumor-derived cell lines from those patients who had received chemotherapy compared to untreated patients *(74,174)*. In addition, individuals who received treatment had significantly shorter survival times than the untreated group suggesting that *MYC* amplification may be a useful negative prognostic indicator for SCLC patients *(174)*.

Conclusions

In summary, cytogenetic analysis has demonstrated that numerous acquired genetic events are involved in the pathogenesis of lung carcinomas. The karyotypes of these neoplasms often have massive changes, even in newly diagnosed primary tumors, but the pattern and biological implications of recurrent chromosome alterations are beginning to emerge. Chromosomal losses are frequently observed, and some of these changes (e.g., deletions of 3p, 5q and 17p in SCLC and 3p, 9p, and 17p in NSCLC) occur at the location of known or suspected tumor suppressor genes, whose loss and/or inactivation may play a fundamental role in lung tumorigenesis. Other alterations (i.e., dmin and hsr) represent cytogenetic manifestations of gene amplification, and the net effect of such changes may be an increase in an oncogene product that provides an added proliferative advantage. Still other chromosomal imbalances, such as gains of chromosome 7 in NSCLC, may have an important, but as yet undetermined role.

It is clear from preliminary investigations that the newer cytogenetic technologies of interphase FISH and CGH will, in conjunction with conventional karyotypic analysis, add to our knowledge of the spectrum of chromosomal alterations in lung cancer. Even though technical advances in cell culture and cytogenetics have improved the quality of chromosome studies in primary NSCLCs, the success rate generally is low, ranging from 33–50% in several recent reports *(80,175)*. Unless the rate of successful cell culture of NSCLCs can be improved, it will not be possible to establish reliable correlations between chromosome alterations and clinicopathological parameters or to use karyotypic analysis routinely in this malignancy. Since interphase cytogenetics and CGH do not require actively dividing cells for analysis, they represent feasible alternative approaches to unravel the patterns and clinical implications of chromosome changes in lung cancer. Moreover, these valuable new technologies complement karyotypic analysis and can provide evidence of aneuploidy even in small or nonsterile specimens, making routine assessment of lung tumors possible. In addition, the detection of genetic heterogeneity within human solid tumors is increased markedly by the application of different types of genetic analysis, including flow cytometry and molecular analyses *(104)*.

The development of new, improved prognostic markers for lung cancer will be an important focus of future research. Current evidence indicates that certain of the molecular alterations observed in lung carcinomas, such as mutations of the *KRAS* gene, hold promise as prognostic indicators. In future studies, it will be important to determine if CGH analysis can uncover alterations that can be correlated with clinical parameters such as metastatic behavior and prognosis. Furthermore, as our awareness of specific recurrent chromosome alterations in lung cancer increases, it should be possible to establish a useful panel of nonisotopic DNA probes to facilitate the rapid diagnostic assessment of lung tumor specimens.

Acknowledgments

This work was supported by NIH grants CA-45745 and CA-06927, NCI-Frederick Subcontract 6S-1602 and by an appropriation from the Commonwealth of Pennsylvania.

References

1. Boring CC, Squires TS, Tong T, Montgomery S: Cancer statistics, 1994. Ca-Cancer J Clinicians 44:7–26, 1994.
2. Aisner J: Lung Cancer. Contemporary Issues in Clinical Oncology, Vol. 3. New York: Churchill Livingstone, 1985.
3. Minna JD, Higgins GA, Glatstein EJ: Cancer of the lung. In: DeVita VT, Hellman S, Rosenberg SA (eds.), Cancer: Principles and Practice of Oncology. Philadelphia: Lippencott, pp. 507–598, 1985.
4. McDowell EM, McLaughlin JS, Merenyi DK, Kieffer RF, Harris CC, Trump BF: The respiratory epithelium. V. Histogenesis of lung carcinomas in the human. J Natl Cancer Inst 61:587–606, 1978.
5. Mitelman F: Catalog of Chromosome Aberrations in Cancer, 4th ed. New York: Liss, 1991.
6. Siegfried JM, Resau J, Miura I, Testa JR: Primary culture of solid lung tumors for chromosomal analysis. In: Adolph, KW (ed.), Advanced Techniques in Chromosome Research. New York: Dekker, pp. 411–425, 1991.
7. Sozzi G, Bertoglio MG, Borrello MG, Giani S, Pilotti S, Pierotti M, Della Porta G: Chromosomal abnormalities in a primary small cell lung cancer. Cancer Genet Cytogenet 27:45–50, 1987.
8. DeFusco PA, Frytak S, Dahl RJ, Weiland LH, Unni KK, Dewald GW: Cytogenetic studies in 11 patients with small cell carcinoma of the lung. Mayo Clin Proc 64:168–176, 1989.

9. Miura I, Graziano SL, Cheng JQ, Doyle LA, Testa JR: Chromosome alterations in small cell lung cancer: frequent involvement of 5q. Cancer Res 52:1322–1328, 1992.

10. Whang-Peng J, Kao-Shan CS, Lee EC, Bunn PA, Carney DN, Gazdar AF, Minna JD: Specific chromosome defect associated with human small-cell lung cancer: deletion of 3p(14–23). Science 215:181, 182, 1982.

11. Morstyn G, Brown J, Novak U, Gardner J, Bishop J, Garson M: Heterogeneous cytogenetic abnormalities in small cell lung cancer cell lines. Cancer Res 47:3322–3327, 1987.

12. Whang-Peng J, Bunn PA Jr, Kao-Shan CS, Lee EC, Carney DN, Gazdar A, Minna JD: A nonrandom chromosomal abnormality, del 3p(14–23), in human small cell lung cancer (SCLC). Cancer Genet Cytogenet 6:119–134, 1982.

13. Wurster-Hill DH, Cannizzaro LA, Pettengill OS, Sorenson GD, Cate CC, Mauer LH: Cytogenetics of small cell carcinoma of the lung. Cancer Genet Cytogenet 13:303–330, 1984.

14. Lee JS, Pathak S, Hopwood V, Tomasovic B, Mullins TD, Baker FL, Spitzer G, Neidhart JA: Involvement of chromosome 7 in primary lung tumor and nonmalignant normal lung tissue. Cancer Res 47:6349–6352, 1987.

15. Viegas-Pequignot E, Flury-Herard A, De Cremoux H, Chlecq C, Bignon J, Dutrillaux B: Recurrent chromosome aberrations in human lung squamous cell carcinomas. Cancer Genet Cytogenet 49:37–49, 1990.

16. Lukeis R, Irving L, Garson M, Hasthorpe S: Cytogenetics of non-small cell lung cancer: analysis of consistent non-random abnormalities. Genes Chromosom Cancer 2:116–124, 1990.

17. Miura I, Siegfried JM, Resau J, Keller SM, Zhou J, Testa JR: Chromosome alterations in 21 non-small cell lung carcinomas. Genes Chromosom Cancer 2:328–338, 1990.

18. Flury-Herard A, Viegas-Pequignot E, De Cremoux H, Chlecq C, Bignon J, Dutrillaux B: Cytogenetic study of five cases of lung adenosquamous carcinomas. Cancer Genet Cytogenet 59:1–8, 1992.

19. Liang JC, Kurzrock R, Gutterman JU, Gallick GE: Trisomy 12 correlates with elevated expression of p21[ras] in a human adenosquamous carcinoma of the lung. Cancer Genet Cytogenet 23:183–188, 1986.

20. Jin Y, Mandahl N, Heim S, Schuller H, Mitelman F: Isochromosomes i(8q) or i(9q) in three adenocarcinomas of the lung. Cancer Genet Cytogenet 33:11–17, 1988.

21. Ronne M, Elberg JJ, Shibasaki Y, Andersen K: A case of squamous cell lung carcinoma with tetrasomy 7 and chromosome 1 C-band polymorphism. Anticancer Res 9:1101–1104, 1989.

22. Pejovic T, Heim S, Orndal C, Jin YS, Mandhal N, Willen H, Mitelman F: Simple numerical chromosome aberrations in well-differentiated malignant epithelial tumors. Cancer Genet Cytogenet 49:95–101, 1990.

23. Johansson M, Jin Y, Heim S, Mandahl N, Hambraeus G, Johansson L, Mitelman F: Pseudodiploid karyotypes in adenosquamous carcinomas of the lung. Cancer Genet Cytogenet 63:95, 96, 1992.

24. Drouin V, Viguie F, Debesse B: Near-haploid karyotype in a squamous cell lung carcinoma. Genes Chromosom Cancer 7:209–212, 1993.

25. Zech L, Bergh J, Nilsson K: Karyotypic characterization of established cell lines and short-term cultures of human lung cancers. Cancer Genet Cytogenet 15:335–347, 1985.

26. Fan Y-S, Li P: Cytogenetic studies of four human lung adenocarcinoma cell lines. Cancer Genet Cytogenet 26:317–325, 1987.

27. Rey JA, Bello MJ, de Campos JM, Kusak ME, Moreno S, Benitez J: Deletion 3p in two lung adenocarcinomas metastatic to the brain. Cancer Genet Cytogenet 25:355–360, 1987.

28. Bello MJ, Moreno S, Rey JA: Involvement of chromosomes 1, 3, and i(8q) in lung adenocarcinoma. Cancer Genet Cytogenet 38:133–135, 1989.

29. Cagle PT, Taylor LD, Schwartz MR, Ramzy I, Elder FFB: Cytogenetic abnormalities common to adenocarcinoma metastatic to the pleura. Cancer Genet Cytogenet 39:219–225, 1989.

30. Kadowaki MH, Ferguson MK: The role of chromosome 3 deletions in lung cancer. Lung Cancer 6:165–170, 1990.

31. Erdel M, Peter W, Spiess E, Trefz G, Ebert W: Karyotypic characterization of established cell lines derived from a squamous cell carcinoma and an adenocarcinoma of human lung cancers. Cancer Genet Cytogenet 49:185–198, 1990.

32. Whang-Peng J, Knutsen T, Gazdar A, Steinberg SM, Oie H, Linnoila I, Mulshine J, Nau M, Minna JD: Non-random structural and numerical chromosome changes in non-small-cell lung cancer. Genes Chromosom Cancer 3:168–188, 1991.

33. Law E, Gilvarry U, Lynch V, Gregory B, Grant G, Clynes M: Cytogenetic comparison of two poorly differentiated human lung squamous cell carcinoma lines. Cancer Genet Cytogenet 59:111–118, 1992.

34. Lukeis R, Ball D, Irving L, Garson OM, Hasthorpe S: Chromosome abnormalities in non-small cell lung cancer pleural effusions: cytogenetic indicators of disease subgroups. Genes Chromosom Cancer 8:262–269, 1993.

35. Testa JR, Siegfried JM, Liu Z, Hunt JD, Feder MM, Litwin S, Zhou J-Y, Taguchi T, Keller SM: Cytogenetic analysis of 63 non-small cell lung carcinomas: recurrent chromosome alterations amid frequent and widespread genomic upheaval. Genes Chromosom Cancer 11:178–194, 1994.

36. Johansson M, Dietrich C, Mandahl N, Hambraeus G, Johansson L, Clausen PP, Mitelman F, Heim S: Karyotypic characterization of bronchial large cell carcinomas. Int J Cancer 57:463–467, 1994.

37. Linnoila I: Pathology of non-small cell lung cancer. New diagnostic approaches. Hematol Oncol Clin North Am 4:1027–1051, 1990.

38. Testa JR, Siegfried JM: Chromosome abnormalities in non-small cell lung cancer. Cancer Res 52:2702–2706, 1992.

39. Testa JR, Graziano SL: Molecular implications of recurrent cytogenetic alterations in human small cell lung cancer. Cancer Detect Prev 17: 267–277, 1993.

40. Graziano SL, Cowan BY, Carney DN, Bryke CR, Mitter NS, Johnson BE, Mark GE, Planas AT, Catino JJ, Comis RL, Poiesz BJ: Small cell lung cancer cell line derived from a primary tumor with a characteristic deletion of 3p. Cancer Res 47:2148–2155, 1987.

41. Graziano SL, Pfeifer AM, Testa JR, Mark GE, Johnson BE, Hallinan EJ, Pettengill OS, Sorenson GD, Tatum AH, Brauch H, Zbar B, Flejter W, Ehrlich GD, Poiesz BJ: Involvement of the *RAF1* locus, at band 3p25, in the 3p deletion of small-cell lung cancer. Genes Chromosom Cancer 3:283–293, 1991.

42. de Leij L, Postmus PE, Buys CH, Elema JD, Ramaekers F, Poppema S, Brouwer M, van der Veen AY, Mesander G, The TH: Characterization of three new variant type cell lines derived from small cell carcinoma of the lung. Cancer Res 45:6024–6033, 1985.

43. Falor WH, Ward-Skinner R, Wegryn S: A 3p deletion in small cell lung carcinoma. Cancer Genet Cytogenet 16:175–177, 1985.

44. Bepler G, Jaques G, Koehler A, Gropp C, Havemann K: Markers and characteristics of human SCLC cell lines. J Cancer Res Clin Oncol 113:253–259, 1985.

45. Naylor SL, Johnson BE, Minna JD, Sakaguchi AY: Loss of heterozygosity of chromosome 3p markers in small-cell lung cancer. Nature 329:451–454, 1987.

46. Brauch H, Johnson B, Hovis J, Yano T, Gazdar A, Pettengill OS, Graziano S, Sorenson GD, Poiesz BJ, Minna J, Linehan M, Zbar B: Molecular analysis of the short arm of chromosome 3 in small-cell and non-small-cell carcinoma of the lung. N Engl J Med 317:1109–1113, 1987.

47. Kok K, Osinga J, Carritt B, Davis MB, van der Hout AH, van der Veen AY, Landsvater RM, de Leij LFMH, Berendsen HH, Postmus PE, Poppema S, Buys CHCM: Deletion of a DNA sequence at the chromosomal region 3p21 in all major types of lung cancer. Nature 330:578–581, 1987.

48. Cavenee WK, Dryja TP, Phillips RA, Benedict WF, Godbout R, Gallie BL, Murphee AL, Strong LC, White RL: Expression of recessive alleles by chromosomal mechanisms in retinoblastoma. Nature 305:779–784, 1983.

49. Ibson JM, Water JJ, Twentyman NM, Rabbitts PH: Oncogene amplification and chromosomal abnormalities in small cell lung cancer. J Cell Biochem 33:267–288, 1987.

50. Sithanandam G, Dean M, Brennscheidt U, Beck T, Gazdar A, Minna JD, Brauch H, Zbar B, Rapp UR: Loss of heterozygosity at the c-*raf* locus in small cell lung carcinoma. Oncogene 4:451–455, 1989.

51. Brauch H, Tory K, Kotler F, Gazdar AF, Pettengill OS, Johnson B, Graziano S, Winton T, Buys CHCM, Sorenson GD, Poiesz BJ, Minna JD, Zbar B: Molecular mapping of deletion sites in the short arm of chromosome 3 in human lung cancer. Genes Chromosom Cancer 1:240–246, 1990.

52. Rabbitts P, Bergh J, Douglas J, Collins F, Waters J: A submicroscopic homozygous deletion at the D3S3 locus in a cell line isolated from a small cell lung carcinoma. Genes Chromosom Cancer 2:231–238, 1990.

53. Yamakawa K, Takahashi T, Horio Y, Murata Y, Takahashi E, Hibi K, Yokoyama S, Ueda R, Takahashi T, Nakamura Y: Frequent homozygous deletions in lung cancer cell lines detected by a DNA marker located at 3p21.3–p22. Oncogene 8:327–330, 1993.

54. Drabkin HA, Mendez MJ, Rabbitts PH, Varkony T, Bergh J, Schlessinger J, Erickson P, Gemmill RM: Characterization of the submicroscopic deletion in

the small-cell lung carcinoma (SCLC) cell line U2020. Genes Chromosom Cancer 5:67–74, 1992.

55. Latif F, Tory K, Modi WS, Graziano SL, Gamble G, Douglas J, Heppell-Parton AC, Rabbitts PH, Zbar B, Lerman MI: Molecular characterization of a large homozygous deletion in the small cell lung cancer cell line U2020: a strategy for cloning the putative tumor suppressor gene. Genes Chromosome Cancer 5:119–127, 1992.

56. Cannizzaro LA, Skolnik EY, Margolis B, Croce CM, Schlesinger J, Huebner K: The human gene encoding phosphatidylinositol-3 kinase associated p85α is at chromosome region 5q12–13. Cancer Res 51: 3818–3820, 1991.

57. Escobedo JA, Navankasattusas S, Kavanaugh WM, Milfay D, Fried VA, Williams LT: cDNA cloning of a novel 85 kD protein that has SH2 domains, and regulates binding of PI3 kinase to the PDGF β-receptor. Cell 65:75–82, 1991.

58. Bishop DT, Westbrook C: Report of the committee on the genetic constitution of chromosome 5. Cytogenet Cell Genet 55:111–117, 1990.

59. Nishisho I, Nakamura Y, Miyoshi Y, Miki Y, Ando H, Horii A, Koyama K, Utsunomiya J, Baba S, Hedge P: Mutations of chromosome 5q21 genes in FAP and colorectal cancer patients. Science 253:665–669, 1991.

60. D'Amico D, Carbone DP, Johnson BE, Meltzer SJ, Minna JD: Polymorphic sites within the *MCC* and *APC* loci reveal very frequent loss of heterozygosity in human small cell lung cancer. Cancer Res 52:1996–1999, 1992.

61. Wieland I, Bohm M, Bogatz S: Isolation of DNA sequences deleted in lung cancer by genomic difference cloning. Proc Natl Acad Sci USA 89:9705–9709, 1992.

62. Motegi T, Komatsu M, Nakazato Y, Ohuchi M, Minoda K: Retinoblastoma in a boy with a de novo mutation of a 13/18 translocation: the assumption that the retinoblastoma locus is at 13q14.1, particularly at the distal portion of it. Hum Genet 60:193–195, 1982.

63. Friend SH, Bernards R, Rogelj S, Weinberg RA, Rapaport JM, Albert DM, Dryja TP: A human DNA segment with properties of the gene that predisposes to retinoblastoma and osteosarcoma. Nature 323:643–646, 1986.

64. Harbour JW, Lai S-L, Whang-Peng J, Gazdar AF, Minna JD, Kaye FJ: Abnormalities in structure and expression of the human retinoblastoma gene in SCLC. Science 241:353–357, 1988.

65. Yokota J, Wada M, Shimosato Y, Terada M, Sugimura T: Loss of heterozygosity on chromosomes 3, 13, and 17 in small-cell carcinoma and on chromosome 3 in adenocarcinoma of the lung. Proc Natl Acad Sci USA 84:9252–9256, 1987.

66. Takahashi T, Nau MM, Chiba I, Birrer MJ, Rosenberg RK, Vinocour M, Levitt M, Pass H, Gazdar AF, Minna JD: p53: A frequent target for genetic abnormalities in lung cancer. Science 246:491–494, 1989.

67. Nigro JM, Baker SJ, Preisinger AC, Jessup JM, Hostetter R, Cleary K, Bigner SH, Davidson N, Baylin S, Devilee P, Glover T, Collins FS, Weston A, Modali R, Harris CC, Vogelstein B: Mutations in the *p53* gene occur in diverse human tumour types. Nature 342:705–708, 1989.

68. Kaufman RJ, Brown PC, Schimke RT: Amplified dihydrofolate reductase genes in unstably methotrexate-resistant cells are associated with double minute chromosomes. Proc Natl Acad Sci USA 76:5669–5673, 1979.

69. Lin CC, Alitalo K, Schwab M, George D, Varmus HE, Bishop JM: Evolution of karyotypic abnormalities and c-*myc* oncogene amplification in human colonic carcinoma cell lines. Chromosoma 92:11–15, 1985.

70. Little CD, Nau MM, Carney DN, Gazdar AF, Minna JD: Amplification and expression of the c-*myc* oncogene in human lung cancer cell lines. Nature 306:194–196, 1983.

71. Nau MM, Brooks BJ, Battey J, Sausville E, Gazdar AF, Kirsch IR, McBride OW, Bertness V, Hollis GF, Minna JD: L-*myc*, a new *myc*-related gene amplified and expressed in human small cell lung cancer. Nature 318:69–73, 1985.

72. Nau MM, Brooks BJ, Carney DN, Gazdar AF, Battey JF, Sausville EA, Minna JD: Human small-cell lung cancers show amplification and expression of the N-*myc* gene. Proc Natl Acad Sci USA 83:1092–1096, 1986.

73. Wong AJ, Ruppert JM, Eggleston J, Hamilton SR, Baylin SB, Vogelstein B: Gene amplification of c-*myc* and N-*myc* in small cell carcinoma of the lung. Science 233:461–464, 1986.

74. Brennan J, O'Connor T, Makuch RW, Simmons AM, Russell E, Linnoila RI, Phelps RM, Gazdar AF, Ihde DC, Johnson BE: *myc* Family DNA amplification in 107 tumors and tumor cell lines from patients with small cell lung cancer treated with different combination chemotherapy regimens. Cancer Res 51:1708–1712, 1991.

75. Elfving P, Lundgren R, Cigudosa JCC, Heim S, Mandahl N, Mitelman F: Trisomy 7 in nonneoplastic kidney tissue cultured with and without epidermal growth factor. Cancer Genet Cytogenet 64:99, 100, 1992.

76. Elfving P, Cigudosa JC, Lundgren R, Limon J, Mandahl N, Kristoffersson U, Heim S, Mitelman F: Trisomy 7, trisomy 10, and loss of the Y chromosome in short-term cultures of normal kidney tissue. Cytogenet Cell Genet 53:123–125, 1990.

77. Dal Cin P, Aly MS, Delabie J, Ceuppens JL, Van Gool S, Van Damme B, Baert L, Van Poppel H, Van den Berghe H: Trisomy 7 and trisomy 10 characterize subpopulations of tumor-infiltrating lymphocytes in kidney tumors and in the surrounding kidney tissue. Proc Natl Acad Sci USA 89:9744–9748, 1992.

78. Pejovic T, Heim S, Mandahl N, Elmfors B, Floderus UM, Furgyik S, Helm G, Willen H, Mitelman F: Trisomy 12 is a consistent chromosomal aberration in benign ovarian tumors. Genes Chromosom Cancer 2:48–52, 1990.

79. Siegfried JM, Ellison DJ, Resau JH, Miura I, Testa JR: Correlation of modal chromosome number of cultured non-small cell lung carcinomas with DNA index of solid tumor tissue. Cancer Res 51:3267–3273, 1991.

80. Siegfried JM, Hunt JD, Zhou J-Y, Keller SM, Testa JR: Cytogenetic abnormalities in non-small cell lung carcinoma: similarity of findings in conventional and feeder cell layer cultures. Genes Chromosom Cancer 6:30–38, 1993.

81. Tsuchiya E, Nakamura Y, Weng S-Y, Nakagawa K, Tsuchiya S, Sugano H, Kitagawa T: Allelotype of non-small cell lung cancer—comparison between loss of heterozygosity in squamous cell carcinoma and adenocarcinoma. Cancer Res 52:2478–2481, 1992.
82. Sato S, Nakamura Y, Tsuchiya E: Difference of allelotype between squamous cell carcinoma and adenocarcinoma of the lung. Cancer Res 54: 5652–5655, 1994.
83. Weston A, Willey JC, Modali R, Sugimura H, McDowell EM, Resau J, Light B, Haugen A, Mann DL, Trump BF, Harris CC: Differential DNA sequence deletions from chromosomes 3, 11, 13, and 17 in squamous-cell carcinoma, large-cell carcinoma, and adenocarcinoma of the human lung. Proc Natl Acad Sci USA 86:5099–5103, 1989.
84. Rabbitts P, Douglas J, Daly M, Sundaresan V, Fox B, Haselton P, Wells F, Albertson D, Waters J, Bergh J: Frequency and extent of allelic loss in the short arm of chromosome 3 in nonsmall-cell lung cancer. Genes Chromosom Cancer 1:95–105, 1989.
85. Viallet J, Minna JD: Dominant oncogenes and tumor suppressor genes in the pathogenesis of lung cancer. Am J Respir Cell Mol Biol 2:225–232, 1990.
86. Olopade OI, Buchhagen DL, Malik K, Sherman J, Nobori T, Bader S, Nau MM, Gazdar AF, Minna JD, Diaz MO: Homozygous loss of the interferon genes defines the critical region on 9p that is deleted in lung cancers. Cancer Res 53:2410–2415, 1993.
87. Kamb A, Gruis NA, Weaver-Feldhaus J, Liu Q, Harshman K, Tavtigian SV, Stockert E, Day RS III, Johnson BE, Skolnick MH: A cell cycle regulator potentially involved in genesis of many tumor types. Science 246: 436–440, 1994.
88. Nobori T, Miura K, Wu DJ, Lois A, Takabayashi K, Carson DA: Deletions of the cyclin-dependent kinase-4 inhibitor gene in multiple human cancers. Nature 368:753–756, 1994.
89. Washimi O, Nagatake M, Osada H, Ueda R, Koshikawa T, Seki T, Takahashi T, Takahashi T: In vivo occurrence of *p16 (MTS1)* and *p15 (MTS2)* alterations preferentially in non-small cell lung cancers. Cancer Res 55:514–517, 1995.
90. Shapiro GI, Edwards CD, Kobzik L, Godleski J, Richards W, Sugarbaker DJ, Rollins BJ, Reciprocal *Rb* inactivation and *p16INK4* expression in primary lung cancers and cell lines. Cancer Res 55:505–509, 1995.
91. Miura I, Resau J, Tomiyasu T, Testa JR: Isochromosome (8q) in four patients with adenocarcinoma of the lung. Cancer Genet Cytogenet 48:203–207, 1990.
92. Yokota J, Wada M, Yoshida T, Noguchi M, Terasaki T, Shimosato Y, Sugimura T, Terada M: Heterogeneity of lung cancer cells with respect to the amplification and rearrangement of *myc* family oncogenes. Oncogene 2:607–611, 1988.
93. Gemma A, Nakajima T, Shiraishi M, Noguchi M, Gotoh M, Sekiya T, Niitani H, Shimosato Y: *myc* family gene abnormality in lung cancers and its relation to xenotransplantability. Cancer Res 48:6025–6028, 1988.

94. Miyaki M, Sato C, Matsui T, Koike M, Mori T, Kosaki G, Takai S, Tonomura A, Tsuchida N: Amplification and enhanced expression of cellular oncogene c-Ki-*ras*-2 in a human epidermoid carcinoma of the lung. Jpn J Cancer Res (Gann) 76:260–265, 1985.

95. Cremer T, Tesin D, Hopman AHN, Manuelidis L: Rapid interphase and metaphase assessment of specific chromosomal changes in neuroectodermal tumor cells by *in situ* hybridization with chemically modified DNA probes. Exp Cell Res 176:199, 200, 1988.

96. van Dekken H, Pizzolo JG, Kelsen DP, Melamed MR: Targeted cytogenetic analysis of gastric tumors by *in situ* hybridization with a set of chromosome-specific DNA probes. Cancer 66:491–497, 1990.

97. Devilee P, Thierry RF, Kievits T, Kolluri R, Hopman AHN, Willard HF, Pearson PL, Cornelisse CJ: Detection of chromosome aneuploidy in interphase nuclei from human primary breast tumors using chromosome-specific repetitive DNA probes. Cancer Res 48:5825–5830, 1988.

98. Hopman AHN, Poddighe PJ, Smeets AW, Moesker O, Beck JLM, Vooijs GP, Ramaekers FCS: Detection of numerical chromosome aberrations in bladder cancer by *in situ* hybridization. Am J Pathol 135:1105–1117, 1989.

99. Waldman FM, Carroll PR, Kerschmann R, Cohen MB, Field FG, Mayall BH: Centromeric copy number of chromosome 7 is strongly correlated with tumor grade and labeling index in human bladder cancer. Cancer Res 51:3807–3813, 1991.

100. Arnoldus EPJ, Noordermeer IA, Peters ACB, Voormolen JHC, Bots GTAM, Rapp AK, van der Ploeg M: Interphase cytogenetics of brain tumors. Genes Chromosom Cancer 3:101–107, 1991.

101. Baretton GB, Valina C, Vogt T, Schneiderbanger K, Diebold J, Löhrs U: Interphase cytogenetic analysis of prostatic carcinomas by use of nonisotopic *in situ* hybridization. Cancer Res 54:4472–4480, 1994.

102. Neubauer S, Liehr T, Tulusan HA, Gebhart E: Interphase cytogenetics by FISH on archival paraffin material and cultured cells on human ovarian tumors. Int J Oncol 4:317–321, 1994.

103. Shah NK, Currie JL, Rosenshein N, Campbell J, Long P, Abbas F, Griffin CA: Cytogenetic and FISH analysis of endometrial carcinoma. Cancer Genet Cytogenet 73:142–146, 1995.

104. Wolman SR, Waldman FM, Balazs M: Complementarity of interphase and metaphase chromosome analysis in human renal tumors. Genes Chromosom Cancer 6:17–23, 1993.

105. El-Naggar AK, van Dekken HD, Ensign LG, Pathak S: Interphase cytogenetics in paraffin-embedded sections from renal cortical neoplasms. Cancer Genet Cytogenet 73:134–141, 1994.

106. Rodriquez E, Mathew S, Mukherjee AB, Reuter VE, Bosl GJ, Chaganti RSK: Analysis of chromosome 12 aneuploidy in interphase cells from human male germ cell tumors by fluorescence in situ hybridization. Genes Chromosom Cancer 5:21–29, 1992.

107. Kim SY, Lee KJ, Hong SC, Han PS, Lee JJ, Cho HJ, Kim AK, Kim JO, Lee MS: Interphase cytogenetics of lung tumors using *in situ* hybridization: numerical aberrations. Korean J Intern Med 9:55–60, 1994.

108. Kallioniemi A, Kallioniemi O-P, Sudar D, Rutovitz D, Gray JW, Waldman F, Pinkel D: Comparative genomic hybridization for molecular cytogenetic analysis of solid tumors. Science 258:818–821, 1992.

109. du Manoir S, Speicher MR, Joos S, Schrock E, Popp S, Dohner H, Kovacs G, Robert-Nicoud M, Lichter P, Cremer T: Detection of complete and partial chromosome gains and losses by comparative genomic *in situ* hybridization. Hum Genet 90:590–610, 1993.

110. Ried T, Petersen I, Holtgreve-Grez H, Speicher MR, Schrock E, du Manoir S, Cremer T: Mapping of multiple DNA gains and losses in primary small cell lung carcinomas by comparative genomic hybridization. Cancer Res 54:1801–1806, 1994.

111. Cher ML, MacGrogan D, Bookstein R, Brown JA, Jenkins RB, Jensen RH: Comparative genomic hybridization, allelic imbalance, and fluorescence *in situ* hybridization on chromosome 8 in prostate cancer. Genes Chromosome Cancer 11:153–162, 1994.

112. Visakorpi T, Kallioniemi AH, Syvanen AC, Hyytinen ER, Karhu R, Tammela T, Isola JJ, Kallioniemi O-P: Genetic changes in primary and recurrent prostate cancer by comparative genomic hybridization. Cancer Res 55:342–347, 1995.

113. Levin NA, Brzoska P, Gupta N, Minna JD, Gray JW, Christman MF: Identification of frequent novel genetic alterations in small cell lung carcinoma. Cancer Res 54:5086–5091, 1994.

114. Speicher MR, Schoell B, du Manoir S, Schrock E, Ried T, Cremer T, Storkel S, Kovacs A, Kovacs G: Specific loss of chromosomes 1, 2, 6, 10, 13, 17, and 21 in chromophobe renal cell carcinomas revealed by comparative genomic hybridization. Am J Pathol 145:356–364, 1994.

115. Kallioniemi A, Kallioniemi O-P, Citro G, Sauter G, DeVries S, Kerschmann R, Caroll P, Waldman F: Identification of gains and losses of DNA sequences in primary bladder cancer by comparative genomic hybridization. Genes Chromosom Cancer 12:213–219, 1995.

116. Kallioniemi A, Kallioniemi O-P, Piper J, Tanner M, Stokke T, Chen L, Smith HS, Pinkel D, Gray JW, Waldman FM: Detection and mapping of amplified DNA sequences in breast cancer by comparative genomic hybridization. Proc Natl Acad Sci USA 91:2156–2160, 1994.

117. Visakorpi T, Hyytinen E, Koivisto P, Tanner M, Keinanen R, Palmberg C, Palotie A, Tammela T, Isola J, Kallioniemi OP: In vivo amplification of the androgen receptor gene and progression of human prostate cancer. Nature Genet 9:401–406, 1995.

118. Tanner MM, Tirkkonen M, Kallioniemi A, Collins C, Stokke T, Karhu R, Kowbel D, Shadravan F, Hintz M, Kuo W-L, Waldman FM, Isola JJ, Gray JW, Kallioniemi O-P: Increased copy number at 20q13 in breast cancer: defining the critical region and exclusion of candidate genes. Cancer Res 54:4257–4260, 1994.

119. Sabiston DC: Carcinoma of the lung. In: Sabiston DC, Spencer FC (eds), Surgery of the Chest. Philadelphia: Saunders, pp. 554–576, 1990.

120. Giedl J, Hohenberger W, Meister R: The pTNM-classification of carcinomas of the lung and its prognostic significance. Thorac Cardiovasc Surg 31:71–75, 1983.

121. Rice TW, Bauer TW, Gephardt GN, Medendorp SV, McLain DA, Kirby TJ: Prognostic significance of flow cytometry in non-small-cell-lung cancer. J Thorac Cardiovasc Surg 106:210–217, 1993.

122. Mountain CF. Assessment of the role of surgery for control of lung cancer. Ann Thorac Surgery 24:365–373, 1977.

123. Cornelisse CJ, van de Velde CJH, Caspers RJC, Moolenaar AJ, Hermans J: DNA ploidy and survival in breast cancer patients. Cytometry 8:225–234, 1987.

124. Friedlander ML, Hedley DW, Tayler IW, Russel P, Coates AS, Tattersall MHN: Influence of cellular DNA content on survival in advanced ovarian cancer. Cancer Res 44:397–400, 1984.

125. Gustafson H, Tribukait B, Esposti PL: The prognostic value of DNA analysis in primary carcinoma *in situ* of the urinary bladder. Scand J Urol Nephrol 16:141–146, 1982.

126. Wolley RC, Schreiber K, Koss LG, Karas M, Sherman A: DNA distribution in human colon carcinomas and its relationship to clinical behavior. J Natl Cancer Inst 69:15–22, 1982.

127. Volm M, Drings P, Mattern J, Sonka J, Vogt-Moykopf I, Wayss K: Prognostic significance of DNA patterns and resistance-predictive tests in non-small cell lung carcinoma. Cancer 56:1396–1403, 1985.

128. Tirindelli-Danesi D, Teodori L, Mauro F, Modini C, Botti C, Cicconetti F, Stipa S: Prognostic significance of flow cytometry in lung cancer. Cancer 60:844–851, 1987.

129. Zimmerman PV, Hawson GAT, Bint MH, Parsons PG: Ploidy as a prognostic determinant in surgically treated lung cancer. Lancet 2:530–533, 1987.

130. Asamura H, Nakajima T, Mukai K, Shimosato Y: Nuclear DNA content by cytofluorometry of stage I adenocarcinoma of the lung in relation to postoperative recurrence. Chest 96:312–318, 1989.

131. Salvati F, Teodori L, Gagliardi L, Signora M, Aquilini M, Storniello G: DNA flow cytometric studies of 66 human lung tumors analyzed before treatment. Prognostic implications. Chest 96:1092–1098, 1989.

132. Dazzi H, Thatcher N, Hasleton PS, Swindell R: DNA analysis by flow cytometry in nonsmall cell lung cancer: relationship to epidermal growth factor receptor, histology, tumor stage and survival. Respir Med 84: 217–223, 1990.

133. Isobe H, Miyamoto H, Shimizu T, Haneda H, Hashimoto M, Inoue K, Mizuno S, Kawakami Y: Prognostic and therapeutic significance of the flow cytometric nuclear DNA content in non-small cell lung cancer. Cancer 65:1391–1395, 1990.

134. Sahin AA, Ro JY, El-Naggar AK, Lee JS, Ayala AG, Teague K, Hong WK: Flow cytometric analysis of the DNA content of non-small cell lung cancer: ploidy as a significant prognostic indicator in squamous cell carcinoma of the lung. Cancer 65:530–537, 1990.

135. Ogawa J-I, Tsurumi T, Inoue H, Shohtsu A: Relationship between tumor DNA ploidy and regional lymph node changes in lung cancer. Cancer 69:1688–1695, 1992.

136. Bunn, PA Jr, Carney DN, Gazdar AF, Whang-Peng J, Matthews MJ: Diagnostic and biological implications of flow cytometric DNA content analysis in lung cancer. Cancer Res 43:5026–5032, 1983.

137. Ten Velde GPM, Schutte B, Vermeulen A, Volovics A, Reynders MMJ, Blijham GH: Flow cytometric analysis of DNA ploidy level in paraffin-embedded tissue of non-small-cell lung cancer. Eur J Cancer Clin Oncol 24:455–460, 1988.

138. Cibas ES, Melamed MR, Zaman MB, Kimmel M: The effect of tumor size and tumor cell DNA content on the survival of patients with stage I adenocarcinoma of the lung. Cancer 63:1552–1556, 1989.

139. van Bodegom PC, Baak JPA, Stroet-van Galen C, Schipper NW, Wisse-Brekelmans ECM, Vanderschueren RGJRA, Wagenaar SSC: The percentage of aneuploid cells is significantly correlated with survival in accurately staged patients with stage I resected squamous cell lung cancer and long-term follow up. Cancer 63:143–147, 1989.

140. Carp NZ, Ellison DD, Brophy PF, Watts P, Chang M-C, Keller SM: DNA content in correlation with postsurgical stage in non-small cell lung cancer. Ann Thorac Surg 53:680–683, 1992.

141. Schmidt RA, Rusch VW, Piantadosi S: A flow cytometric study of non-small cell lung cancer classified as T1N0. Cancer 69:78–85, 1992.

142. Crissman JD, Zarbo RJ, Niebylski CD, Corbett T, Weaver D: Flow cytometric DNA analysis of colon adenocarcinomas: a comparative study of preparatory techniques. Mod Pathol 1:198–204, 1988.

143. Vogelstein B, Fearon ER, Hamilton SR, Kern SE, Preisinger AC, Leppert M, Nakamura Y, White R, Smits AMM, Bos JL: Genetic alterations during colorectal tumor development. N Engl J Med 319:525–532, 1988.

144. Fearon ER, Vogelstein B: A genetic model for colorectal tumorigenesis. Cell 61:759–767, 1990.

145. Johnson B, Brennan JF, Ihde DC, Gazdar AF: *myc* Family DNA amplification in tumors and tumor cell lines from patients with small cell lung cancer. J Natl Cancer Inst Monogr 13:39–43, 1992.

146. Rodenhuis S, Slebos RJC, Boot AJM, Evers SG, Mooi WJ, Wagenaar S-S, Van Bodegom PC, Bos JLP: Incidence and possible clinical significance of K-*ras* oncogene activation in adenocarcinoma of the human lung. Cancer Res 48:5738–5741, 1988.

147. Suzuki Y, Orita M, Shiraishi M, Hayashi K, Sekiya T: Detection of *ras* gene mutations in human lung cancers by single-strand conformation polymorphism analysis of polymerase chain reaction products. Oncogene 5: 1037–1043, 1990.

148. Tateishi M, Ishida T, Mitsudomi T, Kaneko S, Sugimachi K: Prognostic value of c-*erb*B-2 protein expression in human lung adenocarcinoma and squamous cell carcinoma. Eur J Cancer 27:1372–1375, 1991.

149. Pezzella F, Turley H, Kuzu I, Tungekar MF, Dunnill MS, Pierce CB, Harris A, Gatter KC, Mason DY: *Bcl-2* protein in non-small cell lung carcinoma. N Engl J Med 329:690–694, 1993.

150. Fontanini G, Vignati S, Bigini D, Mussi A, Lucchi M, Angeletti CA, Basolo F, Bevilacqua G: Bcl-2 protein: a prognostic factor inversely correlated to p53 in non-small-cell lung cancer. Br J Cancer 71:1003–1007, 1995.

151. Fong KM, Zimmerman PV, Smith PJ: Tumor progression and loss of heterozygosity at 5q and 18q in non-small cell lung cancer. Cancer Res 55:220–223, 1995.

152. Lehman TA, Bennett WP, Metcalf RA, Welsh JA, Ecker J, Modali RV, Ullrich S, Romano JW, Appella E, Testa JR, Gerwin BI, Harris CC: *p53* Mutations, *ras* mutations, and p53-heat shock 70 protein complexes in human lung carcinoma cell lines. Cancer Res 51:4090–4096, 1991.

153. D'Amico D, Carbone D, Mitsudomi T, Nau M, Fedorko J, Russell E, Johnson B, Buchhagen D, Bodner S, Phelps R, Gazdar A, Minna JD: High frequency of somatically acquired p53 mutations in small-cell lung cancer cell lines and tumors. Oncogene 7:339–346, 1992.

154. Carbone DP, Mitsudomi T, Chiba I, Piantadosi S, Rusch V, Nowak JA, McIntire D, Slamon D, Gazdar A, Minna J: p53 Immunostaining positivity is associated with reduced survival and is imperfectly correlated with gene mutations in resected non-small cell lung cancer. Chest 106: 377S–381S, 1994.

155. Chiba I, Takahashi T, Nau MM, D'Amico D, Curiel DT, Mitsudomi T, Buchhagen DL, Carbone D, Piantadosi S, Koga H, Reissman P, Slamon D, Holmes E, Minna J: Mutations in the *p53* gene are frequent in primary, resected non-small cell lung cancer. Oncogene 5:1603–1610, 1990.

156. Suzuki H, Takahashi T, Kuroishi T, Suyama M, Ariyoshi Y, Takahashi T, Ueda R: *p53* mutations in non-small cell lung cancer in Japan: association between mutations and smoking. Cancer Res 52:734–736, 1992.

157. Quinlan DC, Davidson AG, Summers CL, Warden HE, Doshi HM: Accumulation of p53 protein correlates with a poor prognosis in human lung cancer. Cancer Res 52:4828–4831, 1992.

158. Horio Y, Takahashi T, Kuroishi T, Hibi K, Suyama M, Niimi T, Shimokata K, Yamakawa Y, Nakamura Y, Ueda R, Takahashi T: Prognostic significance of *p53* mutations and 3p deletions in primary resected non-small cell lung cancer. Cancer Res 53:1–4, 1993.

159. Ebina M, Steinberg SM, Mulshine JL, Linnoila RI: Relationship of *p53* overexpression and up-regulation of proliferating cell nuclear antigen with the clinical course of non-small cell lung cancer. Cancer Res 54:2496–2503, 1994.

160. Mitsudomi T, Oyama T, Kusano T, Osaki T, Nakanishi R, Shirakusa T: Mutations of the *p53* gene as a predictor of poor prognosis in patients with non-small-cell lung cancer. J Nat Cancer Inst 85:2018–2023, 1993.

161. Passlick B, Izbicki JR, Haussinger K, Thetter O, Pantel K: Immunohistochemical detection of P53 protein is not associated with a poor prognosis in non-small-cell lung cancer. J Thorac Cardiovasc Surg 109:1205–1211, 1995.

162. Morkve O, Halvorsen OJ, Stangeland L, Gulsvik A, Laerum OD: Quantitation of biological tumor markers (p53, c-*myc*, Ki-67 and DNA

ploidy) by multiparameter flow cytometry in non-small-cell lung cancer. Int J Cancer 52:851–855, 1992.

163. Reynolds SH, Anna CK, Brown KC, Wiest JS, Beattie EJ, Pero RW, Iglehart D, Ander son MW: Activated protooncogenes in human lung tumors from smokers. Proc Natl Acad Sci USA 88:1085–1089, 1991.

164. Selbos RJC, Kibbelaar RE, Dalesio O, Kooistra A, Stam J, Meijer CJLM, Wagenaar SS, Vanderschueren RGJRA, van Zandwijk N, Mooi WJ, Bos JL, Rodenhuis S: K-*RAS* oncogene activation as a prognostic marker in adeno-carcinoma of the lung. N Engl J Med 323:561–565, 1990.

165. Mitsudomi T, Steinberg SM, Oie HK, Mulshine JL, Phelps R, Viallet J, Pass H, Minna JD, Gazdar AF: *ras* Gene mutations in non-small cell lung cancers are associated with shortened survival irrespective of treatment intent. Cancer Res 51:4999–5002, 1991.

166. Rodenhuis S, Slebos RJC: Clinical significance of *ras* oncogene activation in human lung cancer. Cancer Res 52:2665S–2669S, 1992.

167. Slamon DJ, Clark GM, Wong SG, Levin WJ, Ullrich A, McGuire WL: Human breast cancer: correlation between relapse and survival with ampli-fication of the *HER-2/neu* oncogene. Science 235:177–182, 1987.

168. Wright C, Angus B, Nicholson S, Sainsbury RC, Cairns J, Gullick WJ, Kelly P, Harris AL, Wilson Horne CH: Expression of c-*erb*B-2 oncoprotein: a prognostic indicator in human breast cancer. Cancer Res 49:2087–2090, 1989.

169. Tsuda H, Hirohashi S, Shimosato Y, Tanaka Y, Hirota T, Tsugane S, Shiraishi M, Toyoshima K, Yamamoto T, Terada M, Sugimura T: Immunohistochemical study on overexpression of c-*erb*B-2 protein in human breast cancer: its correlation with gene amplification and long-term survival of patients. Jpn J Cancer Res 81:327–332, 1990.

170. Kern JA, Schwartz DA, Nordberg JE, Weiner DB, Greene MI, Torney L, Robinson RA: p185[neu] Expression in human lung adenocarcinomas predicts shortened survival. Cancer Res 50:5184–5191, 1990.

171. Kern JA, Slebos RJ, Top B, Rodenhuis S, Lager D, Robinson RA, Weiner D, Schwartz DA: c-*erb*B-2 Expression and codon 12 K-*ras* mutations both pre-dict shortened survival for patients with pulmonary adenocarcinomas. J Clin Invest 93:516–520, 1994.

172. Tsujimoto Y, Finger LR, Yunis J, Nowell PC, Croce CM: Cloning of the chromosome breakpoint of neoplastic B cells with the t(14;18) chromosome translocation. Science 226:1097–1099, 1984.

173. Cleary ML, Smith SD, Sklar J: Cloning and structural analysis of cDNAs for *bcl*-2 and a hybrid *bcl*-2/immunoglobulin transcript resulting from the t(14;18) translocation. Cell 47:19–28, 1986.

174. Johnson BE, Ihde DC, Makuch RW, Gazdar AF, Carney DN, Oie H, Russell E, Nau MM, Minna JD: *myc* Family oncogene amplification in tumor cell lines established from small cell lung cancer patients and its rela-tionship to clinical status and course. J Clin Invest 79:1629–1634, 1986.

175. Lukeis RE: Characterisation and significance of chromosome abnormal-ities in non-small cell lung cancer. Thesis. University of Melbourne, p. 150, 1994.

Chapter 12

Cytogenetic Biomarkers in Skin Cancer

Maria J. Worsham, S. David Nathanson, Min Lee, and Sandra R. Wolman

Introduction

Definition of Cell Types

Skin is one of the largest vital organs, covering the human body. The skin is embryologically derived from ectoderm and mesoderm. Epithelial structures emanate from the ectoderm, nerves and melanocytes from the neuroectoderm, and the mesenchymal component from the mesoderm. The skin consists of three layers: a resistant and impermeable outermost layer known as the epidermis; a tough, durable but porous, connective tissue layer called the dermis; and a soft, lipid-rich, deep layer, the subcutis. The cutaneous adnexa (hair follicles, sweat glands) complement the basic function of the skin.

The epidermis is composed of stratified squamous epithelium derived from surface ectoderm. Growth of the epidermis originates from the basal layer; and the next, spinous layer as cells move upward is noted for its complex intercellular bridges. The permeability barrier is established in the next outer, granular layer, and epidermal cells are shed in the outermost cornified layer.

The replication of keratinocytes that occurs in the 1-cell-thick basal layer is in balance with desquamation to maintain normal

From: *Human Cytogenetic Cancer Markers* Edited by S. R. Wolman and S. Sell
Humana Press Inc., Totowa, NJ

thickness of the epidermis *(1)*. Not all cells in the lower epidermis or in the basal layer are mitotically active; 3–5% of basal keratinocytes synthesize DNA at any given time, but only 0–1% of cells are in mitosis. In general, one daughter cell of every cell division leaves the basal layer to differentiate. Even though the mechanism for this emigration is not entirely clear, some evidence implicates active cell motility. It takes approx 30 d for a cell to reach the granular layer from the basal layer, and another 14 d to transit the stratum corneum and desquamate *(2)*. In addition to the keratinocytes, which play the central role in epidermal structure, melanocytes, Merkel cells, and Langerhans cells are also present in the epidermis and contribute to epidermal function.

Many hamartomatous and benign or malignant neoplastic proliferations in the skin show different directions of differentiation, which can be categorized as epidermal, adnexal, and mesenchymal tumors. Many of these tumors are familial, although their modes of transmission are poorly understood.

The Genetic Basis of Cancer

Cancer results from transformation of a normal to a malignant cell, as a consequence of genetic damage as a result of nonlethal mutations of cellular genes. Acquisition of a fully malignant phenotype by normal cells is thought to occur as a result of multiple steps. These steps are usually viewed in terms of "initiation" and "progression," where the important targets of genetic damage are the growth-promoting oncogenes and the growth-inhibiting cancer suppressor genes *(3)*. In a few of the well-characterized neoplasms such as colorectal cancer, at least four mutations appear to be required for transition of normal cells to frank carcinoma. Mutations are attributable to exogenous and endogenous carcinogenic factors, including certain chemicals, radiation, and viruses, or to genetic alteration inherited through the germ line. Cytogenetics lies at the heart of the detection process that pinpoints genetic targets associated with specific cancers. It serves as a homing device, pointing to individual chromosomes and chromosomal bands and permitting resolution down to a region of 2 to 3 million basepairs, which is the smallest deletion visible in the light microscope *(4)*. The resolution gap between cytogenetic techniques and molecular analysis is being bridged by *in situ* hybridization *(5)* and other new methods; *see* Chapters 3 and 4.

Squamous Cell Carcinoma (SCC)

SCC is the most common histologic type of cancer affecting the human body, originating in more anatomical sites than any other form of tumor. It is the common cancer of the lip, oral cavity, pharynx, larynx, bronchi, esophagus, anus, vulva, vagina, cervix, urethra, and penis, and is found occasionally in the bladder and renal pelvis. SCC is often an aggressive cancer; of the 50,000–100,000 new cases each year in the United States, it causes death in more than 50% of the affected individuals *(6)*. SCC comprises 90% of head and neck cancers, the majority of tumors of the esophagus and tracheo-bronchial tree, and 70–90% of cancers of the vulva, vagina, and uterine cervix. It accounts for 20% of skin cancers (approx 79% are basal cell carcinomas and 1% melanomas); and it is important to remember that cancer of the skin, unlike other SCC, is influenced by exposure to sunlight.

In many white populations, nonmelanoma skin cancer of all types is the most common human malignancy *(7–9)*. Precursor lesions of SCC commonly include actinic (caused by short-wavelength—violet, UV, and X—irradiation) keratoses and, less commonly, Bowen's disease of the penis. Although SCCs show some similarities to basal cell carcinoma (BCC), they manifest marked differences in clinical and biologic features *(7,8)*. In the inherited skin-lesion syndromes, such as nevoid BCC (characterized by multiple BCCs) and the Ferguson-Smith syndrome (characterized by multiple self-healing SCCs), progression from *in situ* lesions to invasive tumors occurs at a fairly high rate, as does spontaneous regression of these lesions *(10)*.

Cytogenetic Studies of Neoplastic and Nonneoplastic Cells of the Skin

Few groups have investigated the cytogenetic changes in squamous cells. Cytogenetic studies of 80 short-term cultures of epithelial skin tumors and 27 nonneoplastic skin samples have not yielded consistent patterns of chromosome rearrangements. Of 20 nonneoplastic skin samples that were karyotyped, six skin biopsies were taken from sun-exposed areas, whereas 14 came from other locations *(11)*. Clonal rearrangements were observed in two of the six exposed nonneoplastic sites. None of the nonexposed areas showed clonal aberrations. Nonclonal aberrations, usually in pseudodiploid cells, were present in both exposed and nonexposed sites, and the frequencies of these aberrations were 9 and 3%, respectively. Similarly, of seven samples of nonneoplastic pharyngeal mucosa *(11)*, only one had clonal aberrations, with nonclonal aberrations present in all. A more recent study of eight nonneoplastic skin lesions *(12)* demonstrated nonclonal aberrations in all but one case, with an average of 17% of the cells exhibiting nonclonal anomalies. Thus, both groups found predominantly nonclonal aberrations in the nonneoplastic lesions studied.

The neoplastic skin lesions (six SCCs *in situ*, five keratoacanthomas, and five papillomata) *(11)* revealed clonal aberrations in six of the 16 lesions, with a high frequency of nonclonal aberrations. Sixty-four skin tumors karyotyped from short-term cultures *(11)* showed mainly nonclonal populations similar to those of nonneoplastic skin lesions, and, therefore, perhaps not representative of the tumors. Small pseudodiploid clones with balanced structural rearrangements and a high frequency of cells with nonclonal abnormalities were evident in the skin tumors. Structural rearrangements were somewhat more common in tumor-derived cultures than in those from nonneoplastic biopsies.

Fibroblast cultures established from nonneoplastic skin have demonstrated nonclonal aberrations in a low percentage of cells in connection with chromosome instability analyses *(13–17)*. In fibroblast cultures from patients with inherited disorders predisposing to cancer, such as Werner's syndrome, porokeratosis of Mibelli, and Gorlin syndrome *(18–21a)*, and in cultures approaching senescence *(22)*, increased levels of both nonclonal and clonal aberrations have been detected. Skin fibroblasts exposed to extensive radiation also display an increased number of structural aberrations, with persistence of these rearrangements for several years, accompanied by clonal expansion in some cases *(23–25)*.

Cytogenetic Studies at Noncutaneous Sites

Consistent clonal chromosomal abnormalities have been reported in SCC from sites other than skin. In a study of 15 patients with Barrett's esophagus (metaplasia of the stratified squamous epithelium), clonal loss of the Y chromosome was detected in seven cases and another had a balanced t(3;6) as the only aberration in 20% of the cells analyzed *(26)*. An evaluation of 14 primary explants and cell lines originating from *esophageal* SCCs found common rearrangements of chromosomes 1, 3, 9, and 11, usually resulting in deletions *(27)*. Breakpoints commonly involved 1p34-pter, 3p13, 11q11–q12, 9q11–q12, and the acrocentric centromere regions. An hsr(11)(q12) was observed in three lines. A description of the karyotypes of seven lung SCCs in short-term culture revealed hypotriploid modal numbers, and the common changes were loss of Y, 3p, 5p, 5q, 8p, 10p, and 13, and gain of 1q, 3q, and 7q *(28)*. (A more comprehensive review of lung cancer findings is presented in Chapter 11 of this volume.) We identified several consistent chromosome abnormalities in SCC of the vulva *(29)*. Recurrent losses of chromosome segments included 3p14-cen, 8pter-p11, 22q13.1–q13.2, and the short arm of the inactive X; common chromosome gains involved region 3q25-qter and band 11q21. Recurrent rearrangement breakpoints at 4q31.1–q35 and 5cen-q11.2 probably result in disruption of function. Thus, regions of 3p, 4q, 5q, 8p, 22q, and Xp appear to harbor genes that may be lost in SCC. The regions of gain within 3q and 11q may harbor oncogenes that, when amplified, contribute to the genesis and development of SCC.

Many studies have focused on the clinically important problem of SCC of the head and neck (HNSCC), which encompasses tumors of the oropharynx, larynx, and pyriform sinus. Heo et al. *(30)* reported that 16 HNSCC lines from 13 subjects had an average modal number of 70 for cell lines representing the primary site, but that the mode for cell lines originating from metastatic or recurrent tumors was only 54 chromosomes. Loss of 3p and trisomy 6 were observed in 12 lines each. Jin and coworkers *(31–38)* employed short-term cultures to karyotype 31 HNSCCs. They noted breakpoints at 1p22 in eight tumors and at 11q13 in nine tumors, apparently separating HNSCCs into separate cytogenetic groups based on these breakpoints. An hsr at 11q13 was identified in two cases, and trisomy 7 and loss and gain of the Y were recurring numerical changes. Up to 12 unrelated and cytogenetically abnormal clones were identified in 9 of 31 tumors.

Studies from our laboratory *(39)* characterized the breakpoints, gains, and losses of chromosome material in HNSCC from 29 patients. Karyotypes in one-third of cases were derived from cell lines; in another one-third they were based on direct preparations or early in vitro harvests; and the remaining cases were analyzed from both sources. Some tumors were near diploid and others near tetraploid, but many had mixed populations with diploid, tetraploid, and octoploid subclones representing essentially the same karyotypic pattern. The most frequent changes were deletions. Losses affecting 3p13–p24, 5q12–q23, 8p22–p23, 9p21–p24, and 18q22–q23 were observed in 40–60% of tumors. Loss of the short arm of the inactive X occurred in 70% of tumors from female patients, and loss or rearrangement of the Y occurred in 74% of tumors from male patients. Loss of 18q appeared to be associated with short survival, as did the presence of multiple deletions. Gains (two to five extra copies) of 3q21-qter, 5p, 7p, 8q, and 11q13–q23 were found in 28–38% of tumors. Three tumors had an hsr involving 11q13–q21.

Molecular Genetics of SCC

Molecular investigations of SCC (mainly noncutaneous) have provided evidence of transcriptional activation of the cellular oncogenes *HRAS, KRAS,* and *MYC (40).* The *HST1* gene, localized to band 11q13, was amplified in 40% of esophageal SCCs, and *HST1* and the closely linked *INT2* were coamplified in an SCC of the gall bladder *(41,42).* This coamplification was described as a prognostic factor in SCC of the esophagus *(43).* Amplification of *EGFR* has been reported in several SCCs *(44).* Loss of the p53 locus has been associated with a high frequency of 17p losses in SCC of the esophagus *(45),* and p53 overexpression and p53 mutations have been reported in head and neck cancer *(46,47).* Yokoyama et al. *(48)* described loss of DNA markers spanning most of 3p in lung SCC, and Latif et al. *(49)* reported frequent loss of restriction fragment length polymorphisms (RFLPs) between 3p14 and 3p25 in SCC of the head and neck. Cytogenetic observation of frequent loss of material from 18q was consistent with loss of heterozygosity (LOH) at the *DCC* gene locus in SCC cell lines and fresh tumors *(50).* The cytogenetic observations are also consistent with frequent LOH involving *RB1* and other tumor suppressor loci that have been observed in esophageal SCC *(51,52).*

Clonality of SCC in Perspective

In many other forms of human neoplasia, specific pathologic entities have been associated with certain chromosome rearrangements, suggesting a monoclonal origin. This pattern is apparently lacking in skin tumors. The nonclonal aberrations may be spurious, and clonal rearrangements, when present, may bear no relation to the neoplastic cell population and have little significance for the genesis of these epithelial tumors. On the other hand, these cytogenetic alterations may represent initial responses of the exposed epithelium that are relevant to genetic destabilization. Complex rearrangements, often accompanied by aneuploidy, appear correlated with increasing histologic evidence of malignancy in skin *(53,54)* as they do in other forms of human cancer.

The persistence of multiple unrelated clones is suggestive of a multiclonal origin for skin lesions, which is consistent with the "field cancerization" concept. Slaughter et al., who originated the concept *(55),* observed that 11% of patients with oral cancer had multiple tumors. They postulated that separate primary epithelial cancers could arise independently following a prolonged exposure to carcinogens, and termed this effect field cancerization. Their hypothesis predicts that, if a common carcinogen is involved, second primary cancers or synchronous primary cancers would arise from independent genetic events.

Evidence to support the field cancerization hypothesis was recently provided by mutational analysis *(56).* The presence and exon locations of *TP53* mutations were analyzed in primary head and neck cancers and their corresponding second primaries. Results indicated that mutations were uniformly discordant within individual hosts, supporting the hypothesis that multiple primary cancers of the upper aerodigestive tract arise independently. In a study of a patient with bilateral ovarian tumors, ploidy analysis showed that the tumors had different aneuploid stemlines, indicating independent origins *(57).*

Considerable evidence has favored a polyclonal origin for SCC of the skin in particular because of data from 168 short-term SCC cultures (Table 1). Of these, 46% were monoclonal and 28% were

Table 1
Clonality of HNSCC after Short-Term Culture[a]

# of HNSCCs	One clone	> One clone	Nonclonal[b]/ other[c]	Normal	Refs.
36	12	21	2	1	31–38
1		1			53
1		1			58
3		3			54
1		1			144
1		1			59
10	7		3		143
8	7			1	142
1		1			60
79	36	14		29	58
10	1	2	2	5	145
2	2				61,62
15	15				39
168	80	45	7	36	

[a]Totals appear at bottom of table.
[b]Karyotypic aberrations present in only one cell.
[c]Chromosomal aberrations not interpreted because of poor quality.

polyclonal in origin. Most of the polyclonal tumors were identified by a single group of investigators. More recently, that group presented new evidence favoring the view that monoclonal origin is actually far more common *(63,64)*. The type of culture medium was the key to selection of cells for karyotypic analysis. In their first series, short-term cultures grown in serum-rich media yielded harvests of cytogenetically unrelated clones. Aberrant, random, and unrelated clones, often characterized by pseudodiploid chromosome number, apparently balanced structural aberrations, or simple numerical changes, were observed in SCCs cultured in a medium that supports both epithelial and mesenchymal cells. This medium may have favored the growth of stromal fibroblasts that overgrew the tumor parenchymal cells. Use of MCDB 153 medium, which promotes the growth of keratinocytes and inhibits proliferation of stromal fibroblasts, resulted in marked reduction in the number of unrelated clones within cultures from individual tumors, so that polyclonality was found in 3% of cases *(63)*, and 14% of 44 cases reported still later *(64)*, as opposed to the higher frequency in cultures reported earlier (Table 1). Thus, with culture media that better support the requirements for epithelial cell growth, the predominant findings of random aberrant clones and nonclonal aberrations in noncutaneous SCC have been modified, but the underlying question remains unresolved.

It is tempting to attribute the unrelated clones to stromal derivation, primarily because they do not persist in culture and are reduced in frequency when restricted by media that are more supportive of epithelial cell growth. On the other hand, it is possible that these aberrant clones are representative of tumor epithelium that has reduced viability under these culture conditions.

When we review the cytogenetic data, patterns of alteration appear to differ in squamous cancers depending on location. Although noncutaneous lesions now appear predominantly monoclonal *(63,64)*, the squamous tumors from keratinized skin still yield complex, polyclonal and nonclonal cytogenetic aberrations from direct harvest and short-term cultures. Thus, SCC originating from the external body surface often contain several clones with nonoverlapping patterns of aberrations, whereas those from mucosal surfaces (oral cavity, vulva) generally show monoclonal or related chromosomal aberrations, suggesting single-cell origins.

These differences may reflect etiologic variables in the two subsets of SCC. The major causative factor in SCC of exposed cutaneous sites is UV radiation. The resultant genetic lesion from such exposure is the introduction into DNA of thymine dimers, C $\rightarrow$ T transition-type mutations, and sometimes formation of pyrimidine tracts *(65)*. It is possible that cells carrying these mutations expand initially into unstable, transitory clones, and that eventually the more persistent of those clones become established in culture. In noncutaneous sites, other etiologic agents, such as viruses (vulva) and smoking, tobacco, and betel nut (head and neck SCCs), have been implicated. G-T transversions are characteristic of exposure to carcinogens from tobacco smoke *(66)*, or to hydrogen radicals generated for example by γ-radiation *(67)*.

Although LOH studies appear to support the monoclonality of SCC and basal cell cancers, molecular studies are not ideal for determination of polyclonality because the molecular milieu represents an average of the cell population. We have used fluorescence *in situ* hybridization (FISH) to demonstrate concordance of cytogenetic aberrations *in situ* with those of tumor karyotypes derived from primary cultures from the same region of the tumor *(68)*. Similarly, *in situ* analysis of cutaneous lesions should prove useful for analysis in individual tumor cells of genetic aberrations that would shed light on the clonal status of the lesion.

BCC

BCC is the most common type of skin cancer. It is considered a malignant lesion because of its ability to infiltrate locally, although it rarely metastasizes. Some etiologic factors associated with BCC include light skin color together with prolonged sun exposure, large doses of X-rays, and genetic disorders, such as xeroderma pigmentosum, and Gorlin's syndrome *(69)*.

Cytogenetic analyses of more than 35 BCCs *(70–72)* indicated no clear nonrandom pattern of abnormalities. In one study *(68)*, 8 of 33 BCCs had clonal aberrations that were different in all 8 tumors. In 2 of the 8 BCCs the abnormal clones were unrelated, and in 23 of 33 BCCs nonclonal aberrations were observed, the latter usually in the form of apparently balanced translocations. Multiple unrelated clones and both clonal and nonclonal aberrations were also reported in two other studies *(71,72)*. The presence of multiple unrelated clones in some BCCs, like the data reported above for SCC, is suggestive of a polyclonal origin. Those BCCs with only clonal aberrations, albeit appearing monoclonal, may also reflect clonal convergence, with the selection of one clonal population of cells over time. The only consistent numerical changes that have emerged include +12, +18, –X, and –Y, changes that are known to be associated with other types of neoplasia. Of the structural aberrations seen, only del(9)(q22) has been consistently associated with neoplasia *(73)*.

At the molecular level, LOH studies of 11 BCCs in a Japanese population indicated LOH at 9q31 in two of five informative cases *(73)*. Additional evidence of 9q loss was reported in larger case series *(74,75)*, and the nevoid basal cell carcinoma syndrome (Gorlin syndrome) gene is tentatively localized to 9q. Loss of 9p, on the other hand, was found in only 4 of 33 BCCs, and LOH for 1q in 6 of 43 tumors. More recently, a gene *(ESS1)* predisposing to the development of multiple, invasive but self-healing skin tumors (squamous cell epitheliomata) has been shown by multipoint linkage analysis to lie in the 9q22.2–q31 region *(76)*. Both Gorlin's syndrome and multiple self-healing squamous epitheliomata present with multiple cutaneous tumors, despite differences in the morphology and clinical course of the skin lesions. It is possible that different mutations in the same gene may be responsible for the two conditions, a question that may be resolved by more detailed mapping of the disease loci.

Clinically, pathologically, and biologically, BCC and SCC present as separate entities, although a genetic basis for these differences is unknown. Both tumor types are keratinocyte-derived, but differ in their histological progression and metastatic potential *(77)*. Cytogenetic and molecular data suggest that the patterns and extent of chromosome loss differ between BCC and SCC. In contrast to the tightly localized loss in BCCs at 9q, SCCs show more widespread chromosomal LOH that involve 9p (41%), 13q (46%), 17p (33%), 17q (33%), and 3p (23%). The increases in cytogenetic aberrations and LOH in SCC may reflect the metastatic capability and more aggressive clinical nature of SCC in comparison to BCC.

Cutaneous Malignant Melanoma (CMM)

The global incidence of CMM is increasing dramatically *(78,79)*. The lifetime risk in the United States of a diagnosis of melanoma is now estimated at 1.25% for males and 1.01% for females *(6)*. Approximately 50% of melanomas occur in individuals less than 55 yr of age *(80)*, with a higher incidence in males than females.

Although the etiologic factors leading to the development of melanoma are not entirely understood, three factors appear to play major roles. First, clinical and epidemiological studies indicate that sunlight is a critical etiologic factor in the development of melanoma *(80)*. Careful case control studies demonstrate that intermittent high exposure to sunlight during childhood leads to significantly higher incidence of melanoma in adults *(81,82)*. Human melanocytes are exposed to ultraviolet (UV) light in sun light, in which UV-B (wavelengths of 290–320 nm) is the biologically most active component *(80)*. UV radiation produces many alterations in the skin, induces or exacerbates many skin diseases *(83)*, increases genetic instability by damaging DNA *(84,85)*, inhibits the endogenous antioxidant system *(86,87)*, alters proto-oncogene and tumor suppressor gene expression *(88)*, acts as a growth factor or growth factor modulator *(89)*, and suppresses cell-mediated immune responses *(90,91)*. However, there is no direct experimental evidence in humans for a causal relation between sunlight exposure and melanoma development; most experiments on UV radiation of skin have utilized keratinocytes.

The second and related factor is the degree of skin pigmentation. The 10-fold higher incidence of melanoma in Whites vs Blacks indicates a strong protective effect of skin pigmentation against melanoma in exposed sites *(92)*.

The third etiologic factor identified in melanoma is hereditary. Clark and Greene in 1978 *(93)* described two families that showed a strong genetic susceptibility to melanoma. Association of cutaneous melanomas with clinically atypical skin moles (dysplastic nevi), segregating in an autosomal dominant fashion, has been confirmed by several other groups. Eight to 10% of all melanoma cases are believed to be familial *(94)*.

Tumor Progression in the Melanocyte System

Melanocytes are pigmented cells located in the basal layer of the epidermis, the bulb of hair sheaths, the choroid of the eye, certain mucous membranes, and the leptomeninges *(95)*. They are neuroectodermal in origin, leaving the neural crest soon after fertilization and migrating through the embryonal dermis to reach the epidermis. Immature precursor cells (melanoblasts) possess premelanosomes (melanosome precursors lacking melanin), and this pattern may also be found in melanocytic tumors. Thus, tumors may arise from any point in cell migration and may be pigmented or may lack pigmentation.

The clinical and histopathological features of tumor progression in the human melanocytic system have been well documented *(96–98)*. Melanoma can develop from precursor or mature melanocytes and progress through different stages from benign nevi (congenital or acquired) *(98)* to dysplastic lesions. Melanocytic nevi are fairly ubiquitous in humans, appearing first in early childhood, reaching a maximum count in young adults and declining in older adults *(80)*. Progression from ordinary to dysplastic nevi is uncommon, and progression beyond benign lesions is even more rare. It has recently been estimated that only one melanoma arises from about 110,000 original nevi *(80)*.

The clinical features of nevi are defined in terms of size, profile, border, and color *(99,100)*. Dysplastic nevi are usually larger than 5 mm in diameter, with a macular component, irregular borders, and heterogeneous colors. Histologically, atypical melanocytes are often surrounded in the dermis by lymphocytes. Early malignant stages include *in situ* melanomas and radial growth phase (RGP) melanomas that are similar histologically to *in situ* melanomas except that individual melanocytic cells have invaded the dermis.

Invasive primary melanomas are currently classified into four subtypes *(101)*:

1. Superficial spreading melanoma, the most common of the four subtypes, can be located at any anatomic site;
2. Nodular melanoma, an elevated or polypoid lesion with uniform pigmentation, is frequently accompanied by ulceration;
3. Lentigo maligna is a macular lesion on sun-exposed skin (head, neck), often found in patients with *in situ* or RGP melanoma; and

4. Acral lentiginous melanoma presents as a darkly pigmented, flat-to-nodular lesion on palms or soles, or subungually.

An investigation of sites of melanoma metastasis revealed that 18% disseminated only to the regional lymph nodes, whereas 39% showed initial dissemination to regional lymph nodes, followed by hematogenous metastases, and 43% showed blood vessel metastases without apparent involvement of the lymphatic system *(97)*. Lung, brain, and liver are preferred sites of distant metastasis, although metastatic melanoma can be found in virtually any anatomic site.

Genetics of CMM

Tumor progression in the melanocytic system is the result of a progressive acquisition of genetic defects *(102–104)* that are presumed to be fundamental to the pathology of CMM. These defects are detectable by alterations in ploidy or karyotype, and as molecular lesions. Cytogenetics, familial linkage studies, LOH analyses, and fusion between normal and malignant cells have all contributed significantly to the identification of chromosomal regions presumed to harbor "melanoma-associated" oncogenes or tumor suppressor loci.

DNA Ploidy

Histological, statistical, antigenic, and clinical analyses, as well as in vitro model systems, show that at least five steps are needed for progression from a diploid human melanocyte to an aneuploid metastatic melanoma cell *(96,105,106)*. Several indicators are commonly used to predict the clinical course of CMM, including Breslow thickness *(107)*, Clark level *(108)*, histopathologic parameters *(109)*, and DNA ploidy *(110)*. The use of DNA ploidy as a predictor of outcome in CMM is supported by data showing that aneuploid melanotic tumors are usually associated with a worse prognosis than near-diploid tumors. DNA ploidy and S-phase fraction appear to be independent predictors of clinical outcome *(110)*.

Cytogenetic Aberrations

In CMM, studies of multiple tumors (usually metastases or a primary and a series of metastases) derived from individual patients have been useful in predicting the timing of events during melanoma progression *(102,104,111)*. Because metastases are the sources of many observations, identical genetic alterations in all cells of a metastasis are interpreted as resulting from a single event in the primary lesion. Consistently aberrant regions or loci in two or more independent sets of multiple metastases can point to initiating events whereas those that occur in only a subset of related tumors are thought to represent late alterations. Cytogenetic reports from many independent studies, dating from 1973–1991, indicate that rearrangements of 1p, 6q, 7, and 9p are common in CMM, and that those of chromosomes 2, 3, 10, and 11 are less frequent.

Chromosome 1

Rearrangements of chromosome 1 were detected in 53/58 (82%) of advanced melanomas *(111–113)*, in most cases involving a deletion or rearrangement of 1p12–22. Linkage analysis points to the terminal portion of 1p (1p36) in at least some forms of familial melanoma *(112)*. LOH studies corroborate 1p involvement in 60% of metastatic melanomas *(114)*. Both LOH and cytogenetic data describe frequent alterations of 1p in metastatic tumors that are rare in precursor or primary lesions *(111,114)*, leading to the conclusion that involvement of 1p is a late event.

Two genes on distal 1p, *TCL5* and *TP58*[clk-1], have been implicated in melanoma progression *(115,116)*. Rearrangement of *TCL5* was reported in a melanoma cell line, but it is unclear whether *TCL5* is over- or underexpressed in melanomas. The p58[clk-1] protein kinase gene, located more distal on 1p36, codes for a protein related to cell-division control *(116)*, and functional analyses suggest a tumor suppressor role for this gene *(111)*. Other neural-crest-derived tumors also exhibit alterations in this region of 1p. The region of the p58[clk-1] gene shows the strongest linkage in the familial melanoma cases mapped to 1p *(112)*.

Chromosome 6

Chromosome 6 is rearranged in about 64% of CMM. Both LOH and somatic cell hybrid studies point to a 6q tumor suppressor gene in melanoma development *(111)*. In metastatic melanomas, about 40–50% of all instances of LOH were detected on chromosome 6, most frequently at 6q22–q27 *(117)*. In addition, the technique of microcell fusion, used to introduce a normal chromosome 6 into melanoma cell lines, resulted in diminution of their tumorigenic potential *(118)*. Rearrangements at 6q22, the locus of the c-*myb* oncogene, have been detected in two independent studies *(119,120)*, but appear to be rare. Because 6q deletions or rearrangements are not found consistently in premalignant lesions, primary tumors, or multiple specimens from single patients, this region is unlikely to be involved in early melanoma progression, but may play a role in late tumor growth or invasion.

Chromosome 7

Polysomy of chromosome 7 in CMM is frequent (noted in 61% of all melanomas), and well-documented in later stage or metastatic melanoma *(121)*. An experimental model of melanoma in the swordtail platyfish implicates a tumor suppressor gene *Tu* as responsible for the tumor phenotype *(122)*. *Tu* encodes a receptor tyrosine kinase homologous to the human epidermal growth factor (EGF) receptor, which maps to a chromosomal region 1p12–13 that is frequently rearranged in melanoma *(102)*. Expression of the EGF receptor in human melanoma cells correlates with increased dosage of chromosome 7 *(123)*. Recently, invasion and metastasis genes on chromosome 7 *(124)* have been identified that add further credence to the role of chromosome 7 in melanoma development.

Chromosome 9

Cytogenetic abnormalities of 9p occur in 44% of melanoma cases *(125)*. Karyotypes of nevi and dysplastic nevi revealed that chromosome 9 was involved most frequently. Markers on 9p21 in a series of melanoma tumors and cell lines demonstrated 86% LOH *(125)*, a frequency much higher than that seen for either 1p or 6q. Homozygous deletions observed in two unrelated melanomas resulted in narrowing the critical region to 2–3 Mb within 9p21. LOH at 9p21 has been demonstrated in a broad spectrum of tumors, and several genes relevant to cell proliferation have already been identified in this region (e.g., p15, p16).

Chromosomes 2, 3, 10, and 11

The long arm of chromosome 10, at 10q24–q26, may harbor a locus for a gene or genes involved in early stages of melanoma development. Studies on dysplastic nevi with early stages of melanocytic neoplasia reported multiple alterations of 10q. One of 10 dysplastic nevi had a t(9;10)(p24;q24); of three complex melanomas, one had loss of chromosome 10, and another had an add(10)(q26) *(126)*. Other cases showed loss of one or more copies of chromosome 10, and one case had a complex rearrangement involving chromosomes 5, 6, and 10, with breakpoints at 10q23 and q25. The region of 10q24–q26 also has a high frequency of LOH in 76% of metastatic melanoma *(127)*. Rearrangements of chromosomes 2, 3, and 11 have also been reported in from 32 to 39% of CMM *(128)*.

Identification of Defects in Known Oncogenes and Tumor Suppressor Genes in CMM

The rapidly growing body of molecular data suggests a broad array of disturbances in CMM involving oncogenes, tumor suppressor genes, transcriptional regulators, growth factors, genes that control phosphorylation of proteins, and genes that control entry into the cell cycle. At present, there appears to be little correspondence between cytogenetic abnormalities and the molecular aberrations that have been identified.

Mutations in the three functional members of the *RAS* proto-oncogene family, *HRAS* (11p), *NRAS* (1p), and *KRAS* (12p), are the most common specific gene defects in both primary and metastatic melanomas *(128)*. The frequency of *RAS* point mutations is approx 24% in cultured melanomas and 12% in noncultured primary and metastatic melanomas. More than 90% of these mutations occurred in codon 61 of the *NRAS* gene.

Approximately 15% of melanomas harbor mutations in the *TP53* tumor suppressor gene (Albino et al., personal communication). Deregulated expression of various members of the *FOS* and *JUN* families of transcriptional activators *(129)*, and of growth factors bFGF, TGFβ2, TGFα, PDGFA, melanocyte growth-stimulating activity (MGSA), aFGF, FGF-5, PDGFB, and interleukins-1α, -a, and -1β have been reported in subsets of melanomas *(129,130)*.

The proto-oncogene *KIT* on 4q is an example of a receptor-type protein tyrosine kinase, which, together with its ligand, plays an essential role in the normal growth and differentiation of melanocytes *(131,132)*. Loss of either the c-*kit* protein product or its ligand may contribute to disruptions in differentiation and homeostatic mechanisms controlling melanocytes. Another member of the tyrosine kinase growth-factor gene family, similar to *KIT*, is *MET* that has been shown to be downregulated or lost in CMM *(128,130)*.

At present, the precise biochemical and biological roles of each of these genes in the pathogenesis and progression of CMM remain to be defined.

Merkel Cell Carcinoma (MCC)

MCC is a rare cutaneous neoplasm, also known as trabecular carcinoma *(133)* or primary neuroendocrine carcinoma of the skin. The function and ancestry of Merkel cells are not known, but they are believed to be mechanoreceptors of neuroendocrine origin with the ability to release various polypeptides. MCC is a very aggressive carcinoma, frequently metastatic at the time of detection (65%), with high recurrence rates (30–40%) and poor survival when metastatic *(134)*. Histologically, MCC presents as irregular collections of hyperchromatic, pleomorphic cells with virtually no cytoplasm. In differential diagnosis, therefore, it must be distinguished from neoplasms such as metastatic small-cell carcinoma of the lung, lymphoma *(135)*, and other uncommon small-cell tumors (neuroblastoma, primitive neuroectodermal tumor, and metastatic Ewing's sarcoma). Immunohistochemical stains and ultrastructural analysis reveal characteristic staining with antibodies against neurofilaments and cytokeratin *(133)*.

About 25 cases of MCC have been analyzed cytogenetically. The inherently high mitotic rate is permissive of cytogenetic analysis from primary MCCs, obviating the need for cell culture. Alterations of chromosome 1, including deletion, translocation, or trisomy, were common in 16 of 21 reported primary and metastatic MCCs *(136–140)*, and LOH of distal 1p in three metastatic MCCs *(141)* is suggestive of a late event in tumor progression, as it is in other solid tumors. Nonclonal numerical and structural aberrations were found in the remaining 5 metastatic MCCs. Loss of the Y chromosome was the only consistent clonal change in one primary tumor; Y loss has been reported in other neoplasms of neural crest origin or neuroendocrine differentiation (small-cell lung carcinoma, Ewing's tumor, meningioma, and melanoma).

Some Intriguing Observations

Cytogenetic studies have been valuable in illustrating differences in epithelial neoplasms with regard to site. The presence of multiple unrelated clones and lack of consistent patterns of chromosomal aberrations, in epithelial neoplasms from sun-exposed sites, support a field cancerization effect. In SCC of unexposed sites, clonal and subclonal proliferations appear to predominate, pointing to a monoclonal origin for these neoplasms. Moreover, the consistent, nonrandom genetic changes that have emerged in these subsets of tumors appear dependent on the site of the unexposed epithelial milieu.

These differences may be related to differing etiological agents. UV radiation in sunlight, acting via the introduction of pyrimidine tracts, may contribute to genome destabilization and great genetic variability in lesions of the skin. In contrast, SCC of mucosal surfaces, for which smoking has been a major risk factor, are likely to be mediated by gene transversions rather than transitions, suggesting that the type of mutation may determine different mechanisms of tumor development.

SCCs and BCCs, although both are keratinocyte-derived, show marked differences in biological behavior *(77)*. SCCs are faster growing lesions, often aggressive tumors with metastatic potential. BCCs, on the other hand, are more slowly growing, locally invasive tumors that rarely metastasize. These two biologically different keratinocyte-derived neoplasms show distinct genetic differences. BCCs are characterized by fewer chromosomal aberrations, whereas SCCs typically present with great chromosomal complexity. A single predominant chromosomal site (9q) is involved in BCC, whereas multiple, consistent regions of genomic loss and gain have been implicated in SCC from different tissues. Although the frequency of p53 mutations appears similar in BCC and SCC, LOH for the 17p allele is relatively infrequent in BCC. Overall, the increased genetic deviation from normal in SCC, as compared to BCC, mirrors the biological deviance.

In contrast, CMM is exemplary of a tumor type that has been carefully investigated at the chromosomal and molecular genetic levels. The cytogenetic landmarks were critical for location of several oncogenes and tumor suppressor genes associated with melanoma progression. Knowledge of other molecular alterations including mutations in *RAS* and *TP53*, and of the recently discovered role of the tyrosine kinase gene C-*KIT* in melanoblast migration, should help to integrate information on the genes responsible for melanoma formation. It is interesting that similarities have emerged among the neural-crest-derived tumors such as melanoma (1p11–p22), neuroblastoma (1p31-pter), and MCC (distal 1p). This region carries many genes involved in control of cellular growth and in differentiation of cells derived from the neural crest.

The diverse genetic alterations found in tumors of the skin reflect, in specificity and extent, the diversity in their cells of origin, their anatomic locations and consequent exposures to mutagens, and the differentiation pathways of the tumor stem cells.

References

1. Penneys NS, Fulton JE, Weinstein GD, et al.: Location of proliferating cells in human epidermis. Arch Dermatol 101:323–327, 1970.
2. Halprin KM: Epidermal turnover time. A reexamination. Br J Dermatol 86:14–19, 1972.
3. Fearon ER, Vogelstein B: A genetic model for colorectal tumorigenesis. Cell 61:759–767, 1990.
4. Ledbetter DH, Cavanee WK: Molecular cytogenetics: Interface of cytogenetics and monogenic disorders. In: Schriver CR. Beaudet AL. Sly WS. Valle D. (eds.), The Metabolic Basis of Inherited Disease, Sixth ed. New York: McGraw-Hill, pp. 343–371, 1989.
5. Pardue ML, Gall JG: Molecular hybridization of radioactive DNA to the RNA of cytological preparations. Proc Natl Acad Sci USA 64:600–604, 1969.
6. SEER Cancer Statistics Review, 1973–1991. National Institutes of Health. National Cancer Institute, Bethesda, MD, June 1994.
7. Kwa RE, Campana K, Moy RL: Biology of cutaneous squamous cell carcinoma. J Am Acad Dermatol 26:1–26, 1992.
8. Miller SJ: Biology of basal cell carcinoma (Part 1). J Am Acad Dermatolol 24:1–13, 1991.
9. Miller SJ: Biology of basal cell carcinoma (Part 2). J Am Acad Dermatol 24:161–175, 1991.
10. Marks R, Rennie G, Selwood TS: Malignant transformation of solar keratoses to squamous cell carcinoma. Lancet 1:795, 796, 1988.
11. Mertens F, Jin Y, Heim S, Mandahl N, Honsson N, Mertens O, Persson B, Salemark L, Wennerberg J, Mitelman F: Clonal structural chromosomal aberrations in nonneoplastic cells of the skin and upper aerodigestive tract. Genes Chromosome Cancer 4:235–240, 1992.

12. Pavarino EC, Antonio JR, Pozzeti EM, Larranaga A, Tajara EH: Cytogenetic study of neoplastic and nonneoplastic cells of the skin. Cancer Genet Cytogenet 85:16–19, 1995.

13. Hoehn H. Bryant EM, Au K, Norwood TH, Boman H, Martin GM: Variegated translocation mosaicism in human skin fibroblast cultures. Cytogenet Cell Genet 15:282–298, 1982.

14. Littlefield LG, Mailhes JB: Observations of de novo clones of cytogenetically aberrant cells in primary fibroblast cell strains from phenotypically normal women. Am J Hum Genet 27:190–197, 1975.

15. Harnden DG, Benn PA, Oxford JM, Taylor AMR, Webb TP: Cytogenetically marked clones in human fibroblasts cultured from normal subjects. Somat Cell Genet 2:55–62, 1976.

16. Salk D, Au K, Hoehn H, Martin GM: Cytogenetics of Werners's syndrome cultured skin fibroblasts: variegated translocation mosaicism. Cytogenet Cell Genet 30:92–107, 1981.

17. Mertens F, Johansson B: No increased chromosome breakage in skin fibroblasts from patients with musculoskeletal sarcoma. Clin Genet 34: 20–25, 1988.

18. Happle R, Hoehn H: Cytogenetic studies on cultured fibroblast-like cells derived from basal cell carcinoma tissue. Clin Genet 4:17–24, 1973.

19. Taylor AMR, Harnden DG, Fairburn EA: Chromosomal instability associated with susceptibility to malignant disease in patients with porokeratosis of Mibelli. J Natl Cancer Inst 51:371–378, 1973.

20. Salk D: Werner's syndrome. A review of recent research with an analysis of connective tissue metabolism, growth control of cultured cels, and chromosomal aberrations. Hum Genet 62:1–5, 1982.

21. Scappaticci S, Fraccaro M, Orecchia G: Multiple clonal chromosome abnormalities ina superficial basal cell epithelioma. Cancer Genet Cytogenet 42:309–311, 1989.

21a. Scappaticci S, Lambiase S, Fraccaro M, Orecchi G: Cancer Genet Cytogenet 43:249, 250, 1989.

22. Benn PA: Specific chromosome aberrations in senescent fibroblast cell lines derived from human embryos. Am J Human Genet 28:465–473, 1976.

23. Visfeldt J: Clone formation in tissue culture. Experience from long-term cultures of irradiated human skin. Acta Pathol Microbiol Scand 68: 305–312, 1966.

24. Bigger TRL, Savage JRK, Watson GE: A scheme for characterizing ASG banding and an illustration of its use in identifying complex chromosomal rearrangements in irradiated human skin. Chromosoma 39:297–309, 1972

25. Savage JRK, Bigger TRL: Aberration distribution and chromosomally marked clones in x-irradiated skin. In: Evans HJ, Lloyd DC, (eds), Mutagen-Induced Chromosome Damage in Man. Edinburgh U.K. Edinburgh University, pp. 155–169, 1978.

26. Garewal HS, Sampliner R, Liu Y, Trent JM: Chromosomal rearrangements in Barrett's esophagus. A premalignant lesion of esophageal adenocarcinoma. Cancer Genet Cytogenet 42:281–286, 1989.

27. Whang-Peng J, Banks-Schlegel SP, Lee EC: Cytogenetic studies of esophageal carcinoma cell lines. Cancer Genet Cytogenet 45:101–120, 1990.

28. Viegas-Pequignot E, Flury-Herard A, De Cremoux H, Chlecq C, Bignon J, Dutrillaux G: Recurrent chromosome aberrations in human lung squamous cell carcinomas. Cancer Genet Cytogenet 49:37–49, 1990.

29. Worsham MJ, Van Dyke DL, Grenman SE, Grenman R, Hopkins MA, Roberts JA, Gasser KM, Schwartz DR, Carey TE: Consistent chromosome abnormalities in squamous carcinoma of the vulva. Genes Chromosomes Cancer 3:420–432, 1991.

30. Heo DS, Snyderman C, Gollin SM, Pan S, Walker E, Deka R, Barnes EL, Johnson JT, Herberman RB, Whiteside TL: Biology, cytogenetics, and sensitivity to immunological effector cells of new head and neck squamous cell carcinoma lines. Cancer Res 49:5167–5175, 1989.

31. Jin Y, Heim S, Mandahl N, Biorklund A, Wennerberg J, Mitelman F: Multiple apparently unrelated clonal chromosome abnormalities in a squamous cell carcinoma of the tongue. Cancer Genet Cytogenet 32:93–100, 1988.

32. Jin Y, Mandahl N, Heim S, Biorklund A, Wennerberg J, Mitelman F: Unique karyotypic abnormalites in a squamous cell carcinoma of the larynx. Cancer Genet Cytogenet 30:177–179, 1988.

33. Jin Y, Mandahl N, Heim S, Biorklund A, Wennerberg J, Mitelman F: t(6;7)as the sole chromosomal anomaly in a vocal cord carcinoma. Cancer Genet Cytogenet 32:305–307, 1988.

34. Jin Y, Heim S, Mandahl N, Biorklund A, Wennerberg J, Mitelman F: Inversion inv(14)(p15q26) in a squamous cell carcinoma of the hypopharynx. Cancer Genet Cytogenet 36:233–234, 1988.

35. Jin Y, Heim S, Mandahl N, Biorklund A, Wennerberg J, Mitelman F: Multiple clonal chromosome aberrations in squamous cell carcinoma of the larynx. Cancer Genet Cytogenet 44:209–216, 1990.

36. Jin Y, Heim S, Mandahl N, Biorklund A, Wennerberg J, Mitelman F: Unrelated clonal chromosome aberrations in carcinomas of the oral cavity. Genes Chromosome Cancer 1:209–215, 1990.

37. Jin Y, Higashi K, Mandahl N, Heim S, Wennerberg J, Bioklund A, Dictor M, Mitelman F: Frequent rearrangement of chromosomal bands 1p22 and 11q13 in squamous cell carcinomas of the head and neck. Genes Chromosome Cancer 2:198–204, 1990.

38. Pejovic T, Heim S, Orndal C, Jin Y, Mandahl N, Willen H, Mitelman F: Simple numerical chromosome aberrations in weli-differentiated malignant epithelial tumors. Cancer Genet Cytogenet 49:95–101, 1990.

39. Van Dyke DL, Worsham MJ, Benninger MS, Krause CJ, Baker SR, Wolf GT, Drumheller T, Tilley BC, Carey TE: Recurrent cytogenetic abnormalities in squamous cell carcinomas of the head and neck region. Genes Chromosome Cancer 9:192–206, 1994.

40. Spandidos DA, Lamothe A, Field JK: Multiple transcriptional activation of cellular oncogenes in human head and neck solid tumours. Anticancer Res 5:221–224, 1985.

41. Tsuda T, Nakatani H, Matsumura T, Yoshida K, Tahara E, Nishihira T, Sakamoto H, Yoshida T, Terada M, Sugimura T: Amplification of the hst-1 gene in human esophageal carcinomas. Jpn J Cancer Res 79:584–588, 1988.
42. Tsuda T, Nakatani H, Tahara E, Sakamoto H, Terada M, Sugimura T: HST1 and INT2 gene coamplification in a squamous cell carcinoma of the gall bladder. Jpn J Clin Oncol 19:26–29, 1989.
43. Kitagawa Y, Ueda M, Ando N, et al.: Significance of int-2/hst-1 coamplification as a prognostic factor in patients with esophageal squamous carcinoma. Cancer Res 51:1504–1508, 1991.
44. Yamamoto T, Kamata N, Kawano H, et al.: High incidence of amplification of epidermal growth factor receptor gene in human squamous carcinoma cell lines. Cancer Res 46:414–416, 1986.
45. Wagata T, Ishizaki K, Imamura M, Shimada Y, Ikenaga M, Tobe T: Deletion of 17p and amplification of the int-2 gene in esophageal carcinomas. Cancer Res 51:2113–2117, 1991.
46. Dolcetti R, Doglioni C, Maestro R, Gasporotto D, Barzan L, Pastore A, Romanelli M, Boiocchi M: p53 overexpression is an early event in the development of human squamous-cell carcinoma of the larynx-genetic and prognostic implications. Int J Cancer 52:178–182, 1992.
47. Somers KD, Merrick MA, Lopez ME, Incognito LS, Schechter GL, Casey G: Frequent p53 mutations in head and neck cancer. Cancer Res 52:5997–6000, 1992.
48. Yokoyama S, Yamakawa K, Tsuchiya E, Murata M, Sakiyama S, Nakamura Y: Deletion mapping on the short arm of chromosome 3 in squamous cell carcinoma and adenocarcinoma of the lung. Cancer Res 52:873–877, 1992.
49. Latif F, Fivash M, Glenn G, Tory K, Orcutt ML, Hampsch K, Dellisio J, Lerman M, Cowan J, Beckett M, Weichselbaum R: Chromosome 3p deletions in head and neck carcinomas: statistical ascertainment of allelic loss. Cancer Res 52:1451–1456, 1992.
50. Kelker W, Van Dyke DL, Worsham MJ, Christopherson PL, James CD, Conlon MR, Carey TE: Loss of 18q and homozygosity for the DCC locus: possible markers for clinically aggressive squamous cell carcinoma. Anti Cancer Res: in press.
51. Boynton RF, Huang Y, Blount PL, Reid BJ, Raskind WH, Haggitt RC, Newkirk C, Resau JH, Yin J, McDaniel T, Meltzer SJ: Frequent loss of heterozygosity at the retinoblastoma locus in human esophageal cancers. Cancer Res 51:5766–5769, 1996.
52. Huang Y, Boynton RF, Blount PL, Silverstein RJ, Yin J, Tong Y, McDaniel TK, Newkirk C, Resau JH, Sridhara R, Reid BJ, Meltzer SJ: Loss of heterozygosity involves multiple tumor suppressor genes in human esophageal cancers. Cancer Res 52:6525–6530, 1992.
53. Heim S, Mandahl N, Mitelman F: Genetic convergence and divergence in tumor progression. Cancer Res 48:5911–5916, 1988.
54. Heim S, Mertens F, Jin Y, Mandahl N, Johansson B, Biorklund A, Wennerberg J, Jonsson N, Mitelman F: Diverse chromosome abnormalities

in squamous cell carcinoma of the skin. Cancer Genet Cytogenet 39: 69–76, 1989.

55. Slaughter DP, Southwick HW, Smejkal W: "Field cancerization" in oral stratified squamous epithelium: clinical implications of multicentric origin. Cancer 6:963–968, 1953.

56. Chung KY, Mukhopadhyay T, Kim J, Casson A, Ro JY, Goepfert H, Hong WK, Roth JA: Discordant p53 gene mutations in primary head and neck cancers and corresponding second primary cancers of the upper aerodigestive tract. Cancer Res 53:1676–1683, 1993.

57. Smit VT, Cornelisse CJ, De Jong D, et al.: Analysis of tumor heterogeneity in a patient with synchronously occurring female genital tract malignancy by DNA flow cytometry, DNA fingerprinting, and immunohistochemistry. Cancer 62:1146–1152, 1988.

58. Mertens F, Heim S, Jin Y, Johansson B, Mandahl N, Biorklund A, Wennerberg J, Jonsson N, Mitelman F. Basosquamous papilloma-a benign epithelial skin tumor with multiple cytogenetic clones. Cancer Genet Cytogenet 37:235–239, 1989.

59. Therapel SA, Lester EP: Two simple translocations in a primary squamous cell carcinoma of the head and neck. Cancer Genet Cytogenet 47:131–134, 1990.

60. Sen P: Chromosome 9 anomalies as the primary clonal alteration in a case of squamous cell carcinoma of the epiglottis. Cancer Genet Cytogenet 66:23–27, 1993.

61. Worsham MJ, Benninger MJ, Zarbo RJ, Carey TE, Van Dyke DL: Deletion 9p22-pter and loss of Y as primary chromosome abnormalities in a squamous cell carcinoma of the vocal cord. Genes Chrom Cancer 7:158–164, 1993.

62. Worsham MJ, Carey TE, Benninger MJ, Gasser KM, Kelker W, Zarbo RJ, Van Dyke DL: Clonal cytogenetic evolution in a squamous cell carcinoma of the skin from a xeroderma pigmentosum patient. Genes Chrom Cancer 7:158–164, 1993.

63. Jin Y, Mertens F, Mandal N, Heim S, Olegard C, Wennerberg J, Biorklund A, Mitelman F: Chromosome abnormalities in eighty-three head and neck squamous cell carcinomas: influence of culture conditions on karyotypic pattern. Cancer Res 53:2140–2146, 1993.

64. Jin Y, Mertens F, Jin C, Akervall J, Wennerberg J, Gorunova L, Mandahl N, Heim S, Mitelman F: Non random chromosome abnormalities in short-term cultured primary squamous cell carcinomas of the head and neck. Cancer Res 55:3204–3210, 1995.

65. Zeigler A, Leffell, DJ, Kumala S, Sharma H, Gailani M, Simon JA, Halperin AJ, Baden HP, Shapiro, PE, Bale AE, Brash DE: Mutation hotspots due to sunlight in the p53 gene of nonmelanoma skin cancers. Proc Natl Acad Sci USA 90:4216–4220, 1993.

66. Chiba T, Takahashi T, Nau MM, D'Amico D, Curiel DT, Mitsudomi T, Buchhagen DL, Carbone D, Piantadosi S, Koga H, Reissman PT, Slamon D, Holmes EC, Minna JD: Mutations in the p53 gene are frequent in primary resected, non-small cell lung cancer. Oncogene 5:1603–1610, 1990.

67. Braun JE, Wanamarta AH, van den Akker E, Lafleur MV, Tetel J: C/G to A/T transversion represent the main type of mutation induced by Y-irradiation in double-stranded M13mp1 ODNA in a nitrogen-saturated solution. Mutat Res 289:255–263, 1993.

68. Worsham MJ, Wolman SR, Carey TE, Zarbo RJ, Benninger MS, Van Dyke DL: Common clonal origin of synchronous primary head and neck squamous cell carcinomas: analysis by tumor karyotypes and fluorescence in situ hybridization. Hum Pathol 26:251–261, 1995.

69. Lever, WF, Schaumburg-Lever G: Histopathology of the skin, 7th ed. Philadelphia, PA: Lippincott, 1990.

70. Mertens F, Heim S, Mandahl N, Johansson B, Mertens O, Persson B, Lasemark L, Wennerberg J, Jonsson N, Mitelman F: Cytogenetic analysis of 33 basal cell carcinomas. Cance Res 51: 954–957, 1991.

71. Kawasaki RS, Caldeira LF, Andre FS, Gasques JAL, Castilho WH, Bozola AR, Thome JA, Tajara EH: Multiple cytogenetic clones in a basal cell carcinoma. Cancer Genet Cytogenet 54:33–38, 1991.

72. Kawasaki-Oyama RS, Andre FS, Caldeira LF, Castilho WH, Gasques JAL, Bozola AR, Thome JA, Tajara EH: Cytogenetic findings in two basal cell carcinomas. Cancer Genet Cytogenet 73:152–156, 1994.

73. Konishi K, Yamanishi K, Ishizaki K, Yamada K, Saburo K, Yasuno H: Analysis of p53 mutations and loss of heterozygosity for loci on chromosome 9q in basal cell carcinoma. Cancer Lett 9:67–72, 1994.

74. Quinn AG, Sikkink S, Rees JL: Basal cell carcinomas and squamous cell carcinomas of human skin show distinct patterns of chromosome loss. Cancer Res 54:4756–4759, 1994.

75. Gailani MR, Bale SJ, Leffell DJ, DiGiovanna JJ, Peck GL, Poliak S, Drum MA, Pastakia B, McBride OW, Kase R, Greene M, Mulvihill JJ, Bale AE: Developmental defects in Gorlins syndrome related to a putative tumour suppressor gene on chromosome 9. Cell 69:111–117, 1992.

76. Goudie DR, Yuille, Leversha MA, Furlong RA, Carter NP, Lush MJ, Affara NA, Ferguson-Smith MA: Multiple self-healing squamous epitheliomata (ESS1) mapped to chromosome 9q22–q31 in families with common ancestry. Nat Genet 3:165–169, 1993.

77. Yuspa SH, Diugosz AA: Cutaneous carcinogenesis: natural and experimental In: Goldsmith LA. (ed.), Physiology, Biochemistry and Molecular Biology of the Skin. New York: Oxford University, pp. 1365–1400, 1991.

78. Boyle P, Maisonneuve P, Dore JF: Epidemiology of malignant melanoma. Br Med Bull 51:523–547, 1995.

79. Lee JA: Trends in melanoma incidence and mortality. Clin Dermatol 10:913, 1992.

80. Rigel DS: Epidemiology and prognostic factors in malignant melanoma. Ann Plas Surg 28:7–8, 1992.

81. Gallagher RP, Mclean DI, Yang CP, Coldman AJ, Silver HK, Spinelli JJ, Beagrie M: Suntan, sunburn, and pigmentation factors and the frequency of acquired melanocytic nevi in children. Similarities to melanoma: the Vancouver mole study. Arch Dermatol 126:770–776, 1990.

82. Osterlink A, Tucker MA, Stone BJ, Jensen OM: The Danish case-control study of cutaneous malignant melanoma. II. Importance of UV light exposure. Int J Cancer 42:319–324, 1988.

83. Elwood JM: Melanoma and ultraviolet irradiation. Clin Dermatol 10: 41–50, 1992.

84. Cifone MA, Fidler IJ: Increasing metastatic potential is associated with increasing genetic instability of clones isolated from murine neoplasms. Proc Natl Acad Sci USA 78:6949–6952, 1981.

85. Megidish T, Mazurek N: A mutant protein kinase C that can transform fibroblasts. Nature 342–807–811, 1989.

86. Fuchs J, Packet L: Ultraviolet irradition and the skin antioxidant system. Photodermatol Photoimmunol Photomed 7:90–92, 1990.

87. Rabiloud T, Asselilneau D, Miquel C, Calvayrac R, Darmon M, Vuillaume M: Deficiency in catalase activity correlates with the appearance of tumor phenotype in human keratinocytes. Int J Cancer 45:952–956, 1990.

88. Ronai AZ, Okini E, Weinstein IB: Ultraviolet light induces the expression of oncogenes in rat fibroblast and human keratinocytes. Oncogene 2:201–204, 1988.

89. Penn I: Ultraviolet light and skin cancer. Immunol Today 6:206–207, 1985.

90. Noonan FP, DeFablo EC: Ultraviolet B dose response curves for local and systemic immunosuppression are identical. Photochem Photobiol 52: 801–810, 1990.

91. Kripke MI: Ultraviolet radiation and tumor immunity. J Reticuloendothel Soc 22:217–222, 1977.

92. Crombie IK: Racial differences in melanoma incidence. Br J Cancer 40:185–193, 1979.

93. Clark WH Jr, Reimer RR, Greene M, Ainsworth AM, Mastrangelo MJ: Origin of familial malignant melanomas from heritable melanocytic lesions. Arch Dermatol 114:732, 1978.

94. Goldstein AM, Tucker MA: Genetic epidemiology of familial melanoma. Dermatol Clin 13:605–612, 1995.

95. Herlyn M: Molecular and Cellular Biology of Melanoma. Austin, TX: Landes, 1993.

96. Clark WH Jr, Elder DE, Guerry DIV, Epstein MN, Greene MH, Van Horn M. A study of tumor progression: the precursor lesions of superficial spreading and nodular melanoma. Hum Pathol 15:1147–1165, 1984.

97. Clark WH Jr, Tumor progression and the nature of cancer. Br J Cancer 64:631–644, 1991.

98. Elder DE, Clark WH Jr, Glenitsas R, Guerry DIV, Halpern AC: The early and intermediate precursor lesions of tumor progression in melanocytic systems: Common acquired nevi and atypical (dysplastic) nevi. Sem Diagnostic Pathol 1993.

99. National Institutes of Health: Precursors to malignant melanoma. National Institutes of Health, Oct. 24–26, 1983. Am J Dermatol 6:169–174, 1984.

100. Elder DE, Greene MH, Guerry DIV, Kraemer KH, Clark WH Jr: The dysplastic nevus syndrome: our definition. Am J Dermatol 4:455–460, 1982.

101. NIH Consensus Development Panel on Early Melanoma: Diagnosis and treatment of early melanoma. JAMA 268:1314–1319, 1992.
102. Balaban GB, Herlyn M, Clark WH Jr, Nowell PC: Karyotypic evolution in human malignant melanoma. Cancer Genet Cytogenet 19:113–122, 1986.
103. Richmond A, Fine R, Murray D, Lawson DH, Priest JH: Growth factor and cytogenetic abnormalities in cultured nevi and malignant melanomas. J Invest Dermatol 86:295–302, 1986.
104. Pedersen MI, Wang N: Chromosomal evolution in the progression and metastasis of human malignant melanoma. Cancer Genet Cytogenet 41:185–201, 1989.
105. Kath R, Rodeck U, Menssen HD, et al.: Tumor progression in the human melanocytic system. Anticancer Res 9:865–872, 1989.
106. Elder DE, Rodeck U, Thurin J, et al.: Antigenic profile of tumor progression stages in human melanocytic nevi and melanomas. Cancer Res 49: 5091–5096, 1989.
107. Breslow A: Thickness cross-sectional areas and depth of invasion in the prognosis of cutaneous melanoma. Ann Surg 172:902–907, 1970.
108. Clark WH, From L, Bernardino EA, Mihm MC: The histogenesis and biologic behavior of primary humn malignant melanomas of the skin. Cancer Res 29:705, 1969.
109. Clark WH, Elder DE, Guerry D, et al.: Model predicting survival in stage 1 melanoma based on tumor progression. J Natl Cancer Inst 81:1893, 1989.
110. Herzberg AJ, Kerns BJ, Horowitz MJ, Seigler HF, Kinney RB: DNA ploidy of malignant melanoma determined by image cytometry of fresh frozen and paraffin-embedded tissue. J Cutan Pathol 18:440–448, 1991.
111. Fountain JW, Bales SJ, Housman DE, Dracopoli NC: Genetics of melanoma. In: Franks LM (ed.), Cancer Survey: Advances and Prospects in Clinical, Epidemiological and Laboratory Oncology. London: Oxford University, Press; pp. 645–671, 1990.
112. Bales SJ, Dracopoli NC, Tucker MA, et al.: Mapping the gene for hereditary cutaneous malignant melanoma-dysplastic nevus to chromosome 1p. N Engl J Med 320:1367–1372, 1989.
113. Parmiter AH, Nowell PC: The cytogenetics of human malignant melanoma and premalignant lesons. In: Nathanson L. (ed.), Malignant melanoma: Biology, Diagnsois, and Therapy. Boston, MA: Kluwer Academic, pp. 47–61, 1988.
114. Dracopoli NC, Harnett P, Bale SJ, et al.: Loss of alleles from the distal short arm of chromosome 1 occurs late in melanoma tumor progression. Proc Natl Acad Sci USA 86:4614–4618, 1989.
115. Finger LR, Kagan J, Christopher G, et al.: Involvement of the TCL5 gene on human chromosome 1 in T- cell leukemia and melanoma. Proc Natl Acad Sci USA 86:5039–5043, 1989.
116. Eipers PG, Barnoski BL, Han J, Carroll AJ, Kidd VJ: Localization of the expressed human p58 protein kinase chnDmosomal gene to chromosome 1p36 and a highly related sequence to chromosome 1 5. Genomics 11: 621–629, 1991.

117. Millikin D, Meese E, Vogelstein B, Witkowski C, Trent J: Loss of heterozygosity for loci on the long arm of chromosome 6 in human malignant melanoma. Cancer Res 51:5449–5453, 1991.
118. Trent JM, Meyskens FL, Salmon SE, et al.: Relation of cytogenetic abnormalities and clinical outcome in metastatic melanoma. N Engl J Med 322:1508–1511, 1990.
119. Linnenbach AJ, Huebner K, Reddy EP, et al.: Structural alteration in the MYB protooncogene and deletion within the gene encoding alpha-type protein kinase C in human melanoma cell lines. Proc Natl Acad Sci USA 85:74–78, 1988.
120. Meese E, Meltzer PS, Witkowski CM, Trent JM: Molecular mapping of the oncogene myb and rearrangements in malignant melanoma. Genes Chromosome Cancer 1:88–94, 1989.
121. Koprowski H, Herlyn M, Balaban G, Parmiter A, Ross A, Nowell P: Expression of the receptor for epidermal growth factor correlates with increased dosage of chromosome 7 in malignant melanoma. Somat Cell Mol Genet 11:297–302, 1985.
122. Wittbrodt J, Adam D, Malitscheck B, Maueler W, Raulf F, Telling A, Robertson SM, Schartl M: Novel putative receptor tyrosine kinase encoded by the melanoma-inducing *Tu* locus in *Xiphophorus*. Nature 341:414–421, 1989.
123. Balaban G, Herlyn M, Guerry D IV, Bartolo R, Koprowski H, Clark WH Jr, Nowell PC: Cytogenetics of human malignant melanoma and premalignant lesions. Cancer Genet Cytogenet 11:429–439, 1984.
124. Collard JG, van de Poll M, Scheffer A, et al.: Localization of genes involved in invasion and metastasis on human chromosome 7. Cancer Res 47:6666–6670, 1987.
125. Fountain JW, Karayiorgou M, Ernstoff MS, et al.: Homozygous deletions within human chromosome band 9p21 in melanoma. Proc Natl Acad Sci USA 89:10,557–10,561, 1992.
126. Parmiter AH, Balaban G, Clark WH Jr, Nowell PC: Possible involvement of the chromosome region 10q24–q26 in early stages of melanocytic neoplasia. Cancer Genet Cytogenet 30:313–317, 1988.
127. Dracopoli NC, Houghton AN, Old LJ: Loss of polymorphic restriction fragments inmalignant melanoma: implications for tumor heterogeneity. Proc Natl Acad Sci USA 82:1470–1474, 1985.
128. Albino A, Fountain JW: Molecular genetics of human malignant melanoma. Cancer Treatment Res 65:201–255, 1993.
129. Yamanishi DT, Buckmeier JA, Meyskens FL Jr: Expression of c-jun, jun-B, and c-fos protooncogenes in human primary melanocytes and metastatic melanoma. J Invest Dermatol 97:349–353, 1991.
130. Halaban R, Moellmann G: Proliferation and malignant transformation of melanocytes. Crit Rev Oncog 2:247–258, 1991.
131. Chabot B, Stephenson DA, Chapman VM, Nesmer P, Bernstein A: The proto-oncogene c-kit encoding a transmembrane tyrosine kinase receptor maps to the mouse W locus. Nature 335:88, 89, 1988.

132. Geissler EN, Ryan MA, Housman DE: The dominant-white spotting (W) locus of the mouse encodes the c-kit proto-oncogene. Cell 55;185–192, 1988.
133. Toker C: Trabecular carcinoma of the skin. Arch Dermatol 105: 107–110, 1972.
134. Andrew KE, Silvers DN, Lattes R: Merkel cell carcinoma. In: Friedman RJ, Rigel DS, Kopf AW, et al. (eds.). Cancer of the Skin. New York: Saunders, pp. 228–294, 1991.
135. Ratner D, Nelson BR, Brown MD, Hohnson TM: Merkel cell carcinoma. J Am Acad Dermatol 29:143–156, 1993.
136. Mercer D, Brander P, Liddell K: Merkel cell carcinoma: the clinical course. Ann Plast Surg 25:136–141, 1990.
137. Johansson L, Tenvall J, Akeman M: Immunohistochemical examination of 25 cases of Merkel cell carcinoma: a comparison with small cell carcinoma of the lung and oesophagus, and review of the literature. Acta Pathol Microbiol Immunol Scand 98:741–752, 1990.
138. Kusyk CJ, Romsdahl MM: Cytogenetic studies of a Merkel cell carcinoma. Cancer Genet Cytogenet 20:311–316, 1986.
139. Smadja N, de Gramont A, Gonzalez-Canali G, Louvet EW, Krulik M: Cytogenetic study of a bone marrow metastatic Merkel cell carcinoma. Cancer Genet Cytogenet 51:85–87, 1991.
140. Sandbrick F, Muler L, Fiebig HH, Kovacs F: Short communication: Deletion 7q, trisomy 6 and 11 in a case of Merkel cell carcinoma. Cancer Genet Cytogenet 33:305–309, 1988.
141. Harnett PR, Kearsley JH, Hayward NK, et al.: Loss of allelic heterozygosity on distal chromosome 1p in Merkel cell carcinoma: a marker of neural crest origin? Cancer Genet Cytogenet 54:109–113, 1991.
142. Osella P, Carlson A, Wyandt H, Milunsky A: Cytogenetic studies of eight squamous cell carcinomas of the head and neck: deletion of 7q, a possible primary chromosomal event. Cancer Genet Cytogenet 59:73–78, 1992.
143. Zaslav AL, Stamberg J, Steinberg BM, Lin YJ, Abramson A: Cyotgenetic analysis of head and neck carcinomas. Cancer Genet Cytogenet 56: 181–187, 1991.
144. Pejovic T, Heim S, Orndal C, Jin Y, Mandahl N, Willen H, Mitelman F: Simple numerical chromosome aberrations in well-differentiated malignant epithelial tumors. Cancer Genet Cytogenet 49:95–101, 1990.
145. Owens W, Fild JK, Howard PJ, Stell PM: Multiple cytogenetic aberrations in squamous cell carcinomas of the head and neck. Oral Oncol Eur J Cancer 28B:1721, 1992.

Chapter 13

Brain Tumors

Joan Rankin Shapiro and Adrienne C. Scheck

Introduction

Tumors of the central nervous system (CNS; brain and spinal cord) are devastating diseases that are most often accompanied by a poor prognosis. Primary brain tumors can occur at all ages, but most frequently cluster within two distinct peaks of age incidence. In adults the peak occurs at 55–65 yr of age, and in children from ages 3–12 (Fig. 1). With the assistance of better imaging devices, approx 15,000 new cases of adult CNS tumors are diagnosed each year *(1)*, and approx 11,000 deaths per year are attributed to these neoplasias. Whereas pediatric brain tumors are less numerous, with approx 1200 new cases each year *(2)*, they are now the leading cause of death from cancer in children. Brain tumors affect the sexes differently. Glioma, the most common CNS tumor in adults, affects more males than females, and the reverse is true for meningiomas.

Cancer is a multiple-step process in which the tumor cells acquire a series of genetic lesions. In leukemia *(3)* and lymphoma *(4)*, many of these steps have been defined at cytogenetic and molecular levels. Although solid tumors have generally lagged behind in this regard, significant advances in defining the genetic lesions associated with different stages of neoplasia have been made in several

From: *Human Cytogenetic Cancer Markers*   Edited by S. R. Wolman and S. Sell
Humana Press Inc., Totowa, NJ

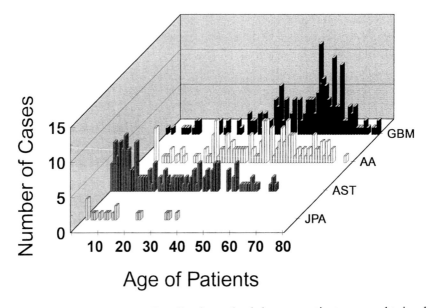

Fig. 1. Age at onset of pediatric and adult astrocytic tumors obtained from the 525 cases included in this study. The pediatric population includes ages 0.1 mo to 18 yr of age and the adult population spans 19–80 yr of age. AA, anaplastic astrocytoma; AST, astrocytoma; GBM, glioblastoma multiforme; JPA, juvenile pilocytic astrocytoma.

tumor systems (5–8). Several factors contribute to the difficulties of such analyses of solid tissues, namely, availability of tissue, problems in obtaining direct preparations on informative samples, and the inherent heterogeneity of tumors (9), which is a major problem in malignant gliomas (10). Further complicating the detection of specific nonrandom chromosome changes in solid tumors are issues of consistency of histological assessment and grading. Despite these difficulties, genetic analyses of both adult and pediatric brain tumors continue to be reported. This chapter reviews the cytogenetic and molecular abnormalities associated with different histological types and grades of adult and pediatric brain tumors of the CNS.

Brain Tumor Classification

The establishment of a histological diagnosis for brain tumors is necessary both to guide therapeutic decisions and to accurately interpret research data and the results of clinical trials. Historically, gliomas have been classified based on their resemblance to normal adult cells. They were divided into many histological categories with names and prognoses determined by cytological similarities to stages of cellular differentiation during embryogenesis *(11)*. Kernohan and Sayre *(12)* later introduced a grading system based on the identification of features of anaplasia, such as necrosis, frequency of mitosis, and loss of cellular differentiation. A number of systems that were based on either three- or four-tiered grading of malignancy followed this model *(13)*. It is important that an investigator know the grading system used in the diagnosis of each sample so that laboratory results can be compared; several excellent reference texts are available and should be referred to when reporting experimental data *(14,15)*.

The term "brain tumor" includes a large variety of histologically different tumors *(14)* ranging from the benign, noninvasive tumor such as the meningioma, to the highly aggressive and invasive mass characteristic of glioblastoma multiforme. Gliomas are the most common type of adult brain tumor (70%). They arise from transformation of glial cells, namely astrocytes, oligodendrocytes, and ependymal cells. The term glioma, therefore, is the general term for a group of glial tumors, i.e., astrocytic tumors (astrocytoma, anaplastic astrocytoma, and glioblastoma multiforme), oligodendroglioma and ependymoma. Brain tumors can also be composed of two cell types, and these are referred to as mixed tumors. Such tumors can be a mixture of two different glial cells, e.g., astrocytoma-oligodendroglioma or ependymoma-oligodendroglioma, or they can be composed of two different tissue types, e.g., gliosarcoma, which is a mixture of transformed glial cells and transformed mesenchymal cells (endothelial, meningeal and/or, smooth muscle cells). Each of these tumor types has a broad range of phenotypes depending on its degree of malignancy. Grades I through IV are used to characterize the degree of aggressive and invasive behavior of these tumor types, ranging from low-grade (I and II) tumors such as the astrocytoma, oligodendroglioma, and ependymoma to the more malignant (grades III and IV) anaplastic astrocytoma, anaplastic oligodendroglioma, anaplastic ependymoma, and glioblastoma multiforme. The many different types of brain tumors and the inconsistency of grading systems are the basis of confusion in the literature when attempts are made to correlate genetic alterations with specific brain lesions. Moreover, since the neuropathologist is frequently requested to make such diagnoses on needle biopsies or on small, potentially nonrepresentative tumor samples *(16)*, the original diagnosis may not be identical to the final diagnosis.

Because of the number of histologically distinct tumor types and controversies regarding grading systems, a brief introduction concerning the histology of individual subtypes of brain tumor precedes the relevant cytogenetic and molecular data in each section. Although detailed molecular descriptions are beyond the scope of this chapter, specific molecular data that relate to cytogenetic results are included. Insufficient data on cytogenetic and molecular analyses preclude mention of many rare brain tumors, and only tumors for which five or more cases have been reported were included herein. Similarly, we have excluded discussion of all recurrent tumors and those cases where patients had received adjuvant therapy (irradiation and/or chemotherapy) in order to focus on chromosome analysis of primary brain tumors.

Astrocytic Tumors

Three major classifications of astrocytic tumors exist, the astrocytoma, the anaplastic astrocytoma, and the glioblastoma multiforme, each defined by specific histological criteria and grading. Unlike many of the other brain tumors described subsequently, the histopathologic evaluation of the astrocytic tumors is prognostic. In addition, there is good correlation between increasing grades of malignancy and the age of onset as illustrated in Fig. 1.

Adult vs Pediatric Astrocytic Tumors

Adults and children frequently develop the same types of tumors; however, several differences are notable other than histology between most adult and pediatric tumors. One such difference is the predilection to specific locations in the brain. Adult brain tumors commonly develop supratentorially within the cortical, subcortical, and basal ganglia regions. In contrast, approx 60% of pediatric tumors develop in the infratentorial cavity within the cerebellum, pons, and brainstem *(17)*. In addition, the incidence of particular tumor types varies significantly between the adult and pediatric population. For example, astrocytic tumors, oligodendrogliomas, and ependymomas, are the most common tumors of adults. Whereas children can develop these tumors, they more commonly develop juvenile pilocytic astrocytomas and a group of tumors called primitive neuroectodermal tumors (PNET), discussed under embryonal tumors. The PNET tumors constitute a large group of pediatric embryonal tumors of which the most common type is the medulloblastoma, which accounts for 20–25% of all childhood tumors *(2)*. Another important difference between adult and pediatric malignancies is their response to therapy *(2)*. Extensive resection, irradiation and chemotherapy in adult patients with a diagnosis of malignant CNS tumors improve survival only modestly *(18)*, whereas pediatric malignancies tend to be more responsive to treatment, especially chemotherapy *(19)*. This has suggested to some investigators that the differential responsiveness observed between adult and pediatric tumors reflects biological differences, even when the tumors appear histologically to be of the same type and grade.

Adult Astrocytic Tumors

Astrocytomas

Astrocytomas are a group of low-grade tumors (grades I and II) that may be further defined as pilocytic, fibrillary, protoplasmic, or gemistocytic. The juvenile pilocytic astrocytoma (grade I) is a tumor that affects the young (first and second decades of life) (Fig. 1), with a predilection for the cerebellum and the region of the third ventricle, the optic nerves, and the thalamus. Juvenile pilocytic astrocytomas are more common than either the protoplasmic or gemistocytic subtypes, but are less common than the fibrillary astrocytoma that comprises 10–15% of the astrocytic tumors in adults. Young adults, generally between the ages of 20 and 40, have the highest incidence of low-grade fibrillary astrocytoma. Although this is generally a slow growing tumor, it is not benign because of its invasive quality and location. Fibrillary astrocytomas may occur anywhere in the brain; however, they are most prevalent in the cerebral hemispheres. This tumor infiltrates neighboring normal brain tissue, although nuclear atypia and mitotic activity are absent from the histology. These tumors will generally progress to more malignant tumors over a period of several years.

Low-grade tumors are difficult to study. One reason is the lack of availability of tissue. Patients diagnosed with low-grade tumors frequently do not undergo surgical resections, and only a needle biopsy is performed for confirmation of diagnosis. Another difficulty is that the tumor masses are frequently admixtures of normal reactive cells and tumor cells. The proportion of normal cells to tumor cells can greatly influence the results of cytogenetic and molecular analyses *(20,21)*. In addition, tumors may appear as mixtures of histologically different grades of tumor. Small nonrepresentative biopsies can, therefore, significantly alter the assignment of tumor grade. It has been demonstrated that incorrect diagnoses are more frequent with examination of needle biopsies than with examination of tissue from subtotal resections *(22,23)*. These problems are reflected in questions as to whether low-grade gliomas are cytogenetically normal with molecular genetic lesions, and whether specific numerical abnormalities reflect a specific pathway of tumor evolution *(24)*. Resolution of these questions is likely to come from combined cytogenetic, molecular cytogenetic, and molecular biological analyses.

Many investigators combine grade I and II tumors under the common term of astrocytoma, making it difficult to determine the genetic alterations that contribute to the formation of pilocytic tumors. We have identified five adult pilocytic (grade I) astrocytomas from the literature that had not received previous adjuvant therapy *(25–27)*. Figure 2, top panel, defines the loss and gain of whole chromosomes associated with this limited number of cases and Fig. 3 details the clonal breakpoints.

Earlier cytogenetic reviews of the astrocytoma literature, which combined grade I and grade II tumors, identified the gain of chromosome 7 and loss of chromosomes 10, 22, and a single sex chromosome. Structural abnormalities were infrequent, and when observed, they most often involved chromosomal arms 1p and 9p *(28,29)*. We have been able to identify 68 primary astrocytomas (grades I and II) from among the cases reported as direct preparations or early passage cells that received no treatment prior to cytogenetic analysis *(25,27,30–40)*. These 68 tumors include only astrocytomas from patients ages 19 or older (Fig. 1), 45 from males, and 23 from females. Twenty-six of the 68 cases reported normal karyotypes as

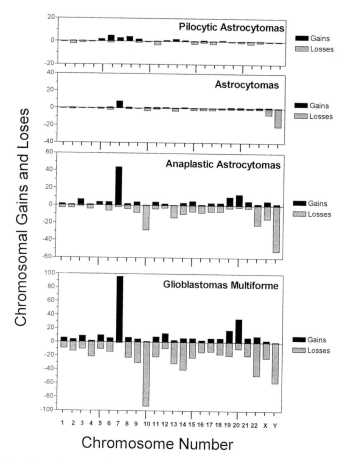

Fig. 2. Clonal numerical chromosome changes in adult astrocytic tumors: five cases of adult pilocytic astrocytoma, 68 cases of astrocytoma, 127 cases of anaplastic astrocytoma, and 198 cases of GBM.

the only finding. Whole chromosome losses and gains in these 68 cases are illustrated in Fig. 2, second panel. The most common chromosome abnormality was the loss of a single sex chromosome (X or Y) in 25 of 68 cases. Twenty of the male samples had lost a Y chromosome, and it was the sole abnormality in 14 of these 20 cases. Five of the cases from females had lost an X chromosome as the only clonal abnormality. Chromosome 7 was the only chromosome gained in this group of adult astrocytomas. Of the eight cases with chromosome 7 aneuploidy, it was the sole clonal abnormality in two cases and the other five cases contained additional clonal numerical and/or structural abnormalities. In contrast to previous reviews, this larger survey of grade I and II astrocytomas suggests that loss of chromosome 10 is infrequent, and loss of chromosome 22 is rare.

Figure 3 illustrates the identified breakpoints associated with the astrocytic tumors. Most of the changes in low-grade astrocytomas are numerical changes rather than structural rearrangements. Only chromosome 1 had more than three breakpoints on the same chromosome.

A comparison of the cytogenetic data with the molecular data obtained from astrocytomas demonstrates the utility of performing molecular analyses in concert with cytogenetic techniques. This is most evident for chromosome 17. Although the cytogenetic data have not displayed loss, gain, or structural rearrangement of chromosome 17 in adult astrocytomas *(27,30–46)*, molecular investigations have demonstrated that the principle genetic lesions in these low-grade tumors are mutations of p53, with or without loss of heterozygosity (LOH) *(42,44,45,47–54)*. Furthermore, although the vast majority of published data show no molecular changes associated with chromosomes other than 17 in low-grade astrocytomas *(38,55,56)*, sporadic reports of a few astrocytomas substantiate LOH on chromosome 1 *(42,57,58)*, chromosome 3 *(59–61)*, chromosome 10 *(62)*, or chromosome 22 *(63)*. Each LOH is a probable site for tumor suppressor genes. The data suggest that two tumor suppressor genes exist on chromosome 10, one located on the p arm and the other on the q arm *(35,59,64)*. The retinoblastoma (Rb) locus that maps to 13q14 is also deleted in a small number of astrocytomas *(47)*. Likewise, the neurofibromatosis gene (NF2), which maps to 22q12, was considered the likely responsible gene for the observed LOH on 22q; however, recent data do not support a role for this gene in astrocytomas since the NF2 gene appears to be intact *(65)*. It is, however, likely that an additional tumor suppressor gene on chromosome 22 lies more distal to NF2 *(31)*. Increased expression of the platelet-derived growth factor receptor α (PDGFR-α) that maps to

Fig. 3. *(opposite page)* Identified clonal chromosome breakpoints involved in structural rearrangements in: 5 pilocytic astrocytomas (✳), 68 astrocytoma (●), 125 anaplastic astrocytomas (○), and 180 GBM (▲).

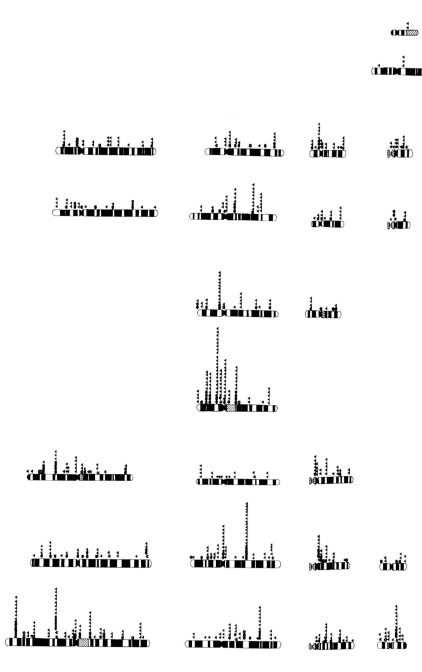

Fig 3.

chromosome 4 has been reported *(66)*. Unfortunately, numerous unsubstantiated reports that concern genetic alterations in astrocytomas have led to a generally held notion that grade II astrocytoma formation is accompanied by loss of genetic material from 13q, 17p, 22q and overexpression of PDGFR-α and PDGF-A. There is clearly a need for careful evaluation of the published data with respect to genetic changes in different grades of gliomas and generalization of results obtained from isolated tumors.

Anaplastic Astrocytomas

It is generally accepted that many of the anaplastic astrocytomas develop from low-grade astrocytomas *(14,16)*, although some evidence indicates that these tumors may arise *de novo (51)*. Although no sharply defined histological criteria separate astrocytomas from anaplastic astrocytomas, the latter are distinguished by higher cell density and mitotic activity, early or focal contrast enhancement, and greater nuclear polymorphism with multinucleation, lobulation, and angulation. The nuclear/cytoplasmic ratio is also increased, but the astrocytic character is still evidenced by fibrillar eosinophilic cytoplasm and the presence of processes.

Anaplastic astrocytomas are found in both young and old patients, with the peak incidence occurring in the mid-50s, as illustrated by the 127 primary, untreated cases depicted in Fig. 1. In contrast to astrocytomas, in which more than half of the cases reported had normal banded karyotypes, only 10 of the 127 (7%) anaplastic astrocytomas had a normal banded karyotype. The gain and loss of specific chromosomes is depicted in Fig. 2, showing that the pattern of gain and loss attributed to astrocytomas (panel 2) is more clearly reflected in the anaplastic astrocytomas (panel 3). Chromosome 7 is frequently gained, with less frequent gain of chromosomes 19 and 20. Loss of chromosomes 10, 22, and a single sex chromosome are also prominent, with fewer instances of loss of chromosomes 13 and 14.

Two chromosome changes, the gain of chromosome 7 *(32,67)* and loss of a sex chromosome *(68)*, have been the center of considerable controversy. Some investigators have reported that these chromosome changes occur in normal tissue, and that the sex chromosome loss is age related. It should be noted, however, that the tissue referred to as "normal" in these studies was, in fact, taken from patients undergoing craniotomy for a diagnosis of glioma. The other patients whose cells did not show trisomy 7 had hematoma (three patients) or meningioma (one patient), although several of the otherwise-normal cultures were mosaic for loss of a sex chromosome. A series of articles followed that demonstrated that normal brain does not have abnormalities of chromosome 7 *(69–72)* or the Y chromosome *(73,74)*.

Of the 127 cases of anaplastic astrocytoma we reviewed, only 2 cases gained chromosome 7 as the only clonal abnormality. Thirty-seven other cases demonstrated aneuploidy of chromosome 7 in addition to other clonal numerical and/or structural aberrations. The loss of a sex chromosome was more frequently an isolated clonal abnormality. For example, 82 of the 127 tumors were from male patients. Of these, 47 demonstrated Y chromosome loss and in 24 of these cases it was the only clonal abnormality. The remaining 23 cases included loss of a Y chromosome among other clonal aberrations. Two of the 45 female cases showed loss of a single X chromosome as the only clonal abnormality. Six additional cases were missing an X chromosome in addition to other clonal abnormalities. The remaining cases contained a spectrum of numerical and/or structural aberrations. The loss of chromosome 10 was observed in 29 of the 127 cases. In 3 cases it was the sole abnormality and in 26 other cases additional clonal abnormalities accompanied chromosome 10 loss. Loss of chromosome 22 displayed a similar pattern; of the 23 cases only 2 examples were confined to chromosome 22 loss and the remaining 21 contained additional clonal abnormalities.

Structural abnormalities were more frequent on the p arms of chromosomes 1, 3, and 9 (1p32, 1p36, 3p21, 9p21, and 9p22) as indicated by the open circles in Fig. 3. Similar clusters were also observable on the q arms of chromosomes 6 and 7 (6q21 and 7q22). Chromosomal bands 5p13, 15q11, 17p11, and 19q12.1, each have three breakpoints in common; all other chromosomes appear to have breaks at various places along the length of their chromosome. These data have served as a guide for many molecular studies.

Several molecular analyses have indicated that >30% of anaplastic astrocytomas have mutation and/or deletion of the p53 gene (17p13.1) *(42–45,47,49,52,53,55,62,75–79)*. However, it was difficult to understand why aberrations of the p53 gene were identified in <50% of samples if this gene was indeed critical for tumor evolution. A possible explanation came from combined molecular and cytogenetic analyses. Reifenberger et al. *(80)* and Raffel et al. *(81)* demonstrated that a region on chromosome 12 (12q13–14) is amplified in 15% of WHO grade III (anaplastic astrocytoma) and IV (glioblastoma multiforme) tumors. These amplified tumors showed a high incidence of LOH on adjacent 12q loci, data corresponding to results reported for testicular germ cell and other solid tumors *(81)*. A number of genes map to this region, three of which are frequently amplified; the murine double minute 2 *(MDM2)*, CDK4, and *SAS*. *MDM2* codes for a cellular protein that complexes with the p53 tumor suppressor gene product and inhibits its function. *MDM2* is amplified in a subset of gliomas *(80,81)* that typically have neither loss nor mutation of p53, thus providing a mechanism by which glioma cells can escape p53-mediated growth regulation in the absence of direct genetic inactivation of p53. Several investigators have demonstrated homozygous loss of 9q21 in gliomas *(82–85)*, and the gene mapped to this region is now called the multiple tumor suppressor 1 *(MTS-1)*. It encodes an inhibitor of cyclin-dependent kinase 4 *(86–89)*, again suggesting an alternative genetic mechanism leading to the same biological result, in this case, increased CDK4. Another LOH on chromosome 19q has been observed by several investigators, although the putative tumor suppressor gene has not yet been identified *(35,90–94)*. As illustrated in Fig. 3, each of these loci is a breakpoint in anaplastic astrocytomas. More recently, the allelic status of chromosome 1 has been analyzed. A region spanning 1p36–p32, which is involved by numerous deletions and translocations, demonstrates frequent LOH *(58,94,95)*. The sampling of anaplastic astrocytomas is small and the LOH detected in this region may be more important in another group of brain tumors, the oligodendrogliomas. Another chromosome region in which allelic loss has been detected is chromosome 11p15 → pter *(96,97)*. The chromosomal region at 3p21 is also a common site of deletion and translocation, but no allelic loss has yet been established for this chromosome (Fig. 3).

Glioblastomas Multiforme (GBM)

The peak age incidence for the GBM is in the mid-60s (Fig. 1). The GBM is the most malignant of the astrocytic tumors and the mean survival time of patients with this diagnosis is approx 1 yr *(2)*. This tumor is highly infiltrative, producing undifferentiated elements as a dominant feature, with high mitotic activity and necrosis. Vascular proliferation may also be evident, and the bromodeoxyuridine/Ki-67 labeling index is high. Although genetic instability in this tumor results in complex, nonuniform genetic changes, malignant gliomas of the astrocytic series show several significant nonrandom chromosome changes. One hundred and ninety-eight cases of GBM were identified for this review *(10,25,27,30,35,37–39,98–106)*. The most frequent numerical chromosome changes are gain of chromosomes 7 and 20, and the loss of chromosomes 10, 22, and a single sex chromosome *(10,25,27,28,30,31,72,74,100,107–109)*. The gain of chromosome 20 is more evident in GBM than in anaplastic astrocytoma. Chromosome losses are more prevalent than gains, with added loss of whole chromosomes 9, 13, and 14. The proportion of tumors in males with loss of a single sex chromosome is approximately the same as in anaplastic astrocytomas. Of the 58 cases with loss of the Y chromosome, it was the only abnormality in half the cases, whereas the remaining cases lost a Y in addition to other clonal abnormalities.

Structural abnormalities within glioblastomas are notably increased as illustrated in Fig. 3. The most frequent abnormalities occur in chromosomal arms 9p, 9q, 1p, and 6q *(16,25,100)*. Rearrangement involving chromosome 9 is clustered around two breakpoints, 9p12 and 9q11. On chromosome 1 breakpoints occur at chromosome bands 1p36 and 1p22.1, and on chromosome 6 at band 6q23.1. Less frequent but clustered breakpoints occur at chromosomal loci 3p21, 7q11 and 7q22, 10p11, 11q22, 15q11, 17p11, and 19q13. Although it has been reported that about half of the malignant gliomas contain double minutes (dmin) *(10,28,100)*, in this review of primary untreated GBM, we found an incidence of 25%. Also differing from the less malignant tumors is the increase in cases reporting marker chromosomes (30%). Because markers may represent selective retention of specific genes, it is important to assess their origin with fluorescent *in situ* hybridization (FISH) techniques.

The largest body of molecular data for astrocytic tumors has been obtained from the GBM. The frequency of p53 mutation and/or alellic loss is approximately the same in GBMs as in anaplastic astrocytomas, supporting the hypothesis that this DNA lesion occurs early in the evolution of gliomas *(47)*. Additional support derives from a study in which clonal expansion of a p53 mutation was demonstrated in the recurrent tumor *(43)*. Other significant genetic lesions involve chromosome 7, which is overrepresented in the majority of GBM (Fig. 2, bottom panel). The genes encoding the epidermal growth factor receptor (EGFR) and the PDGF-A map to chromosome 7 at positions 7p13–p11 and 7q11–13, respectively. Both genes are amplified and/or overexpressed in GBMs *(66,103,110–113)*. EGFR amplification and/or gene rearrangement, occurring in 40–60% of GBMs, is frequently associated with the expression of truncated forms of the message and protein. PDGF overexpression is less frequent, but its autocrine regulation suggests that, like EGFR, it could provide a selective growth advantage to tumor cells.

Significant loss of the whole chromosome 10 (Fig. 2, bottom panel) was reported in approx 50% of the tumors reviewed, but alellic loss from 10p and 10q is even more common, occurring in 70–80% of the tumors. Although the identity of specific putative tumor suppressor gene(s) remains unknown, loss of at least two independent regions from chromosome 10 has been demonstrated, suggesting the existence of more than one tumor suppressor gene *(47,59,64,114,115)*. More recently, some investigators have attempted to subdivide patients with GBMs, assuming that different pathways are dependent on the genetic defects acquired in the formation of GBMs. They suggest that tumors whose progression is stepwise from low grade to more malignant anaplastic astrocytoma and then to GBM have a p53 mutation followed by alellic loss of chromosome 10. In contrast, GBMs that arise *de novo* demonstrate alellic loss on chromosome 10 and amplification of EGFR *(53,114, 116)*. Other workers have attempted to determine whether subsets of the genetic lesions are prognostically significant *(117)*.

One is still confronted with the problem of understanding those tumors that do not appear to have the aforementioned genetic lesions. An obvious source of such confounding data is tumor heterogeneity that can be demonstrated by histology, cytogenetics, and molecular techniques. Data to support the hypothesis that some genetic alterations may actually presage the frank appearance of histological markers has been obtained from regional analyses of cytogenetic characteristics *(20)*, flow cytometric analysis of ploidy and S-phase fraction *(20)*, LOH analysis *(118)*, and comparisons of primary and recurrent tumor from the same patient *(119)*.

An additional explanation for the lack of uniformity with respect to the presence of specific genetic lesions requires an understanding of the biology of the tumor system. The presence or absence of a gene, chromosome, or chromosomal locus provides a clue as to the function that is missing or aberrant in a cell. However, any aberrant phenotype may be the result of different mechanisms rather than being mediated by a single gene. An example of this can be seen in the allelic loss associated with 9p. The p16 protein is mapped to this region, and acts as a cell cycle inhibitor of cyclin-dependent kinase 4; however, recent studies have shown that aberrant cell cycle control may arise from many different genetic lesions including amplification of *MDM2* or CDK4 (chromosome 12), and mutation of p53 (chromosome 17). Thus, an understanding of the genetic lesions leading to tumor formation is likely to require the collaborative efforts of cytogeneticists, molecular geneticists, and molecular biologists.

Pediatric Astrocytic Tumors

Pediatric astrocytic tumors differ from adult astrocytic tumors in that they are more frequently identified in the cerebellum, pons, and brain stem, and the incidence in males is equal to that found in females. Children can develop highly malignant and invasive tumors, such as the GBM, but the most common astrocytic neoplasm in children is the juvenile pilocytic (grade I) astrocytoma. The pilocytic astrocytoma is considered a tumor of the young and is referred to as the juvenile pilocytic astrocytoma (JPA), although as indicated earlier, some adults can develop this neoplasm. The cytogenetic and molecular literature will in some instances separate this tumor from other astrocytomas. In other studies, many tumors included in the astrocytoma category may, in fact, be JPAs.

Astrocytomas

Figure 1 illustrates the incidence of astrocytic tumors within the pediatric age range. The JPA are distributed over the same range

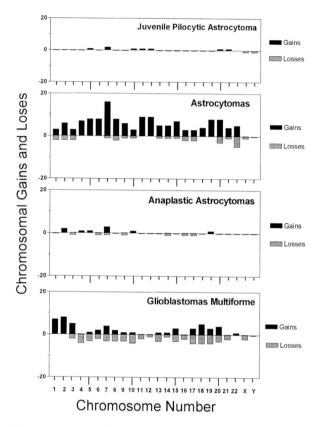

Fig. 4. Clonal numerical chromosome changes in pediatric astrocytic tumors: 16 cases of adult pilocytic astrocytoma, 99 cases of astrocytoma, 17 cases of anaplastic astrocytoma, and 16 cases of GBM.

as the group designated astrocytomas. JPA are low-grade (grade I) tumors characterized by the presence of Rosenthal fibers. Most often these tumors are slow growing and associated with >5-yr survival. Only 16 primary untreated pilocytic cases have been reported in the cytogenetic literature *(25,26,33,34,101,120)*. Nine of these 16 cases had diploid normal Giemsa (G)-banded karyotypes, and the other 7 cases contained additional numerical and/or structural abnormalities (Fig. 4, top panel, and Fig. 5). No single numerical or structural aberration was common among these cases, although 2 cases, 1 male and 1 female, each involved the loss of a single sex chromosome as the only clonal abnormality.

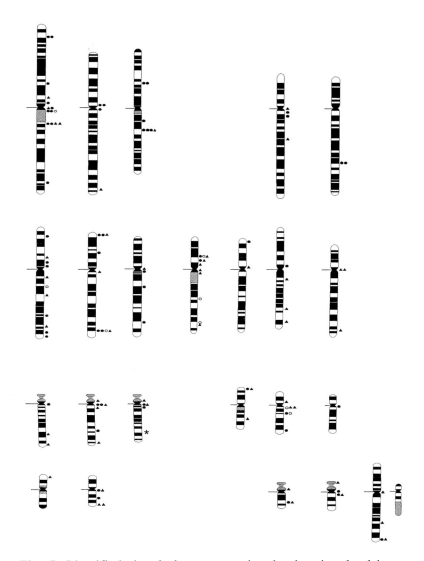

Fig. 5. Identified clonal chromosome breakpoints involved in structural rearrangements in 16 pilocytic astrocytomas (✳), 99 astrocytomas (●), 16 anaplastic astrocytomas (○), 16 GBM (▲).

Ninety-nine primary untreated pediatric astrocytomas (grade II) were identified for review *(26,27,31,34,36,40,101,105,120–127)*. More than half of these cases (60 of 99) were reported as normal diploid G-banded karyotypes; the remaining cases had one or more clonal abnormalities. Notable among the 53 female and 46 male cases was the absence of missing sex chromosomes. Only 1 of the 53 female patients had a missing X chromosome as the sole clonal abnormality and two additional cases (1 female, 1 male) were missing a sex chromosome in addition to other clonal abnormalities. Also in contrast to adult tumors, the pediatric astrocytomas tended to show gain of whole chromosomes (Fig. 4, second panel). Although gain of chromosome 7 was almost twice as frequent as gain of any other chromosome, only a single case showed trisomy of chromosome 7 as the only clonal abnormality.

The breakpoints among the pediatric astrocytomas were most numerous on chromosomes 1, 3 and 6 (Fig. 5). No cluster of breakpoints to particular bands were evident, although many breakpoints were identical to those observed in adult astrocytic tumors.

Only a few investigations have included JPA tumors in their restriction fragment length polymorphism (RFLP) analyses *(26,27, 62,114,128–130)*. In each study, the tissues analyzed displayed constitutional heterozygosity at one or more loci, but demonstrated rare allelic loss. One molecular analysis of 20 JPA for allelic loss on chromosome 17p detected two regions of loss in 6 tumors; 1 in the telomeric region (17p13.3) and 1 centromeric to p53 (17p13.1) *(129)*. Clinical correlation between those tumors demonstrating 17p allelic loss and tumor recurrence was found. Since the p53 gene may be rendered nonfunctional by mutation with or without allelic loss, or may be inactivated by the overexpression of the protein encoded by the *MDM2* gene, further investigation is needed to determine whether functional loss of p53 is predictive of clinical course. Studies of allelic loss in fibrillary astrocytomas are discussed in the section on adult astrocytomas.

Anaplastic Astrocytomas

Anaplastic astrocytomas are generally rare in children, and only 16 published cases met the criteria for inclusion in this review *(27,40,121,124,127)*. Fifty percent of the cases were recorded as normal G-banded karyotypes, and the remaining 8 contained numerical and/or structural abnormalities (Fig. 4, third panel, and Fig. 5). Loss and gain of whole chromosomes appeared to be random in this small sample, unlike results observed in the adult population (Fig. 2, third panel). Because only a few breakpoints were identified in these tumors, no specificity of chromosome or clustering of breakpoints could be determined. However, the few rearranged chromosomes recorded had breakpoints similar to those found in adult astrocytic tumors.

Molecular analyses of pediatric astrocytomas were also very limited *(62,114,129,130)*. Although several studies detected only rare allelic loss of p53, one report differed in detecting allelic loss of 17p in 5 of 7 anaplastic samples, using multiple probes that spanned the p arm *(129)*. The most common site of loss was telomeric in all 5 pediatric anaplastic tumors. Moreover, all 5 recurred within 4 yr, again suggesting that lesions in 17p are early events in the evolution of astrocytic tumors.

GBM

The GBM is a rare tumor in individuals under 18 yr of age, with only 16 cases identified in the cytogenetic literature *(27,40, 120,124,126,127)*. This is a highly malignant tumor in children, as it is in adults, that carries a poor prognosis. One notable difference in the cytogenetics of pediatric GBM (Fig. 4, bottom panel) is that, unlike the astrocytomas and anaplastic astrocytomas, only 3 of the 16 cases showed a normal diploid G-banded karyotype. The remaining 13 cases had extensive numerical and/or structural rearrangements with marker chromosomes in addition to multiple sideline clones and/or dmin. Losses and gains of whole chromosomes appeared random, as in the less malignant pediatric astrocytic tumors. One notable difference is the absence of karyotypes demonstrating loss of a sex chromosome.

Even though structural rearrangements were more numerous in pediatric GBMs than in either the pediatric astrocytomas or anaplastic astrocytomas (Fig. 5), no clustering of breakpoints at specific chromosome bands was evident. The distribution and location of many of the identified breakpoints were similar to those observed in adult astrocytic tumors.

Investigations of pediatric GBMs for p53 mutation have demonstrated allelic loss of 17p and p53 gene alterations in the majority of cases *(46,129,131)*. In one study, loss of 10q was noted in about half of the samples, although the concurrent amplification of EGFR observed in adults was not found *(131)*.

Some investigators contend that these results suggest that high-grade pediatric tumors share similarities with the GBMs of young adults, whereas other investigators suggest that fundamental differences between adult and pediatric tumors are reflected in both the cytogenetic and molecular results. For example, p53 mutations range from 15% in adult, low-grade tumors to 38% in high-grade tumors, but such mutations are rare in pediatric tumors, accounting for only 1–2% of the tumors examined. Thus, additional studies are required to resolve these issues, most appropriately those incorporating cytogenetic as well as molecular analyses.

Other Astrocytic Neoplasms

Cytogenetic studies of the infrequent astrocytic variant tumors number four or fewer analyzed cases.

Xanthoastrocytoma

This lesion generally arises in the temporal or parietal lobes and usually forms cysts with mural nodules. The tumor is generally associated with an abrupt interface with normal brain. It can be densely cellular, and shows four characteristic features; pleomorphic cells, lipidization of astrocytes, foci of perivascular lymphocytes, and abundance of reticulin. Analyses of this tumor are limited to a few case reports *(25)*.

Gliomatosis Cerebri

This neoplasm remains problematic, as it is a highly infiltrative astrocytic neoplasm like the GBM. It differs from the GBM in that it lacks a necrotic glioblastomatous epicenter. Only two cytogenetic studies of this rare tumor have been reported *(124,132)*.

Giant Cell Astrocytomas (Tuberous Sclerosis)

Distinguished by its "giant" cells, this tumor lacks the vascular proliferation, necrosis, and pseudo palisading associated with GBM. Several reports have included examples of this lesion *(25,*

38,100). Each of these tumors is considerably more rare than the aforementioned astrocytic tumors. Until more cases are accrued for cytogenetic and molecular analyses, the data are insufficient for discussion.

Tumors of Ependyma and Related Cells

Ependymoma

Each of the ventricles of the brain and spinal canal is covered with ciliated epithelium. This layer of cells is embryologically related to glia; when ependymal cells become transformed they frequently express this glial heritage by acquiring a more astrocytic morphology. Ependymomas are most common in the first two decades of life. These tumors are more clearly defined from surrounding brain than other gliomas, although they sometimes demonstrate anaplasia. Historically, the term ependymoblastoma was used to refer to the anaplastic ependymoma, but now that term carries a specific reference to embryonal tumors. There is no apparent correlation between histologic grade and survival, as there is for the astrocytic tumors. The incidence of ependymomas is slightly higher in males than females.

Twenty-nine primary untreated adult ependymomas *(25,26,31, 34,101,133–135),* and 46 pediatric ependymomas *(25,31,34,39,40, 101,120,121,124,125,127,133–140)* have been analyzed by cytogenetics. The only substantial loss and gain of whole chromosomes is loss of chromosome 22 (Fig. 6). Neither adult nor pediatric tumors recorded excessive loss of sex chromosomes. Only 2 of 44 adult male cases showed Y chromosome loss and in 4 of 31 female cases (2 adult and 2 pediatric) an X chromosome was lost in addition to other clonal abnormalities.

The most numerous breakpoints were 7q32 and 9p22 in adult ependymomas and 11q13 and 22q13.1 for pediatric ependymomas (Fig. 7). Two groups have reported allelic loss in ependymomas. One study reported single instances of loss on 1q, 2p, 3p, 4p, 5p, 7p, 10p, 11p, 13q, and 18q in 6 ependymomas *(26),* and the second observed allelic loss on 13q (2 of 4 tumors), 14q (1 of 4 tumors), 17p (1 of 4 tumors) and 22q (3 of 4 tumors) *(128).* These discordant

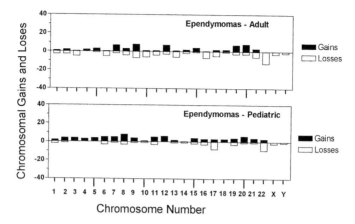

Fig. 6. Clonal numerical chromosome changes in 29 adult cases of ependymoma and 46 cases of pediatric ependymomas.

observations may reflect the use of different probes. Although the sampling of ependymomas was small, several cytogenetic and molecular investigations are suggestive of a tumor suppressor gene on chromosome 22. It is well known that the NF2 gene is localized to chromosome 22 and that neurofibromatosis patients tend to develop multiple ependymomas *(16)*. One group has detected mutations in the NF2 gene in ependymomas, further supporting this gene as a contributory factor in tumor formation *(65)*. Mutations and/or deletions of p53 have not been found *(48)*, although a single patient with a p53 germline mutation (Li-Fraumeni Syndrome) developed an intracranial ependymoma *(141)*. Clearly, more studies are needed to determine the genetic aberrations specific and important to this tumor type.

Choroid Plexus Papilloma

This is a rare neoplasm that occurs most frequently during the first decade of life and only rarely in adults. It mimics its parental tissue in secreting cerebrospinal fluid and is, therefore, a reason for the development of hydrocephalus. The cells of the tumor are strikingly normal in appearance and essentially free of mitotic activity, so that only the crowding of cells provides identification of its neoplastic nature. Six cases of choroid plexus papilloma have been

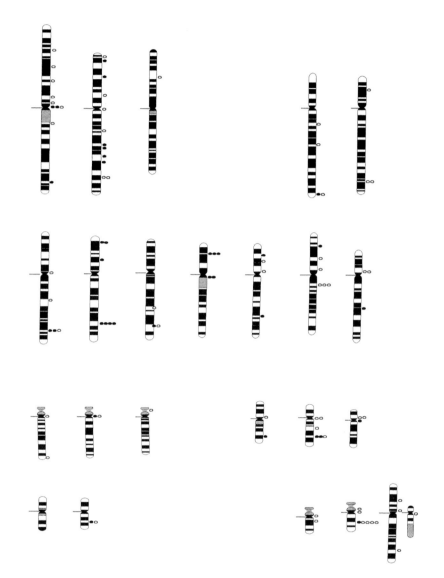

Fig. 7. Identified clonal chromosome breakpoints involved in structural rearrangements in 29 adult ependymomas (●) and 46 pediatric ependymomas (○).

reported *(34,40,120,124,142,143)*, of which three had normal diploid G-banded karyotypes and the remaining three contained clonal numerical and structural aberrations. No informative molecular studies have been performed.

Oligodendroglioma

Oligodendrogliomas

The oligodendroglial cell produces the myelin in the CNS and tumors of this cell type account for 10% of the gliomas diagnosed. This tumor is more associated with adults than children and is considered slow growing. The locations of oligodendrogliomas relate roughly to the amount of white matter in the different lobes of the brain. Although these tumors arise in white matter, they tend to infiltrate the cerebral cortex more than do astrocytomas of similar grade. Features similar to those in astrocytomas, namely, cell density, mitotic activity, and necrosis, are used to grade these tumors. However, the correlation of these markers with survival is controversial. With increasing anaplasia, the tumors become more astrocytic in appearance and develop necrosis. Totals of 46 adult *(25–27,30, 31,34,38,101,104)* and eight pediatric cases *(25,26,30,34)* were identified in which no treatment preceded chromosome analysis, nor was there any astrocytic or ependymal component of the histology. Nineteen of the 46 adult cases and 5 of the 8 pediatric cases had normal G-banded karyotypes. Losses and gains of whole chromosomes were limited, with sex chromosome loss notable in 19 of 46 adult samples (Fig. 8). The loss of a sex chromosome was the only clonal abnormality in 12 of the 19, and was added to other clonal abnormalities in the remaining 7 cases. In the pediatric oligodendrogliomas only 1 of the 8 cases lost a Y chromosome as the sole clonal abnormality. Chromosome 7 was the most frequently gained chromosome, but chromosome 7 was also lost, and study of more cases may demonstrate that this result was random.

Mixed Tumors

Oligodendrogliomas may show regional or diffuse mixture with astrocytic cells. The term "mixed glioma" is reserved for tumors with two distinct populations of glial cells, but the proportion of cells in the mixture can vary considerably and is, therefore, a frequent point of disagreement. The combination observed most frequently in a mixed tumor includes fibrillary astrocytes and oligodendrocytes. Mixtures of astrocytes and ependymal cells can occur, but this tumor

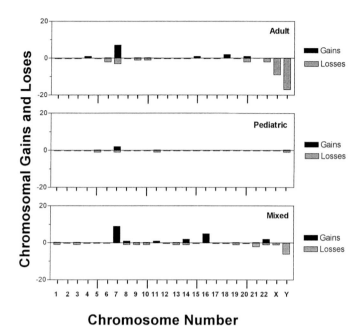

Chromosome Number

Fig. 8. Clonal numerical chromosome changes in 45 adult cases of oligodendroglioma, 8 cases of pediatric oligodendroglioma, and 26 cases of mixed oligodendroglioma.

is rare and difficult to separate from ependymal tumors that have begun to acquire astrocytic phenotypes, as discussed earlier. In the 22 mixed gliomas we reviewed, whole chromosome gains and losses were similar to those of oligodendrogliomas without an astrocytic component (Fig. 8, bottom panel) *(20,25,27,31,34,35,38,100)*. Sex chromosomes were most frequently lost, the Y more often than the X chromosome. Chromosome 7 was most frequently gained, although this group of tumors appears to have gained chromosome 16 as well.

The breakpoints associated with the identified aberrant chromosomes in oligodendrogliomas (adult and pediatric) and mixed oligodendrogliomas were scattered (Fig. 9). Chromosome 1 had the greatest number of breaks, but no clustering of breaks to a specific chromosome 1 band was noted.

Although occasional loss of 19q was reported in primary anaplastic astrocytomas, GBMs, and one exceptional adult case of pilocytic astrocytoma (Fig. 3), such loss was less frequently

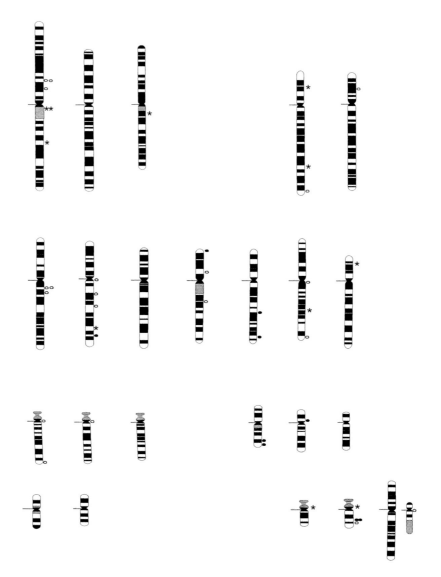

Fig. 9. Identified clonal chromosome breakpoints involved in structural rearrangements in 45 adult cases of oligodendroglioma (●), 8 cases
of pediatric oligodendroglioma (✳), and 26 cases of mixed oligodendroglioma (adult and pediatric) (○).

observed in oligodendrogliomas and mixed oligodendrogliomas. Of
the adult cases reported, only 2 of the 45 oligodendrogliomas
showed whole chromosome 19 loss; however, neither the 45 adult

oligodendrogliomas nor the 22 mixed oligodendrogliomas-astrocytomas demonstrated a single deletion or breakpoint on chromosome 19 *(20,25,26,30,31,34,35,38,101,104)*.

Molecular analyses have been more informative in this regard, as several reports describe allelic losses on 1p and 19q *(26,35)*, preferentially for oligodendrogliomas *(58,90,144,145)*. A putative tumor suppressor gene has been mapped to 19q13.3, telomeric to D19S219 *(145)*. In addition, occasional tumors appear to have mutations in the p53 gene *(48)*. Other allelic deletions that correspond to known chromosomal deletions in astrocytic tumors *(128)* have not been identified in oligodendrogliomas *(146)*. Little other information is available on these tumors.

Ganglion Cell Tumors

Ganglion tumors, also called ganglioglioma or gangliocytoma, are neoplasms that contain mature neurons. Such tumors arise in the cerebellum, brain stem, and spinal cord and are generally associated with childhood. These tumors are distinctive from normal brain because the neoplastic neurons will vary in size and shape as well as spatial distribution. One study of 14 gangliogliomas included 11 with normal diploid G-banded karyotypes and 3 with abnormal stem lines without discernible selection for specific chromosome abnormality *(40)*.

Embryonal Neoplasms

PNET

This group of tumors lacks distinctive cytologic features to assist in classification. Most of these tumors are composed largely of undifferentiated cells. Some neuropathologists use location to assist in tumor classification and designate a small-cell cerebellar tumor as a medulloblastoma and a similar neoplasm in the pineal region a pineoblastoma; other neuropathologists classify these tumors by histology alone and call all such tumors PNET, irrespective of location. The nomenclature for this group of tumors continues to generate considerable controversy. Both systems have been used to classify samples for cytogenetic study. Thus, some studies refer to an embryonal tumor as medulloblastoma and others call the same tumor a PNET. In this chapter we use the designation of PNET. The cerebellar PNET (medulloblastoma) is the most common tumor of children and has a peak incidence during the first two decades of life. Four histologic patterns are recognized, one in which only undifferentiated cells are present, the second with neuroblastic features, the third with a nodular pattern, and the fourth a tumor with glial differentiation.

Although neuroblastomas can be found in the cerebral hemisphere, usually before the age of 2, most of the neuroblastomas studied by cytogenetic analysis have originated outside the CNS and are not discussed further. The embryonal ependymoblastoma is a histologically distinct, aggressive neoplasm, occurring in children and sometimes congenital. The prospect for long-term survival is poor.

One hundred and twenty-six primary untreated cases of PNET were identified for review *(40,120,121,124,125,127,147–155)*. The majority of patients were below the age of 10 and the tumors originated from 66 males and 60 females. Thirty percent of the cases contained only normal G-banded karyotypes. Cases with gain and loss of whole chromosomes are illustrated in Fig. 10. Chromosome 7 was more frequently gained than any other chromosome, whereas loss was greatest for chromosomes 8 and 11. Loss of a sex chromosome was accompanied by additional clonal abnormalities in both males and females. The most frequent nonrandom structural abnormality was the i(17q) in 29% of the PNET tumors. Less frequent were marker chromosomes and double minutes (found in 10 and 6%, respectively). The breakpoints associated with 126 cases of PNET are illustrated in Fig. 11. Most notable is the breakpoint for chromosome 17 that contributes to the formation of i(17q) *(151)*. The only other cluster of breaks was on chromosome 11 at band 11p11.

Molecular analyses of medulloblastomas have focused on gene amplification and allelic loss. Amplification of c-*myc* *(155,156)* and N-*myc* *(155)* have been observed. The frequency of amplification approximates that of dmin. Allelic losses have been observed for 6q, 11p15, 16q, and 17p *(128,152,156–162)*. The most prevalent allelic loss, from 17p, is consistent with formation of the i(17q) observed in 30% of these tumors by cytogenetic analysis. Few mutations have

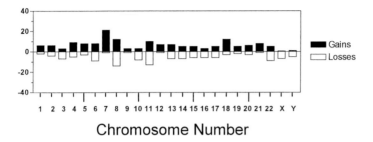

Fig. 10. Clonal numerical chromosome changes in 126 cases of PNET.

been found in the p53 gene *(157,161)*, although another gene more distal to p53 may be the critical gene for PNETs *(152,160)*. This hypothesis is supported by studies that have detected 17p telomeric losses in cases where heterozygosity of p53 was retained *(152,160)*. The chromosome arm, 17p, is of continuing interest because allelic loss in this region is predictive of poor prognosis for pediatric patients *(158)*. Investigation of the potential role of the tumor suppressor gene *MTS1/CDKN2* (9p21) in PNETs revealed no allelic loss or mutation of this gene *(163)*.

Brain Tumors that Result from Mesenchymal Tissues

Gliosarcoma

Gliomas frequently generate reactive responses causing vascular cells, vascular adventitia, and fibroblasts of the meninges to undergo cell division. In most instances this proliferation is benign, but occasionally these processes become transformed and contribute to a neoplasm containing transformed cells of both glial and mesenchymal origins. These tumors are difficult tumors to analyze cytogenetically unless the tumor cells are cloned directly from the freshly resected tumor. Without cloning, it is not possible by morphology or intermediate filament staining to determine whether a chromosome abnormality is from the glial or the sarcomatous component. However, once a clonal cytogenetic abnormality has been identified, it is possible to use FISH on the paraffin-embedded original tumor tissue to determine if the chromosome abnormality is associated with

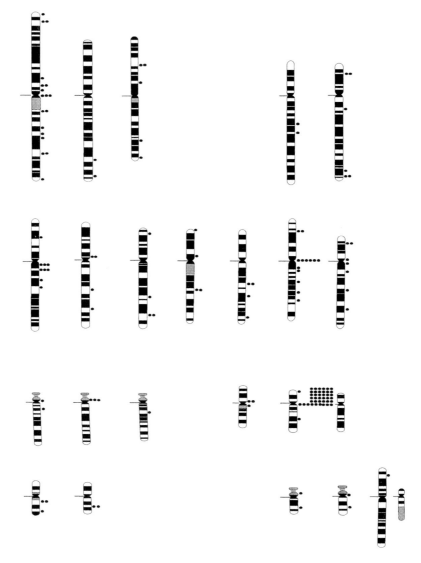

Fig. 11. Identified clonal chromosome breakpoints involved in structural rearrangements in 126 cases of PNET (●).

the glial or sarcomatous component, or both. Cytogenetic analyses of six gliosarcomas from patients ranging in age from 33–80 *(25,98, 100,127)* were identified in the literature. Four of the six cases gained chromosome 7, and three of the six lost chromosome 10. Structural abnormalities were frequent, and involved chromosome 9 in five of the six cases; although three of the five had translocations of chromosome 9, the breakpoints were different in each case. Molecular results other than occasional allelic loss and mutation of the p53 gene have not been reported *(77,78)*.

Rhabdoid Tumors

This rare pediatric tumor of the CNS is basically indistinguishable from its renal counterpart. The cells are epithelial in nature and this distinguishes the tumor from gemistocytic astrocytoma. Eight cases with cytogenetic studies have been reported *(120,124,164–166)*, and seven of the eight either lost chromosome 22 or had a deletion of chromosome 22, del(22)(q13.1).

Meningiomas

Meningiomas have been studied extensively, yet no one of the three layers of meninges has been singled out as the tumor-forming component. Meningiomas comprise approx 15% of all primary brain tumors *(16)*. Spinal cord meningiomas are less common, but still constitute the largest group of tumors in this region. Meningiomas develop in the middle decades of life, predominantly in women (Fig. 12). Such tumors are rare in children, accounting for <2% of intracranial tumors. Familial occurrence is infrequent, and is largely associated with von Recklinghausen's disease. The current grading system recognizes three grades of meningiomas; benign (grade I), atypical (grade II), and anaplastic (grade III). The benign tumors represent about 94% of meningiomas, with 5% atypical and 1% anaplastic *(14,16)*. The atypical and anaplastic meningiomas pose greater risks of recurrence and prognostic markers indicating those at risk would be helpful in selection of appropriate patient treatment. Meningiomas can occur almost anywhere in the brain, with the greatest incidence in the cerebral convexities. The rarest site is the pineal region.

This review identified 355 meningiomas *(30,32,127,167–181)*, only 3 of which were in the pediatric population *(120,124,182)*. Thirty-two percent of these tumors had a normal G-banded karyotype (122 of 383 cases). The most common nonrandom chromosome loss was chromosome 22. It was reported in 195 cases (51%

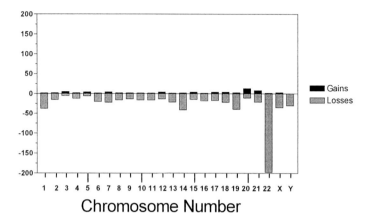

Fig. 12. Clonal numerical chromosome changes in 355 meningiomas (352 adults and 3 pediatric cases).

of the analyzed tumors). Loss of chromosome 22 was the only clonal abnormality in 55 cases, whereas in the other 140 it was added to other clonal numerical and structural abnormalities. As illustrated in the gain/loss chart (Fig. 12), meningiomas tend to lose rather than gain chromosomes. Less frequent than loss of chromosome 22 were losses of whole chromosomes 1, 14, 19, and a sex chromosome.

Structural abnormalities were common in many cases, often associated with more aggressive tumors *(174)*. The breakpoints are illustrated in Fig. 13. Chromosomes 1, 14, 19, and 22 were most frequently rearranged and several prevalent breakpoints were noted. Loss of 22q regions by deletion and/or translocation was relatively common.

The NF2 gene has been localized to chromosome 22 *(183)*, and neurofibromatosis patients tend to develop multiple meningiomas. Molecular genetic studies have verified a close association between allelic loss and mutation in the NF2 gene in approx 57% of meningiomas *(184–187)*. However, several inconsistent findings have emerged. For example, hyperdiploid and pseudodiploid meningiomas retained heterozygosity *(173)*, and allelic loss from some tumors occurred between 22q12.3 and the telomere, a region not associated with the NF2 gene *(63)*. Cytogenetic analyses also suggested that chromosome 22 loss was not the only relevant chromo-

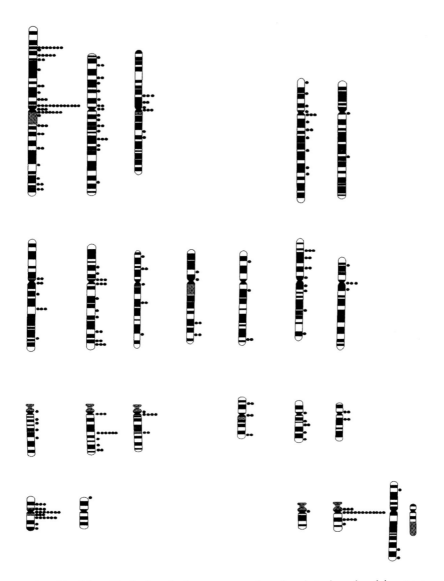

Fig. 13. Identified clonal chromosome breakpoints involved in structural rearrangements in 261 meningiomas (●) (259 adults and 2 pediatric cases).

some abnormality in this tumor *(174)*. More recent molecular investigations have identified deletions of 1p and 10q *(188–190)*, and 14q *(191)*. These deletions have appeared in tumors with more aggressive phenotypes.

Neoplasms of the Pineal Region

Germ Cell Tumors

The most frequent tumor of the pineal region is the germ cell tumor, identical to gonadal neoplasms and classified according to the same criteria used for testicular or ovarian germ cell tumors. The pineal tumors are most common in males and present in the first three decades of life. Germ cell tumors are divided into two major groups, the germinoma (most common) and the embryonal carcinoma. The embryonal carcinoma is further subtyped as: yolk sac carcinoma, choriocarcinoma, immature teratoma, and mature teratoma. The immature teratoma occurs at about twice the frequency of the mature teratoma.

Although germinomas are clinically more common, only 3 cases have been analyzed cytogenetically *(40,120,192)*, whereas 21 cases of embryonal carcinoma have been studied *(40,121,124,125,164,193–197)*. Of the latter, 7 cases were reported to have normal karyotypes and 14 cases contained numerical and/or structural abnormalities. No preferential loss or gain of chromosomes was found, nor was there specificity for structural rearrangement.

Craniopharyngiomas

Craniopharyngiomas are epithelial neoplasms that are primarily located in the sellar region of the brain and only rarely arise elsewhere. They comprise 2–3% of all intracranial growths and most often appear in the first two decades of life. Cytogenetic analyses have been performed on 10 cases, 7 of which had normal G-banded karyotypes *(30,34,40,120)*.

Intracranial Schwann Cell Neoplasms

Schwannomas (Neurilemomas)

The most common intracranial Schwann cell neoplasm is localized to the eighth cranial nerve and less frequently to the fifth cranial nerve. The acoustic neuroma is derived from Schwann cells enveloping the vestibular branch of the eighth nerve. Most tumors are sporadic, but bilateral tumors occur and are an indication of familial predisposition *(16)*. The greatest incidence occurs between the third and sixth decades of life. Cytogenetic and molecular studies *(198–200)* have demonstrated that some 40% of sporadic acoustic neuromas have allelic losses on chromosome 22 and that the loss maps closely to the NF2 gene *(201)*. Most recently, a report has documented inactivating mutations of the NF2 gene in 3 of 11 schwannomas, further suggesting a role of the NF2 gene in the pathogenesis of this tumor type *(202)*.

Summary

At present, no single karyotypic abnormality defines any one type or grade of brain tumor. The majority of metaphases in lower grade adult tumors (pilocytic and astrocytomas) are generally diploid or near-diploid. When abnormalities are found, they are frequently the simple numerical changes of chromosome 7 gain and sex chromosome loss (Fig. 2). The same changes are prevalent in more anaplastic astrocytomas as well. Significant loss of chromosome 10, and a tendency for gain of chromosomes 19 and 20, and for loss of chromosomes 13 and 22, are the other common findings. Clonal structural aberrations are present in anaplastic astrocytomas, but both numerical (Fig. 2) and structural (Fig. 3) abnormalities are far more frequent in the most malignant astrocytic tumor, the GBM. Less common tumors, such as ependymomas (Fig. 6) and oligodendrogliomas (Fig. 8) have shown a high proportion of karyotypically normal cells, but the cytogenetic data are limited to relatively few cases. Moreover, analysis of oligodendrogliomas has been hampered by the admixture of astrocytic cells that may account for apparent gain of chromosome 7 in the adult and mixed tumors (Fig. 8).

Abnormalities in pediatric astrocytic tumors (Fig. 4) differ from those in tumors of adults, in that the former infrequently lose sex chromosomes and the only notable polysomy is for chromosome 7. The significance of these findings is debatable because of the limited numbers of cases analyzed. The most common pediatric tumor, the PNET, has been characterized by numerical changes (Fig. 10) and chromosome rearrangements (Fig. 11). One structural change, the i(17p), is frequent and may convey prognostic information *(152)*, an observation that should be expanded by molecular marker studies.

Molecular alterations, with or without cytogenetic abnormalities, have been associated with certain brain tumors. The loss of chromosome 22 observed in meningiomas led to assumptions that the tumor suppressor gene, NF2, was involved in disease progression. However, recent work suggests that NF2 does not play a critical role in meningiomas, underscoring the potential for incorrect molecular marker identification based solely on karyotypic data *(170,191)*. In contrast, amplification and rearrangement of the *EGFR* gene in astrocytic tumors is clinically significant (higher grade tumors) and is clearly associated with visible aberrations of chromosome 7. The utility of this cytogenetic observation in prognostication for gliomas has not been demonstrated conclusively, but the aberrant truncated EGFR product may prove to be a suitable target for therapy. Many of the molecular alterations in brain tumors are not directly attributable to cytogenetic abnormality. For example, we reported reduced expression of the deleted in colon cancer *(DCC)* gene in gliomas *(21)*, apparently associated with higher grade and reduced survival; however, neither LOH for this region nor chromosome 18 anomalies are common in these tumors *(35)*. Further, changes in expression of cell-type specific genes such as myelin basic protein may prove useful in differential diagnosis of the gliomas *(203)*. Many types of genetic and molecular analysis hold promise for improved understanding of the etiology of human brain tumors, and may ultimately prove objective markers for diagnosis, prognostic indicators, and targets for novel therapeutic approaches.

References

1. Mahaley MS Jr, Mettlin C, Natarajan N, Laws ER, Peace BB: National survey of patterns of care for brain-tumor patients. J Neurosurg 71: 826–836, 1989.
2. Shapiro WR, Shapiro JR, Walker RW: Central nervous system. In: Abeloff MD, Armitage JO, Lichter AS, Niederhuber JE (eds.), Clinical Oncology, New York: Churchill Livingstone, pp. 851–912, 1995.
3. Gauwerky CE, Croce CM: Molecular genetics and cytogenetics of hematopoietic malignancies. In: Mendelsohn J, Howley PM, Israel MA,

Liotta LA (eds.), The Molecular Basis of Cancer, Philadelphia, PA: Sauders, pp. 18–31, 1995.

4. Gaidano G, Dalla-Favera R: Molecular biology of lymphoid neoplasms. In: Mendelsohn J, Howley PM, Israel MA, Liotta LA (eds.), The Molecular Basis of Cancer, Philadelphia, PA: Saunders, pp. 251–293, 1995.
5. Fearon ER, Vogelstein B: A genetic model for colorectal tumorigenesis. Cell 61:759–767, 1990.
6. Brodeur GM, Fong CT: Molecular biology and genetics of neuroblastoma. Cancer Genet Cytogenet 41:153–174, 1989.
7. Fong C, White PS, Peterson K, Sapienza C, Cavenee WK, Kern SE, Vogelstein B, Cantor AB, Look AT, Brodeur GM: Loss of heterozygosity for chromosomes 1 or 14 defines subsets of advanced neuroblastomas. Cancer Res 52:1780–1785, 1992.
8. Cavenee WK, Dryja TP, Phillips RA: Expression of recessive alleles by chromosomal mechanisms in retinoblastomas. Nature 305:779–784, 1983.
9. Heppner GH: Tumor heterogeneity. Cancer Res 44:2259–2265, 1984.
10. Shapiro JR, Yung WA, Shapiro WR: Isolation, karyotype, and clonal growth of heterogeneous subpopulations of human malignant gliomas. Cancer Res 41:2349–2359, 1981.
11. Bailey P, Cushing H: A classification of the tumors of the glioma group on a histogenetic basis with a correlated study of prognosis. Philadelphia, PA: Lippincott, 1926.
12. Kernohan JW, Sayre GP: Atlas of tumor pathology: tumors of the central nervous system. Section X. Washington, DC: Fascicle 35, Armed Forces Institute of Pathology, 1952.
13. Bruner JM: Neuropathology of malignant gliomas. Semin Oncol 21:126–138, 1994.
14. Burger PC, Scheithauer BW, Vogel FS: Brain: tumors. In: Burger PC, Scheithauer BW, Vogel FS (eds.), Surgical Pathology of the Nervous System and its Coverings. New York: Churchill Livingstone. pp. 194–404, 1991.
15. Russell DS, Rubinstein LJ: Pathology of Tumors of the Nervous System. Baltimore, MD: Williams & Wilkins, 1989.
16. Daumas-Duport C: Histological grading of gliomas. Curr Opinion Neurol Neurosurg 5:924–931, 1992.
17. Schofield DE: Diagnostic histopathology, cytogenetics, and molecular markers of pediatric brain tumors. Neurosurg Clin North Am 3:723–738, 1992.
18. Shapiro WR: Therapy of adult malignant brain tumors: what have the clinical trials taught us? Semin Oncol 13:38–45, 1986.
19. Israel MA: Molecular biology of childhood neoplasms. In: Mendelsohn J, Howley PM, Israel MA, Liotta LA (eds.), The Molecular Basis of Cancer, Philadelphia, PA: Sauders, pp. 294–316, 1995.
20. Coons SW, Johnson PC, Shapiro JR: Cytogenetic and flow cytometry DNA analysis of regional heterogeneity in a low grade glioma. Cancer Res 55:1569–1577, 1995.
21. Scheck AC, Coons SW: Expression of the tumor suppressor gene DCC in human gliomas. Cancer Res 53:5605–5609, 1993.

22. Glantz MJ, Burger PC, Herndon JE, Friedman AH, Cairncross, JG, Vick NA, Schold SC Jr: Influence of the type of surgery on the histologic diagnosis in patients with anaplastic gliomas. Neurology 41:1741–1744, 1991.
23. Janus TJ, Kyritsis AP, Forman AD, Levin VA: Biology and treatment of gliomas. Ann Oncol 3:423–433, 1992.
24. Louis DN, Gusella JF: A tiger behind many doors: multiple genetic pathways to malignant glioma. Trends Genet 11:412–415, 1995.
25. Jenkins RB, Kimmel DW, Moertel CA, Schultz CG, Scheithauer BW, Kelly PJ, Dewald GW: A cytogenetic study of 53 human gliomas. Cancer Genet Cytogenet 39:253–279, 1989.
26. Ransom DT, Ritland SR, Kimmel DW, Moertel CA, Dahl RJ, Scheithauer BW, Kelly PJ, Jenkins RB: Cytogenetic and loss of heterozygosity studies in ependymomas, pilocytic astrocytomas and oligodendrogliomas. Genes Chromosome Cancer 5:348–356, 1992.
27. Debiec-Rychter M, Alwasiak J, Liberski PP, Nedoszytko B, Babinska M, Mrozek K, Imielinski B, Borowska-Lehman J, Limon J: Accumulation of chromosomal changes in human glioma progression: a cytogenetic study of 50 cases. Cancer Genet Cytogenet 85:61–67, 1995.
28. Bigner SH, Mark J, Bigner DD: Cytogenetics of human brain tumors. Cancer Genet Cytogenet 47:141–154, 1990.
29. Rey JA, Pestaña A, Bello MJ: Cytogenetics and molecular genetics of nervous system tumors. Oncol Res 4:321–331, 1992.
30. Yamada K, Kondo T, Yoshioka M, Oami H: Cytogenetic studies in twenty human brain tumors: association of no. 22 chromosome abnormalities with tumors of the brain. Cancer Genet Cytogenet 2:293–307, 1980.
31. Rey JA, Bello MJ, de Campos JM, Kusak ME, Moreno S: Chromosomal composition of a series of 22 human low-grade gliomas. Cancer Genet Cytogenet 29:223–237, 1987.
32. Heim S, Mandahl N, Jin Y, Stromblad S, Lindstrom E, Salford LG, Mitelman F: Trisomy 7 and sex chromosome loss in human brain tissue. Cytogenet Cell Genet 52:136–138, 1989.
33. Lindstrom E, Salford LG, Heim S, Mandahl N, Stromblad S, Brun A, Mitelman F: Trisomy 7 and sex chromosome loss need not be representative of tumor parenchyma cells in malignant glioma. Genes Chromosome Cancer 3:474–479, 1991.
34. Griffin CA, Long PP, Carson BS, Brem H: Chromosome abnormalities in low-grade central nervous system tumors. Cancer Genet Cytogenet 60:67–73, 1992.
35. Ransom DT, Ritland SR, Moertel CA, Dahl RJ, O'Fallon JR, Scheithauer BW, Kimmel DW, Kelly PJ, Olopade OI, Diaz MO, Jenkins RB: Correlation of cytogenetic analysis and loss of heterozygosity studies in human diffuse astrocytomas and mixed oligo-astrocytomas. Genes Chromosome Cancer 5:357–374, 1992.
36. Thiel G, Lozanova T, Vogel S, Kintzel D, Janisch W, Witkowski R: Age-related nonrandom chromosomal abnormalities in human low-grade astrocytomas. Hum Genet 91:547–550, 1993.

37. Shapiro JR, Pu P, Mohamed AN, Galicich JH, Ebrahim SAD, Shapiro WR: Chromosome number and carmustine sensitivity in human gliomas. Cancer 71:4007–4021, 1993.
38. Magnani I, Guerneri S, Pollo B, Cirenei N, Colombo BM, Broggi G, Galli C, Bugiana O, DiDonato S, Finocchiaro G, Conti AMF: Increasing complexity of the karyotype in 50 human gliomas. Progressive evolution and *de novo* occurrence of cytogenetic alterations. Cancer Genet Cytogenet 75: 77–89, 1994.
39. Yamada K, Kasama M, Kondo T, Shinoura N, Yoshioka M: Chromosome studies in 70 brain tumors with special attention to sex chromosome loss and single autosomal trisomy. Cancer Genet Cytogenet 73:46–52, 1994.
40. Neumann E, Kalousek DK, Norman MG, Steinbok P, Cochrane DD, Goddard K: Cytogenetic analysis of 109 pediatric central nervous system tumors. Cancer Genet Cytogenet 71:40–49, 1993.
41. Bullard DE, Schold SC, Bigner SH, Bigner DD: Growth and chemotherapeutic response in athymic mice of tumors arising from human glioma-derived cell lines. J Neuropathol Exp Neurol 40:410–427, 1981.
42. El-Azouzi M, Chung RY, Farmer GE, Martuza RL, Black PM, Rouleau GA, Hettlich C, Hedley-Whyte ET, Zervas NT, Panagopoulos, K, Nakamura Y, Gusella JF, Seizinger BR: Loss of distinct regions on the short arm of chromosome 17 associated with tumorigenesis of human astrocytomas. Proc Natl Acad Sci USA 86:7186–7190, 1989.
43. Sidransky D, Mikkelsen T, Schwechheimer K, Rosenblum ML, Cavenee W, Vogelstein B: Clonal expansion of p53 mutant cells is associated with brain tumour progression. Nature 355:846,847, 1992.
44. Kraus JA, Bolln C, Wolf HK, Neumann J, Kinderman D, Fimmers R, Forster F, Baumann A, Schlegel U: TP53 Alterations and clinical outcome in low grade astrocytomas. Genes Chromosome Cancer 10:143–149, 1994.
45. Koga H, Zhang S, Kumanishi T, Washiyama K, Ichikawa T, Tanaka R, Mukawa J: Analysis of p53 gene mutations in low- and high-grade astrocytomas by polymerase chain reaction-assisted single-strand conformation polymorphism and immunohistochemistry. Acta Neuropathol (Berl) 87:225–232, 1994.
46. Chen P, Ivarone A, Fick J, Edwards M, Prados M, Israel MA: Constitutional p53 mutations associated with brain tumors in young adults. Cancer Genet Cytogenet 82:106–115, 1995.
47. James CD, Carlbom E, Dumanski JP, Hansen M, Nordenskjold M, Collins VP, Cavenee WK: Clonal genomic alterations in glioma malignancy stages. Cancer Res 48:5546–5551, 1988.
48. Ohgaki H, Eibl RH, Wiestler OD, Yasargil MG, Newcomb EW, Kleihues P: p53 mutations in nonastrocytic human brain tumors. Cancer Res 51:6202–6205, 1991.
49. von Deimling A, Eibl RH, Ohgaki H, Louis DN, von Ammon K, Petersen I, Kleihues P, Chung RY, Wiestler OD, Seizinger BR: p53 Mutations are associated with 17p allelic loss in grade II and grade III astrocytoma. Cancer Res 52:2987–2990, 1992.

50. Ohgaki H, Eibl RH, Schwab M, Reichel MB, Mariani L, Gehring M, Petersen I, Höll T, Wiestler OD, Kleihues P: Mutations of the *p53* tumor suppressor gene in neoplasms of the human nervous system. Mol Carcinogenesis 8:74–80, 1993.

51. Louis DN, Seizinger BR: Genetic basis of neurological tumours. Bailliere's Clin Neurol 3:335–352, 1994.

52. Louis DN, von Deimling A, Chung RY, Rubio M, Whaley JM, Eibl RH, Ohgaki H, Wiestler OD, Thor AD, Seizinger BR: Comparative study of p53 gene and protein alterations in human astrocytic tumors. J Neuropathol Exper Neurol 52:31–38, 1993.

53. Van Meyel DJ, Ramsay DA, Casson AG, Keeney M, Chambers AF, Cairncross JG: p53 mutation, expression, and DNA ploidy in evolving gliomas: evidence for two pathways of progression. J Natl Cancer Inst 86:1011–1017, 1994.

54. Ghosh M, Dinda A, Chattopadhyay P, Sarkar C, Bhatia S, Sinha S: Rearranged p53 gene with loss of normal allele in a low-grade nonrecurrent glioma. Cancer Genet Cytogenet 76:68–71, 1994.

55. Fults D, Brockmeyer D, Tullous MW, Pedone CA, Cawthon RM: p53 mutation and loss of heterozygosity on chromosome 17 and 10 during human astrocytoma progression. Cancer Res 52:674–679, 1992.

56. Cavenee WK: Recessive mutations in cancer predisposition and progression. In: Sudilovsky O (ed.), Boundaries Between Promotion and Progression During Carcinogenesis, New York: Plenum, pp. 171–181, 1991.

57. Venter DJ, Thomas DG: Multiple sequential molecular abnormalities in the evolution of human gliomas. Br J Cancer 63:753–757, 1991

58. Bello MJ, Leone PE, Nebreda P, de Campos JM, Kusak ME, Vaquero J, Sarasa JL, García-Miguel P, Queizan A, Hernández-Moneo JL, Pestaña A, Rey JA: Allelic status of chromosome 1 in neoplasms of the nervous system. Cancer Genet Cytogenet 83:160–164, 1995.

59. Karlbom AE, James CD, Boethius J, Cavenee WK, Collins VP, Nordenskjöld M, Larsson C: Loss of heterozygosity in malignant gliomas involves at least three distinct regions on chromosome 10. Hum Genet 92:169–174, 1993.

60. James CD, Carlbom E, Nordenskjold M, Collins VP, Cavenee WK: Mitotic recombination of chromosome 17 in astrocytomas. Proc Natl Acad Sci USA 86:2858–2862, 1989.

61. James CD, Collins VP: Molecular genetic characterization of CNS tumor oncogenesis. Adv Cancer Res 58:121–142, 1992.

62. Rasheed BKA, McLendon RE, Herndon JE, Friedman HS, Friedman AH, Bigner DD, Bigner SH: Alterations of the *TP53* gene in human gliomas. Cancer Res 54:1324–1330, 1994.

63. Rey JA, Bello MJ, de Campos JM, Vaquero J, Kusak ME, Sarasa JL, Pestaña A: Abnormalities of chromosome 22 in human brain tumors determined by combined cytogenetic and molecular genetic approaches. Cancer Genet Cytogenet 66:1–10, 1993.

64. Steck PA, Ligon AH, Cheong P, Yung WKA, Pershouse MA: Two tumor suppressive loci on chromosome 10 involved in human glioblastomas. Genes Chromosome Cancer 12:255–261, 1995.

65. Rubio M, Correa KM, Ramesh V, MacCollin MM, Jacoby LB, von Deimling A, Gusella JF, Louis DN: Analysis of the neurofibromatosis 2 gene in human ependymomas and astrocytomas. Cancer Res 54:45–47, 1994.

66. Hermanson M, Funa K, Hartman M, Claesson-Welsh L, Heldin C, Westermark B, Nistér M: Platelet-derived growth factor and its receptors in human glioma tissue: expression of messenger RNA and protein suggests the presence of autocrine and paracrine loops. Cancer Res 52:3213–3219, 1992.

67. Humphrey PA, Gangarosa LM, Wong AJ, Archer GE, Lund-Johansen M, Bjerkvig R, Laerum OD, Friedman HS, Bigner DD: Deletion-mutant epidermal growth factor receptor in human gliomas: effects of type II mutation on receptor function. Biochem Biophys Res Commun 178:1413–1420, 1991.

68. Hecht F, Hecht BK, Chatel M, Gaudray P, Turc-Carel C: Nonrandom sex chromosome changes in brain tumors. Cancer Genet Cytogenet 72:160, 1994.

69. Arnoldus EPJ, Noordermeer IA, Peters ACB, Voormolen JHC, Bots GTAM, Raap AK, van der Ploeg M: Interphase cytogenetics of brain tumors. Genes Chromosome Cancer 3:101–107, 1991.

70. Arnoldus EPJ, Wolters LBT, Voormolen JHC, van Duinen SG, Raap AK, van der Ploeg M, Boudewijn Peters AC: Interphase cytogenetics: a new tool for the study of genetic changes in brain tumors. J Neurosurg 76:997–1003, 1992.

71. Bello MJ, de Campos JM, Kusak ME, Vaquero J, Sarasa JL, Petaña A, Rey JA: Ascertainment of chromosome 7 gains in malignant gliomas by cytogenetic and RFLP analyses. Cancer Genet Cytogenet 72:55–58, 1994.

72. Hecht BK, Turc-Carel C, Chatel M, Grellier P, Gioanni J, Attias R, Gaudray P, Hecht F: Cytogenetics of malignant gliomas: I. The autosomes with reference to rearrangements. Cancer Genet Cytogenet 84:1–8, 1996.

73. Jay V, Rutka J, Becker LE, Squire J: Pediatric malignant glioma with tubuloreticular inclusions and MYCN amplification: report of a case with immunohistochemical, ultrastructural, flow cytometric, karyotypic, and Southern blot analysis. Cancer 73:1987–1993, 1994.

74. Hecht BK, Turc-Carel C, Chatel M, Paquis P, Gioanni J, Attias R, Gaudray P, Hecht F: Cytogenetics of malignant gliomas II. The sex chromosomes with reference to X isodisomy and the role of numerical X/Y changes. Cancer Genet Cytogenet 84:9–14, 1996.

75. Fults D, Tippets RH, Thomas GA, Nakamura Y, White R: Loss of heterozygosity for loci on chromosome 17p in human malignant astrocytoma. Cancer Res 49:6572–6577, 1989.

76. Fults D, Pedone CA, Thomas GA, White R: Allelotype of human malignant astrocytoma. Cancer Res 50:5784–5789, 1990.

77. Kyritsis AP, Bondy ML, Xiao M, Berman EL, Cunningham JE, Lee PS, Levin VA, Saya H: Germline p53 gene mutations in subsets of glioma patients. J Natl Cancer Inst 86:344–349, 1994.

78. Frankel RH, Bayona W, Koslow M, Newcomb EW: p53 mutations in human malignant gliomas: comparison of loss of heterozygosity with mutation frequency. Cancer Res 52:1427–1433, 1992.

79. Saxena A, Clark WC, Robertson JT, Ikejiri B, Oldfield EH, Ali IU: Evidence for the involvement of a potential second tumor suppressor gene on chromosome 17 distinct from p53 in malignant astrocytomas. Cancer Res 52:6716–6721, 1992.

80. Reifenberger G, Liu L, Ichimura K, Schmidt EE, Collins VP: Amplification and overexpression of the *MDM2* gene in a subset of human malignant gliomas without *p53* mutations. Cancer Res 53:2736–2739, 1993.

81. Raffel C, Thomas G, Tishler DM, Lassoff S, Allen JC: Absence of p53 mutations in childhood central nervous system primitive neuroectodermal tumors. Neurosurgery 33:301–306, 1993.

82. James CD, He J, Carlbom E, Nordenskjold M, Cavenee WK, Collins VP: Chromosome 9 deletion mapping reveals interferon α and interferon β-1 gene deletions in human glial tumors. Cancer Res 51:1684–1688, 1991.

83. Olopade OI, Jenkins RB, Ransom DT, Malik K, Pomykala H, Nobori T, Cowan JM, Rowley JD, Diaz MO: Molecular analysis of deletions of the short arm of chromosome 9 in human gliomas. Cancer Res 52:2523–2529, 1992.

84. Giese A, Rief MD, Loo MA, Berens ME: Determinants of human astrocytoma migration. Cancer Res 54:3897–3904, 1994.

85. James CD, He J, Collins VP, Allalunis-Turner MJ, Day RS III: Localization of chromosomes 9p homozygous deletions in glioma cell lines with markers constituting a continuous linkage group. Cancer Res 53:3674–3676, 1993.

86. Ueki K, Rubio M-P, Ramesh V, Correa KM, Rutter JL, von Deimling A, Buckler AJ, Gusella JF, Louis DN: *MTS1/CDKN2* gene mutations are rare in primary human astrocytomas with allelic loss of chromosome 9p. Hum Mol Genet 3:1841–1845, 1994.

87. Nobori T, Miura K, Wu DJ, Lois A, Takabayashi K, Carson DA: Deletions of the cyclin-dependent kinase-4 inhibitor gene in multiple human cancers. Nature 368:753–756, 1994.

88. Kamb A, Gruis NA, Weaver-Feldhaus J, Liu Q, Harshman K, Tavtigian SV, Stockert E, Day RS III, Johnson BE, Skolnick MH: A cell cycle regulator potentially involved in genesis of many tumor types. Science 264:436–440, 1994.

89. Ichimura K, Schmidt EE, Yamaguchi N, James CD, Collins VP: A common region of homozygous deletion in malignant human gliomas lies between the IFN a\w gene cluster and the D9S171 locus. Cancer Res 54: 3127–3130, 1994.

90. von Deimling A, Louis DN, von Ammon K, Petersen I, Wiestler OD, Seizinger BR: Evidence for a tumor suppressor gene on chromosome 19q associated with human astrocytomas, oligodendrogliomas, and mixed gliomas. Cancer Res 52:4277–4279, 1992.

91. Ritland SR, Ganju V, Jenkins RB: Region-specific loss of heterozygosity on chromosome 19 is related to the morphologic type of human glioma. Genes Chromosome Cancer 12:277–282, 1995.

92. Rubio M-P, Correa KM, Ueki K, Mohrenweiser HW, Gusella JF, von Deimling A, Louis DN: The putative glioma tumor suppressor gene on chromosome 19q maps between *APOC2* and *HRC*. Cancer Res 54: 4760–4763, 1994.

93. von Deimling A, Negel J, Bender B, Lenartz D, Schramm J, Louis DN, Wiestler OD: Deletion mapping of chromosome 19 in human gliomas. Int J Cancer 57:676–680, 1994.

94. Zagzag D, Friedlander DR, Miller DC, Dosik J, Cangiarella J, Kostianovsky M, Cohen H, Grumet M, Greco MA: Tenascin expression in astrocytomas correlates with angiogenesis. Cancer Res 55:907–914, 1995.

95. Bello MJ, Vaquero J, de Campos JM, Kusak ME, Sarasa JL, Saez-Castresana J, Pestana A, Rey JA: Molecular analysis of chromosome 1 abnormalities in human gliomas reveals frequent loss of 1p in oligodendroglial tumors. Int J Cancer 57:172–175, 1995.

96. Sonoda Y, Iizuka M, Yasuda J, Makino R, Ono T, Kayama T, Yoshimoto T, Sekiya T: Loss of heterozygosity at 11p15 in malignant glioma. Cancer Res 55:2166–2168, 1995.

97. Fults D, Petronio J, Noblett BD, Pedone CA: Chromosome 11p15 deletions in human malignant astrocytomas and primitive neuroectodermal tumors. Genomics 14:799–801, 1992.

98. Bigner SH, Mark J, Mahaley MS, Bigner DD: Patterns of the early, gross chromosomal changes in malignant human gliomas. Hereditas 101:103–113, 1984.

99. Bigner SH, Mark J, Bullard DE, Mahaley MSJ, Bigner DD: Chromosomal evolution in malignant human glioma starts with specific and usually numerical deviations. Cancer Genet Cytogenet 22:121–135, 1986.

100. Bigner SH, Mark J, Burger PC, Mahaley MSJ, Bullard DE, Muhlbaier LH, Bigner DD: Specific chromosomal abnormalities in malignant human gliomas. Cancer Res 48:405–411, 1988.

101. Thiel G, Losanowa T, Kintzel D, Nisch G, Martin H, Vorpahl K, Witkowski R: Karyotypes in 90 gliomas. Cancer Genet Cytogenet 58: 109–120, 1992.

102. Arbit E, Malkin MG, Rosenblum M, Anderson L, Fiola MR, Shapiro JR: Stereotactic implantation of high-activity iodine-125 seeds for the treatment of malignant glioma. Neurosurgery 32:105–110, 1993.

103. Scheck AC, Mehta BM, Beikman MK, Shapiro JR: BCNU-resistant human glioma cells with over-representation of chromosomes 7 and 22 demonstrate increased copy number and expression of platelet-derived growth factor genes. Genes Chromosome Cancer 8:137–148, 1993.

104. Patt S, Thiel G, Maas S, Lozanova T, Prosenc N, Cervos-Navarro J, Witkowski R, Blumenstock M: Chromosomal changes and correspondingly altered protooncogene expression in human gliomas. Value of combined cytogenetic and molecular genetic analysis. Anticancer Res 13:113–118, 1993.

105. Dalrymple SJ, Herath JF, Ritland SR, Moertel CA, Jenkins RB: Use of fluorescence *in situ* hybridization to detect loss of chromosome 10 in astrocytomas. J Neurosurg 83:316–323, 1995.

106. Muleris M, Almeida A, Dutrillaux AM, Pruchon E, Vega F, Delattre JY, Poisson M, Malfoy B, Dutrillaux B: Oncogene amplification in human gliomas: a molecular cytogenetic analysis. Oncogene 9:2717–2722, 1994.
107. Bigner DD, Schold C, Bigner SH, Bullard DE, Wikstrand C: How heterogeneous are gliomas? Cancer Treat Rep 65:45–49, 1981.
108. Zang KD, Fischer H, van der Hout A, Unteregger G, Henn W, Scheffer H, Wollenberg C, Buys CH, Blin N: A human glioblastoma line with karyotypic nullisomy 13 containing several chromosome 13-specific sequences. Cancer Genet Cytogenet 33:127–132, 1988.
109. Rey JA, Bello MJ, de Campos JM, Kusak ME, Ramos C, Benitez J: Chromosomal patterns in human malignant astrocytomas. Cancer Genet Cytogenet 29:201–221, 1987.
110. Arita N, Hayakawa T, Izumoto S, Taki T, Ohnishi T, Yamamoto H, Bitoh S, Mogami H: Epidermal growth factor receptor in human glioma. J Neurosurg 70:916–919, 1989.
111. Malden LT, Novak U, Kaye AH, Burgess AW: Selective amplification of the cytoplasmic domain of the epidermal growth factor receptor gene in glioblastoma multiforme. Cancer Res 48:2711–2714, 1988.
112. Ekstrand AJ, Longo N, Hamid ML, Olson JJ, Liu L, Collins VP, James CD: Functional characterization of an EGF receptor with a truncated extracellular domain expressed in GBMs with EGFR gene amplification. Oncogene 9:2313–2320, 1994.
113. Malden LT, Novak U, Kaye AH, Burgess AW: Selective amplification of the cytoplasmic domain of the epidermal growth factor receptor gene in glioblastoma multiforme. Cancer Res 48:2711–2714, 1988.
114. von Deimling A, von Ammon K, Schoenfeld D, Wiestler OD, Seizinger BR, Louis DN: Subsets of glioblastomas multiforme defined by molecular genetic analysis. Brain Pathol 3:19–26, 1993.
115. Fults D, Pedone C: Deletion mapping of the long arm of chromosome 10 in glioblastoma multiforme. Genes Chromosome Cancer 7:173–177, 1993.
116. von Deimling A, Louis DN, Schramm J, Wiestler OD: Astrocytic gliomas: characterization on a molecular genetic basis. Recent Results Cancer Res 135:33–42, 1994.
117. Leenstra S, Bijlsma EK, Troost D, Oosting J, Westerveld A, Bosch DA, Hulsebos TJM: Allele loss on chromosomes 10 and 17p and epidermal growth factor receptor gene amplification in human malignant astrocytoma related to prognosis. Br J Cancer 70:684–689, 1994.
118. Leenstra S, Troost D, Westerveld A, Bosch DA, Hulsebos TJM: Molecular characterization of areas with low grade tumor or satellitosis in human malignant astrocytomas. Cancer Res 52:1568–1572, 1992.
119. Scheck AC, Shapiro JR, Coons SW, Norman SA, Johnson PC: Biological and molecular analysis of a low grade recurrence of a glioblastoma multiforme. Clin Cancer Res 2:187–199, 1995.

120. Karnes PS, Tran TN, Cui MY, Raffel C, Gilles FH, Barranger JA, Ying KL: Cytogenetic analysis of 39 pediatric central nervous system tumors. Cancer Genet Cytogenet 59:12–19, 1992.
121. Griffin CA, Hawkins AL, Packer RJ, Rorke LB, Emanuel BS: Chromosomal abnormalities in pediatric brain tumors. Cancer Res 48:175–180, 1988.
122. Sawyer JR, Roloson GJ, Hobson EA, Goosen LS, Chadduck WM: Trisomy for chromosome 1q in a pontine astrocytoma. Cancer Genet Cytogenet 47:101–106, 1990.
123. Sawyer JR, Thomas JR, Teo C: Low grade astrocytoma with a complex four-breakpoint inversion of chromosome 8 as the sole cytogenetic aberration. Cancer Genet Cytogenet 83:168–171, 1995.
124. Agamanolis DP, Malone JM: Chromosomal abnormalities in 47 pediatric brain tumors. Cancer Genet Cytogenet 81:125–134, 1995.
125. Fujii Y, Hongo T, Hayashi Y: Chromosome analysis of brain tumors in childhood. Genes Chromosome Cancer 11:205–215, 1994.
126. Sawyer JR, Roloson GJ, Chadduck WM, Boop FA: Cytogenetic findings in a pleomorphic xanthoastrocytoma. Cancer Genet Cytogenet 55:225–230, 1991.
127. Chadduck WM, Boop FA, Sawyer JR: Cytogenetic studies of pediatric brain and spinal cord tumors. Pediatr Neurosurg 92:57–65, 1991.
128. James CD, He J, Carlbom E, Mikkelsen T, Ridderheim PA, Cavenee WK, Collins VP: Loss of genetic information in central nervous system tumors common to children and young adults. Genes Chromosome Cancer 2:94–102, 1990.
129. Bello MJ, de Campos JM, Kusak ME, Vaquero J, Sarasa JL, Pestana A, Rey JA: Molecular analysis of genomic abnormalities in human gliomas. Cancer Genet Cytogenet 73:122–129, 1994.
130. Litofsky NS, Hinton D, Raffel C: The lack of a role for p53 in astrocytomas in pediatric patients. Neurosurgery 34:967–973, 1994.
131. Louis DN, Rubio M, Correa KM, Gusella JF, von Deimling A: Molecular genetics of pediatric brain stem gliomas. Application of PCR techniques to small and archival brain tumor specimens. J Neuropath Exper Neurol 52:507–515, 1993.
132. Hecht BK, Turc-Carel C, Chatel M, Lonjon M, Roche JL, Gioanni J, Hecht F, Gaudray P: Chromosomes in gliomatosis cerebri. Genes Chromosomes Cancer 14:149–153, 1995.
133. Rogatto SR, Casartelli C, Rainho CA, Barbieri-Neto J: Chromosomes in the genesis and progression of ependymomas. Cancer Genet Cytogenet 69:146–152, 1993.
134. Sawyer JR, Sammartino G, Husaom M, Boop FA, Chadduck WM: Chromosome aberrations in four ependymomas. Cancer Genet Cytogenet 74:132–138, 1994.
135. Wernicke C, Thiel G, Lozanova T, Vogel S, Kintzel D, Jänisch W, Lehmann K, Witkowski R: Involvement of chromosome 22 in ependymomas. Cancer Genet Cytogenet 79:173–176, 1995.

136. Cin PD, Sandberg AA: Cytogenetic findings in a supratentorial ependymoma. Cancer Genet Cytogenet 30:289–293, 1988.
137. Weremowicz S, Kupsky WJ, Morton CC, Fletcher JA: Cytogenetic evidence for a chromosome 22 tumor suppressor gene in ependymoma. Cancer Genet Cytogenet 61:193–196, 1992.
138. Sawyer JR, Crowson ML, Roloson GJ, Chadduck WM: Involvement of the short arm of chromosome 1 in a myxopapillary ependymoma. Cancer Genet Cytogenet 54:55–60, 1991.
139. Svard ML, Gilchrist DM: Ependymomas in two sisters and a maternal male cousin with mosaicism with monosomy 22 in tumour. Pediatr Neurosci 15:80–84, 1989.
140. Stratton MR, Darling J, Lantos PL, Cooper CS, Reeves BR: Cytogenetic abnormalities in human ependymomas. Int J Cancer 44:579–581, 1989.
141. Metzger AK, Sheffield VC, Duyk G, Daneshvar L, Edwards MSB, Cogen PH: Identification of a germ-line mutation in the p53 gene in a patient with an intracranial ependymoma. Proc Natl Acad Sci USA 88:7825–7829, 1991.
142. Punnett HH, Tomczak EZ, de Chadarevian JP, Kanev PM: Cytogenic analysis of a choroid plexus papilloma. Genes Chromosome Cancer 10: 282–285, 1994.
143. Mertens F, Heim S, Mandahl N, Mitelman F, Brun A, Strömblad L, Kullendorff C, Donnér M: Recurrent chromosomal imbalances in choroid plexus tumors. Cancer Genet Cytogenet 80:83–84, 1995.
144. Reifenberger J, Reifenberger G, Liu L, James CD, Wechsler W, Collins VP: Molecular genetic analysis of oligodendroglial tumors shows preferential allelic deletions on 19q and 1p. Am J Pathol 145:1175–1190, 1994.
145. Yong WH, Chou D, Ueki K, Harsh GR, von Deimling A, Gusella JF, Mohrenweiser HW, Louis DN: Chromosome 19q deletions in human gliomas overlap telomeric to D19S219 and may target a 425 kb region centromeric to D19S112. J Neuropathol Exp Neurol 54:622–626, 1995.
146. Fuller GN, Bigner SH: Amplified cellular oncogenes in neoplasms of the human central nervous system. Mutat Res 276:299–306, 1992.
147. Vagner-Capodano AM, Zattara-Cannoni H, Gambarelli D, Gentet JG, Genitori L, Lena G, Graziani N, Raybaud C, Choux M, Grisoli F: Detection of i(17q) chromosome by flourescent *in situ* hybridization (FISH) with interphase nuclei in medulloblastoma. Cancer Genet Cytogenet 78:1–6, 1994.
148. Biegel JA, Rorke LB, Janss AJ, Sutton LN, Parmiter AH: Isochromosome 17q demonstrated by interphase fluorescence *in situ* hybridization in primitive neuroectodermal tumors of the central nervous system. Genes Chromosome Cancer 14:85–96, 1995.
149. Stratton MR, Darling J, Cooper CS, Reeves BR: A case of cerebellar medulloblastoma with a single chromosome abnormality. Cancer Genet Cytogenet 53:101–103, 1991.
150. Bigner SH, Mark J, Friedman HS, Biegel JA, Bigner DD: Structural chromosomal abnormalities in human medulloblastoma. Cancer Genet Cytogenet 30:91–101, 1988.

151. Biegel JA, Rorke LB, Packer RJ, Sutton LN, Schut L, Bonner K, Emanuel BS: Isochromosome 17q in primitive neuroectodermal tumors of the central nervous system. Genes Chromosome Cancer 1:139–147, 1989.

152. Biegel JA, Burk CD, Barr FG, Emanuel BS: Evidence for a 17p tumor related locus distinct from p53 in pediatric primitive neuroectodermal tumors. Cancer Res 52:3391–3395, 1992.

153. Latimer FR, Al Saadi AA, Robbins TO: Cytogenetic studies of human brain tumors and their clinical significance I. Medulloblastoma. J Neurol Oncol 4:287–291, 1987.

154. Callen DF, Cirocco L, Moore L: A der(11)t(8;11) in two medulloblastomas. Cancer Genet Cytogenet 38:255–260, 1989.

155. Bigner SH, Friedman HS, Vogelstein B, Oakes WJ, Bigner DD: Amplification of the c-*myc* gene in human medulloblastoma cell lines and xenografts. Cancer Res 50:2347–2350, 1990.

156. Raffel C, Gilles FE, Weinberg KI: Reduction to homozygosity and gene amplification in central nervous system primitive neuroectodermal tumors of childhood. Cancer Res 50:587–591, 1990.

157. Wong AJ, Zoltick PW, Moscatello DK: The molecular biology and molecular genetics of astrocytic neoplasms. Semin Oncol 21:139–148, 1994.

158. Cogen PH: Prognostic significance of molecular genetic markers in childhood brain tumors. Pediatr Neurosurg 17:245–250, 1991.

159. Thomas GA, Raffel C: Loss of heterozygosity on 6q, 16q, and 17p in human central nervous system primitive neuroectodermal tumors. Cancer Res 51:639–643, 1991.

160. Scheurlen WG, Krauss J, Kühl J: No preferential loss of one parental allele of chromosome 17p13.3 in childhood medulloblastoma. Int J Cancer 63:372–374, 1995.

161. Saylors RL, Sidransky D, Friedman HS, Bigner SH, Bigner DD, Vogelstein B, Brodeur GM: Infrequent p53 gene mutations in medulloblastomas. Cancer Res 51:4721–4723, 1991.

162. Cogen PH, Daneshvar L, Metzger AK, Edwards MS: Deletion mapping of the medulloblastoma locus on chromosome 17p. Genomics 8:279–285, 1990.

163. Raffel C, Ueki K, Harsh GR, Louis DN: The multiple tumor suppressor 1/cyclin-dependent kinase inhibitor 2 gene in human central nervous system primitive neuroectodermal tumor. Neurosurgery 36:971–975, 1995.

164. Biegel JA, Rorke LB, Packer RJ, Emanuel BS: Monosomy 22 in rhabdoid or atypical tumors of the brain. J Neurosurg 73:710–714, 1990.

165. Hasserjian RP, Folkerth RD, Scott RM, Schofield DE: Clinicopathologic and cytogenetic analysis of malignant rhaboid tumor of the central nervous system. J Neurol Oncol 25:193–203, 1995.

166. Douglass EC, Valentine M, Rowe ST, Parham DM, Willimas JA, Sanders JM, Houghton PJ: Malignant rhabdoid tumor: a highly malignant childhood tumor with minimal karyotypic changes. Genes Chromosome Cancer 2:210–216, 1990.

167. Mark, J: Karyotype patterns in human meningiomas: a comparison between studies with G- and Q-banding techniques. Hereditas 75:213–220, 1973.

168. Rey JA, Bello MJ, de Campos JM, Benitez J, Ayuso MC, Valcarcel E: Chromosome studies in two human brain tumors. Cancer Genet Cytogenet 8:159–165, 1983.
169. Doco-Fenzy M, Cornillet P, Scherpereel B, Depernet B, Bisiau-Leconte S, Ferre D, Pluot M, Graftiaux J, Teyssier J: Cytogenetic changes in 67 cranial and spinal meningiomas: relation to histopathological and clinical pattern. Anticancer Res 13:845–850, 1993.
170. Deprez RHL, Riegman PH, van Drunen E, Warringa UL, Groen NA, Stefanko SZ, Koper JW, Avezaat CJJ, Mulder PGH, Zwarthoff EC, Hagemeijer A: Cytogenetic, molecular genetic and pathological analyses in 126 meningiomas. J Neuropathol Exp Neurol 54:224–235, 1995.
171. Casalone R, Simi P, Granata P, Minelli E, Giudici A, Butti G, Solero CL: Correlation between cytogenetic and histopathological findings in 65 human meningiomas. Cancer Genet Cytogenet 45:237–243, 1990.
172. Al Saadi A, Latimer F, Madercic M, Robbins T: Cytogenetic studies of human brain tumors and their clinical significance. II. Meningioma. Cancer Genet Cytogenet 26:127–141, 1987.
173. Bello MJ, de Campos JM, Vaquero J, Kusak ME, Sarasa JL, Rey JA, Pestaña A: Chromosome 22 heterozygosity is retained in most hyper-diploid and pseudodiploid meningiomas. Cancer Genet Cytogenet 66:117–119, 1993.
174. Griffin CA, Hruban RH, Long PP, Miller N, Volz P, Carson B, Brem H: Chromosome abnormalities in meningeal neoplasms: do they correlate with histology? Cancer Genet Cytogenet 78:46–52, 1994.
175. Westphal M, Hänsel M, Kunzmann R, Hölzel F, Herrmann H-D: Spectrum of karyotypic aberrations in cultured human meningiomas. Cytogenet Cell Genet 52:45–49, 1989.
176. Vagner-Capodano AM, Grisoli F, Gambarelli D, Sedan R, Pellet W, De Victor B: Correlation between cytogenetic and histopathological findings in 75 human meningiomas. Neurosurgery 32:892–900, 1993.
177. Butti G, Assietti R, Casalone R, Paoletti P: Multiple meningiomas: a clinical, surgical, and cytogenetic analysis. Surg Neurol 31:255–260, 1989.
178. Henn W, Cremerius U, Heide G, Lippitz B, Schröder JM, Gilsbach JM, Büll U, Zang KD: Monsomy 1p is correlated with enhanced *in vivo* glucose metabolism in meningiomas. Cancer Genet Cytogenet 79:144–148, 1995.
179. Schneider BF, Shashi V, von Kap-herr C, Golden WL: Loss of chromosomes 22 and 14 in the malignant progression of meningiomas. Cancer Genet Cytogenet 85:101–104, 1996.
180. Maltby EL, Ironside JW, Battersby RDE: Cytogenetic studies in 50 meningiomas. Cancer Genet Cytogenet 31:199–210, 1988.
181. Katsuyama J, Pappepnhausen PR, Herz F, Gazivoda P, Hirano A, Koss LG: Chromosome abnormalities in meningiomas. Cancer Genet Cytogenet 22:63–68, 1986.
182. Gollin SM, Janecka IP: Cytogenetics of cranial base tumors. J Neurol Oncol 20:241–254, 1994.

183. Rouleau GA, Wertelecki W, Haines JL, Hobbs WJ, Trofatter JA, Seizinger JA, Martuza RL: Genetic linkage of bilateral acoustic neurofibromatosis to a DNA marker on chromosome 22. Nature 329:246–248, 1987.
184. Seizinger BR, De la Monte SM, Atkins L: Molecular genetic approach to human meningioma: loss of genes on chromosome 22. Proc Natl Acad Sci USA 84:5419–5423, 1987.
185. Dumanski JP, Rouleau GA, Nordenskjold M, Collins VP: Molecular genetic analysis of chromosome 22 in 81 cases of meningioma. Cancer Res 50:5863–5867, 1990.
186. Dumanski JP, Carlbom E, Collins VP, Nordenskjöld M: Deletion mapping of a locus on human chromosome 22 involved in the oncogenesis of meningioma. Proc Natl Acad Sci USA 84:9275–9279, 1987.
187. Ruttledge MH, Xie Y-G, Han F-Y, Peyrard M, Collins VP, Nordenskjöld M, Dumanski JP: Deletions on chromosome 22 in sporadic meningioma. Genes Chromosome Cancer 10:122–130, 1994.
188. Lindblom A, Ruttledge M, Collins VP, Nordenskjöld M, Dumanski JP: Chromosome deletions in anaplastic meningiomas suggest multiple regions outside chromosome 22 as important in tumor progression. Int J Cancer 50:391–394, 1994.
189. Bello MJ, de Campos JM, Kusak ME, Vaquero J, Sarasa JL, Pestana A, Rey JA: Allelic loss at 1p is associated with tumor progression of meningiomas. Genes Chromosome Cancer 9:296–298, 1994.
190. Rempel SA, Schwechheimer K, Davis RL, Cavenee WK, Rosenblum ML: Loss of heterozygosity for loci on chromosome 10 is associated with morphologically malignant meningioma progression. Cancer Res 53:2386–2392, 1993.
191. Simon M, von Deimling A, Larson JL, Wellenreuther R, Kaskel P, Waha A, Warnick RE, Tew JM Jr, Menon AG: Allelic losses on chromosomes 14, 10, and 1 in atypical and malignant meningiomas: A genetic model of meningioma progression. Cancer Res 55:4696–4701, 1995.
192. Albrecht S, Armstrong DL, Mahoney DH, Cheek WR, Cooley LD: Cytogenetic demonstration of gene amplification in a primary intracranial germ cell tumor. Genes Chromosome Cancer 6:61–63, 1993.
193. Yu I-T, Griffin CA, Phillips PC, Strauss LC, Perlman EJ: Numerical sex chromosomal abnormalities in pineal teratomas by cytogenetic analysis and fluorescence *in situ* hybridization. Lab Invest 72:419–423, 1995.
194. Hecht F, Grix A, Hecht B, Berger C, Bixenman H, Szucs S, O'Keefe D, Finberg HJ: Direct prenatal chromosome diagnosis of a malignancy. Cancer Genet Cytogenet 11:107–111, 1984.
195. Shen V, Chaparro M, Choi BH, Young R, Bernstein R: Absence of isochromosome 12p in a pineal region malignant germ cell tumor. Cancer Genet Cytogenet 50:153–160, 1990.
196. de Bruin TWA, Slater RM, Defferrari R, van Kessel AG, Suijkerbuijk RF, Jansen G, de Jong B, Oosterhuis JW: Isochromosome 12p-positive pineal germ cell tumor. Cancer Res 54:1542–1544, 1994.

197. Rostad S, Kleinschmidt-DeMasters BK, Manchester DK: Two massive congenital intracranial immature teratomas with neck extension. Teratology 32:163–169, 1985.
198. Seizinger BR, Martuza RL, Gusella JF: Loss of genes on chromosome 22 in human acoustic neuroma. Nature 322:644–647, 1986.
199. Couturier J, Delattre O, Kujas M, Philippon J, Peter M, Rouleau G, Aurias A, Thomas G: Assessment of chromosome 22 anomalies in neurinomas by combined karyotype and RFLP analyses. Cancer Genet Cytogenet 45:55–62, 1990.
200. Rey JA, Bello MJ, de Campos JM, Kusak ME, Moreno S: Cytogenetic analysis in human neurinomas. Cancer Genet Cytogenet 28:187–188, 1987.
201. Wolff RK, Frazer KA, Jackler RK, Lanser MJ, Pitts LH, Cox DR: Analysis of chromosome 22 deletions in neurofibromatosis type 2-related tumors. Am J Hum Genet 51:478–485, 1992.
202. De Vitis LR, Tedde A, Vitelli F, Ammannati F, Mennonna P, Bono P, Grammatico B, Grammatico P, Radice P, Bigozzi U, Montali E, Papi L: Analysis of the neurofibromatosis type 2 gene in different human tumors of neuroectodermal origin. Hum Genet 97:638–641, 1996.
203. Golfinos JG, Norman SA, Coons SW, Spetzler RF, Scheck AC: Expression of the genes encoding myelin basic protein and proteolipid protein in glial tumors. Proc Am Assoc Cancer Res 35:551, 1994.

Chapter 14

Cytogenetic Abnormalities Associated with Endocrine Neoplasia

Stefan K. G. Grebe, Norman L. Eberhardt and Robert B. Jenkins

Introduction

During the past decade, cytogenetic studies of solid human neoplasms have come of age. Although technically more difficult and often ambiguous in comparison with cytogenetic studies of leukemias and lymphomas (1), cytogenetic studies of many solid tumors have yielded valuable insights into tumor pathogenesis and prognosis. In addition, in the last decade we have seen increasing application of molecular genetic techniques to the study of cancer, which has contributed greatly to our understanding of mechanisms controlling cell growth. Specific genetic alterations responsible for the pathogenesis of a number of neoplasms have been identified.

In this chapter, we summarize cytogenetic and molecular genetic studies of endocrine neoplasia. We review those alterations that may be relevant for endocrine cancer development and describe diagnostic and prognostic markers in these tumors. The latter studies are of particular practical interest in endocrine neoplasias because it is frequently difficult to distinguish benign from malignant tumors.

From: *Human Cytogenetic Cancer Markers*   Edited by S. R. Wolman and S. Sell
Humana Press Inc., Totowa, NJ

Parathyroid Tumors

Most endocrine tumors we discuss, including parathyroid neoplasms, occur sporadically as well as in the context of multi-organ family cancer syndromes. For parathyroid tumors, the typical familial syndrome is multiple endocrine neoplasia type 1 (MEN 1) syndrome. Whether sporadic or familial, the vast majority of parathyroid cell proliferations are benign, with histology ranging from hyperplastic-appearing lesions to classical adenomas. It can be difficult to distinguish adenomas from simple hyperplastic lesions, but, by establishing the clonality of a neoplasm, molecular genetic studies can be invaluable in this differential diagnosis *(2)*. Clonal loss of chromosome 11 and loss of heterozygosity (LOH) of the region of the suspected MEN 1 locus are common events in parathyroid adenomas, but not in parathyroid hyperplasias *(2–5)*. Almost all MEN 1-related parathyroid adenomas show LOH of alleles mapped to 11q13 *(6–12)*, although some investigators have not found LOH in a significant fraction of such tumors *(5)*. Whether this difference relates to insensitive detection methods, contamination with normal tissue, or is indicative of involvement of other genes remains to be elucidated.

Sporadic parathyroid tumors also demonstrate LOH of alleles mapped to 11q13 in about 25% of cases *(5)*, and both clonal loss of chromosome 11 *(3)* and rearrangement of the parathyroid hormone locus on 11p15 *(4)* have been reported. In addition, a rearrangement involving chromosome 1, t(1;5)(p22;q32), has been reported in a single sporadic parathyroid adenoma. Genetic analysis of a kindred with hyperparathyroidism-jaw tumor syndrome linked to 1q21–1q31 has suggested the presence of an "endocrine tumor gene" in this region *(13)*. This study suggested that a gene on 1q is involved in tumorigenesis of parathyroid lesions, as well as in other endocrine and nonendocrine neoplasms. Nevertheless, many sporadic parathyroid tumors have no obvious modifications of either the 11q or 1q arms *(5)*. Furthermore, neither cytogenetic nor molecular genetic changes in parathyroid tumors have thus far been correlated with clinical outcome.

Recent interest has been directed toward a candidate oncogene, *PRAD1*, which is localized to chromosome band 11q13. Rearrangements of this gene in a subset of benign parathyroid tumors suggest its possible role in parathyroid tumorigenesis. The same gene has also been implicated in breast cancers and in B-cell lymphoid proliferations with a t(11;14) translocation. A placental cDNA clone corresponding to the *PRAD1* gene encodes a protein of 295 amino acids with sequence similarity to the D1 cyclins *(14)*. D1 cyclins form active complexes with p34/cdc2 protein kinase and are involved in control of cell cycle progression. Single-strand conformational polymorphism (SSCP) analysis of the *PRAD1* gene in 30 primary breast cancers and 25 parathyroid adenomas failed to reveal any tumor-specific mutations *(15)*. However, examination of 48 consecutive cases of infiltrating mammary carcinoma revealed overexpression of the *PRAD1* gene product in 33% of these tumors *(15)*. Accordingly, it is possible that overexpression rather than mutational activation may account for *PRAD1*'s role in breast and parathyroid oncogenesis.

In the case of parathyroid cellular proliferations, the evidence to date indicates that molecular genetic and, to a limited degree, classical cytogenetic studies can be helpful in distinguishing hyperplastic lesions from true neoplasms. However, definitive etiologic and prognostic information has not yet been gained from these approaches. MEN 1 tumors are the obvious exception to this characterization, because these parathyroid tumors characteristically lose at least one allele of the putative 11q13 tumor suppressor gene.

Adrenal Neoplasms and Neuroectodermal Tumors

Adrenal tumors fall into two broad and fundamentally different categories: neoplasms of the adrenal cortex and the adrenal medulla. The former group includes hormonally active and inactive tumors, whereas the latter is comprised of pheochromocytomas and neuroblastomas, both of which are classified as neuroectodermal tumors. The genetics of neuroblastoma is reviewed in Chapter 16.

Most adreno-cortical neoplasms are sporadic, though some occur in the context of MEN 1 or other rare genetic disorders, such as Beckwith-Wiedmann syndrome (BWS—which is associated with Wilm's tumor and other embryonal neoplasms).

Tumors of the adrenal cortex have only rarely been examined by cytogenetic or molecular genetic techniques. The literature is essentially limited to case reports and small case series, all of which have used molecular genetic techniques rather than classical cytogenetic analysis. Interestingly, the limited data available indicate frequent allelic loss from chromosome 11, which harbors the MEN 1 and *WT1* (implicated in the development of Wilm's tumor) genes on its long arm and short arm, respectively. Restriction fragment length polymorphism (RFLP) mapping of nonfunctional adrenal adenomas from patients with BWS has revealed LOH of two nonoverlapping 11p15 regions, both distal to the region of the *WT1* gene, but not at the MEN 1 locus on 11q *(16,17)*.

In contrast, Beckers et al. *(18)* described a patient with MEN 1 with an aldosterone-producing adrenal adenoma and found LOH of the MEN 1 locus at 11q13. Recently, Iida et al. *(19)* screened tumor tissue from nine patients with sporadic aldosterone-producing adrenal tumors and three patients with familial hyperaldosteronism type II for LOH in the region of the presumed MEN 1 locus; they were able to demonstrate allelic loss in 5 of 11 informative cases. In addition, they demonstrated loss of a nearby, nonoverlapping region, suggesting a possible second tumor suppressor gene on 11q. From these studies it appears likely that a gene or genes in the vicinity of the MEN 1 may also be involved in the etiology of sporadic and familial aldosterone-producing adrenal neoplasms. Unfortunately, there is presently no information available on other sporadic adrenocortical tumors.

Another lesion that frequently involves the adrenal cortex, but that is not strictly an endocrine cancer, is represented by the adrenocortical carcinomas arising in patients with the Li-Fraumeni syndrome. Susceptibility for this disease is transmitted as an autosomal dominant trait, and molecular genetic analyses have demonstrated germline mutations of the p53 tumor suppressor gene in many families *(20,21)*. Patients with this disorder are often affected by sarcomas that occur in childhood, and breast cancers in young adult women, as well as adrenocortical carcinomas. In addition, Li-Fraumeni disease is characterized by an increased frequency of cerebral tumors and leukemias. Occasionally, p53 mutations are also observed in sporadic adrenocortical carcinomas *(22)*. However, the reported incidence of p53 mutations of 20% is not unusual for human cancers in general *(23–25)*, and suggests that p53 mutations may not play a primary role in the genesis of sporadic adrenocortical carcinoma.

Tumors of the adrenal medulla have been more thoroughly studied by molecular genetic and cytogenetic methods, chiefly because pheochromocytoma is associated with a number of inherited syndromes, such as neurofibromatosis type 2 (NF2), von Hippel-Lindau disease (VHL), and MEN 2, and because neuroblastoma is a relatively common and often lethal childhood cancer. For VHL and MEN 2, the probable disease-causing genes have been identified by classical molecular genetic analysis and positional cloning. *VHL* is a tumor suppressor gene *(26)* localized to chromosomal region 3p25–p26. Recent evidence indicates that the *VHL* gene product operates by a unique mechanism involving transcription elongation that is mediated by interactions with elongation factors elongin B and C *(27)*. This raises the prospect that *VHL* may control oncogenes that are regulated at the level of elongation such as c-*myc*, L-*myc*, N-*myc*, and c-*fos (28)*. The MEN 2 gene has been shown to be the *RET* proto-oncogene, a member of the tyrosine kinase transmembrane receptor family localized to 10q11.2 *(29)*. It is very likely that the pheochromocytomas in patients with either VHL or MEN 2 result from mutations in their respective predisposing genes.

Interestingly, more than 60% of pheochromocytomas associated with MEN 2 also revealed LOH of alleles mapped to 1p *(30–32)*, suggesting that loss of another tumor suppressor gene at this locus may be a cofactor in the development of pheochromocytomas arising in patients with MEN 2. There is also mounting evidence of involvement of chromosome 1p in childhood neuroblastoma. An alternative possibility is that the primary abnormality in MEN 2 gives rise to generalized genetic instability. The latter is supported by a number of cytogenetic studies that have shown an increased incidence of cytogenetic abnormalities in normal peripheral white blood cells from patients with MEN 2. For example, deletions of 20p12.2 are observed frequently in peripheral blood lymphocytes in MEN 2 patients *(33,34)*. In fact, this finding initially led to the erroneous hypothesis that chromosome 20 was the site of the MEN 2 gene *(35)*.

Widespread genetic alterations are relatively common in sporadic pheochromocytomas. LOH of markers mapped to chromosome

22 has been reported *(36)* and fluorescent *in situ* hybridization (FISH) studies using highly specific pericentromeric DNA probes, have shown high prevalence of numerical chromosome aberrations involving other chromosomes *(37)*. Flow cytometric studies have also reported high frequencies of DNA aneuploidy *(38–41)*, and have tentatively established a correlation between ploidy and prognosis. In contrast to MEN 2-related pheochromocytomas, or pheochromocytomas arising in the context of other well-studied syndromes, no specific primary or secondary cytogenetic or molecular genetic abnormalities have been identified in sporadic cases. However, the degree of genetic disarray may have prognostic implications, probably as a nonspecific marker of (loss of) differentiation. Furthermore, chromosomes 1 and 22 may warrant further study in sporadic pheochromocytoma.

Pituitary Tumors

Pituitary tumors are generally benign adenomas. For the most part their etiology remains obscure. They are classified in a variety of ways, including light microscopic appearance, hormone production, and by ultrastructural features *(42,43)*. Regardless of the classification scheme used, within a given tumor subgroup, as well as between subtypes, a staggering array of variable growth patterns and degrees of differentiation are observed. Classical criteria for malignancy, based on mitotic index, growth pattern, invasiveness, and degree of differentiation, often fail to predict an individual tumor's biological behavior. Even the most aggressive-appearing neoplasms are usually benign. However, a handful of pituitary carcinomas have been described, and a fair proportion of benign adenomas recur after therapy, some displaying extreme invasiveness, with resultant difficulties in management. The failure of classical pathological methods to predict such events is one of the major problems facing pituitary pathology. Genetic methods could potentially aid in categorizing pituitary tumors in a way that correlates more closely to their behavior. Furthermore, such studies may define potential causes for tumor development. However, the benign nature of most pituitary neoplasms has made it difficult to establish short-term cell cultures, leading to a paucity of published cytogenetic studies. The more aggressive tumors that might lend themselves more easily to kary-otyping are often prolactinomas, which are generally no longer treated surgically, and thus tissue for analysis is scarce.

Despite the problems indicated in the preceding paragraph, chromosomally aneuploid pituitary tumors were observed in the 1960s *(44)* and flow-cytometric studies later confirmed the frequent occurrence of DNA aneuploidy in human pituitary adenomas *(45,46)*. In a study of 29 histologically benign hypophyseal tumors, Anniko et al. *(45)* found 12 to have aneuploid DNA content by flow-cytometry. Subsequently, Anniko et al. *(46)* noted that three partic-ularly aggressive pituitary adenomas displayed aneuploidy, although no similar correlation had been observed in their earlier paper and clearly none of the subsequent tumors were malignant. Given that aneuploidy in most solid tumors is associated with clini-cally aggressive malignancy, these findings are somewhat paradox-ical, extending the histopathological difficulties of predicting biological behavior to the cytogenetic level.

As recent methods have evolved to allow the short-term sub-culturing of pituitary tumors, a growing number of karyotypic analyses of pituitary tumors have been performed. Results from these studies further underscore the problem of correlating genetic abnormalities with disease histology. Various cytogenetic abnor-malities have been reported, none of which seems closely related to histology or clinical behavior. In 1986 Rey et al. *(47)* reported a case of a pituitary adenoma with 58 chromosomes and numerical aberra-tions of chromosomes 3, 5, 7, 9, 11, 12, 13, 17, 19, 20, and the gono-somes. Two further cases with simple numerical aberration of chromosomes 4, 9, 20, and Y have since been reported *(48)*, in addi-tion to a case with deletion of chromosomes 18 and 11p *(49)*.

In a more comprehensive study of 18 pituitary neoplasms that were successfully grown in short-term culture, multiple numeric and structural abnormalities were found in 10 adenomas *(50)*. Supporting the results of the earlier DNA-ploidy studies, no correlations between karyotype and invasiveness or morphology could be made, though a tendency for more invasive tumors to be associated with chromosomal abnormalities was noted. In addition, only 3 of 11 hor-monally active tumors (secreting growth hormone and/or prolactin), but 5 of 8 hormonally inactive had normal karyotypes, suggesting that genetic differences may underlie hormonally active and hormonally silent tumors. Chromosomes 1, 4, 7, and 19 were either numerically or structurally abnormal in at least three specimens each, only one tumor with abnormal karyotype did not show involvement of at least one of these chromosomes. Moreover, those that had involvement of chromosome 19 had no abnormalities of chromosomes 1, 4, or 7, suggesting the presence of two distinct groups of tumors with possibly differing etiology.

From the published data it appears that no cytogenetic markers that predict biological behavior of pituitary adenoma can yet be firmly identified. However, further genetic studies of chromosomes 1, 4, 7, 9, and 19 may well yield some clues as to pathogenesis of these neoplasms. In addition, the data that hormonally active tumors are more likely to harbor cytogenetic abnormalities than null-cell tumors need to be confirmed and extended.

Most recently, molecular genetic studies have expanded our understanding of the etiology of pituitary tumors. Based on the incidence of pituitary tumors in patients with MEN 1, a number of sporadic and MEN-related pituitary adenomas have been screened for LOH of this region *(9,51–53)*. It appears that about 30% of MEN 1-associated hypophyseal tumors exhibit LOH of markers mapped to 11q13 and between 10 and 30% of sporadic tumors have genetic losses in this region. Finally, mutations in the growth hormone (GH) releasing hormone-coupled G_α subunit gene (*GSP* oncogene) were identified as the cause of constitutive activation of adenylate cyclase in a small proportion (~30%) of sporadic GH-secreting human pituitary tumors, but this type of mutation appears to be rare in all other pituitary neoplasms *(51,54)*. Whether mutation of *GSP* is necessary or sufficient for adenoma development is not known, and awaits further study. This observation raises the question of whether other point mutations in various proteins that mediate signal transduction pathways may be involved in pituitary neoplasms.

Medullary Thyroid Carcinoma

Medullary thyroid carcinoma (MTC) is a malignant thyroid neoplasm arising from the parafollicular C-cells. C-cells produce calcitonin, which has important hormonal functions in bone mineral metabolism in amphibians, reptiles, and fish. By contrast, in man calcitonin acts largely as a neurotransmitter, and does not appear to have significant hormonal activity, because there is no discernable clinical syndrome associated with loss of C-cell function.

Most cases of MTC are sporadic, but a significant proportion (up to 50% in some populations) occur in the context of either MEN 2 or familial medullary thyroid carcinoma. The latter shares genetic features with MEN 2 and is seen by many as a *form fruste* of the complete MEN 2 syndrome *(55)*. The overwhelming majority of cytogenetic and molecular genetic investigations concern familial and MEN 2-related tumors. Familial MTC and MEN 2-related MTC are both characterized by the almost universal occurrence of mutations in the *RET* proto-oncogene in the paracentromeric region of chromosome 10 *(56)*. Although no other consistent molecular genetic abnormalities have been identified in these familial tumors, several other molecular genetic abnormalities have been found, including LOH of alleles mapped to 1p, 3p, 13q, and 22 *(31,32,57–60)*. The fact that LOH at 1p is common to both sporadic and MEN-related pheochromocytomas suggests that this locus may encompass a gene serving as a cofactor in MEN 2 development or, alternatively, the development of tumors derived from neuroectodermal tissue in general. However, 1p loss abnormalities are far from universal in MEN 2-related MTC *(61)*. Furthermore, most molecular genetic studies in familial and MEN 2-related MTC have been biased toward chromosomal sites known or suspected to be abnormal in a significant proportion of MEN 2 patients. Hence, a positive detection bias seems likely. Classical cytogenetic studies also support the relatively infrequent occurrence of major genetic rearrangements in familial MTC, although, as summarized by Cooley et al. *(62)*, structural and numerical abnormalities involving 1p, 3p, 5q, 7p, 7q, 8, 9, 10, 11p, 12, 14, 17p, 22, and X have been reported in a number of primary tumor specimens and MTC cell lines. None of these abnormalities was consistently found in all tumors, suggesting that they may well represent epiphenomena, or, in the case of tumor cell lines, culture artifacts. Very little is known about molecular and cytogenetic changes in sporadic MTC. Interestingly, approx 20% of patients with sporadic MTC have apparent new germline mutations in *RET (56)*, thus giving rise to new families with familial MTC or MEN 2.

Neither patients with familial nor with sporadic MTC have evidence of a generalized increased in chromosomal fragility, as has been observed in patients with MEN 2-related pheochromocytomas. In a study of 18 sporadic, 7 familial, and 7 MEN-related MTC cases, no increase in the proportion of abnormal karyotypes in peripheral lymphocytes was observed *(63)*. Similarly, in another study, none of 26 individuals with MTC from 5 families with MEN 2 showed any greater chromosomal instability in peripheral blood lymphocytes than did healthy control subjects *(61)*. In addition to reducing the role that chromosomal instability may play in the etiology of MTC, these results also suggest that the role of chromosomal instability in MEN 2 patients with pheochromocytoma should be viewed with skepticism.

In summary, beyond the important elucidation of the *RET* oncogene as the major common molecular factor in familial and MEN 2-related MTC, and the potential role of 1p in familial MTC progression, cytogenetic and molecular genetic studies have thus far failed to provide additional clues to medullary carcinoma tumorigenesis. Unfortunately, no important prognostic markers have been identified, in part because of the relative rarity of this tumor. Additional sporadic and inherited tumors must be studied to achieve further insight into MTC etiology and to also identify potential prognostic markers.

Nonmedullary Primary Thyroid Tumors

Nonmedullary thyroid tumors in the widest sense comprise all thyroid neoplasms derived from follicular epithelium, as well as the various sarcomas, lymphomas, and other miscellaneous tumors including metastases that involve the gland. However, only those tumors arising from glandular epithelial tissue are considered to be "endocrine neoplasms" and these tumors are the focus of this section.

Benign and malignant thyroid neoplasms are by far the most common endocrine tumors, outnumbering all other endocrine cancers combined, by an order of magnitude. Although not generally lethal, because of their increased frequency, thyroid malignancies kill far more people than tumors of all other endocrine organs.

Consequently, there is a strong perceived clinical need for reliable prognostic staging systems. Furthermore, well-differentiated follicular thyroid carcinomas can be difficult to distinguish from benign adenomas, particularly on cytological examination. Since the latter has become the first line diagnostic procedure for thyroid nodules, a reliable test to distinguish follicular adenomas from follicular carcinomas is needed.

As a consequence of all the aforementioned factors, a much greater literature exists on genetic abnormalities in thyroid tumors than for most other endocrine tumors. To a limited degree the results of this research have been helpful in addressing certain diagnostic and prognostic questions, and are beginning to provide insight into the mechanisms involved in thyroid tumorigenesis. However, the data accumulated so far have also shown a bewildering array of abnormalities, making it difficult to pinpoint the most important genetic abnormalities in these tumors.

As in many other endocrine neoplasms, abnormal cellular DNA content is not uncommon in thyroid tumors. DNA cytometric analyses have shown rates of DNA aneuploidy between 12 and 68%, depending on tumor type (64). Follicular thyroid cancers (FTC) show higher rates of aneuploidy than papillary tumors (PTC) (64), and when analyzed for potential prognostic significance, DNA aneuploidy seems to be particularly important in the oxyphilis (Hürthle cell) variant of FTC. However, the clinical utility of DNA content measurements is much less in other thyroid cancers and the occurrence of aneuploid cellular DNA content in benign follicular adenomas (65) limits the usefulness of flow cytometry in the differential diagnosis of follicular thyroid adenomas vs carcinomas.

More specific analysis of chromosome abnormalities by karyotyping has also shown a wide range of abnormalities in all types of benign and malignant thyroid tumors. This raises the question of whether a continuum between benign and malignant follicular thyroid tumors exists, with gradual transitions from benign hyperplasia to adenoma and finally to carcinoma. Indeed, when one compares benign hyperplasia, adenomas, PTC, FTC, and poorly differentiated carcinomas, chromosomal abnormalities become increasingly more common in each of these groups.

Benign Nodules and Follicular Adenomas

Numerical chromosome aberrations have even been discovered in benign hyperplastic thyroid nodules *(66)* and structural abnormalities involving translocations of chromosome 19 have also been observed in histologically simple benign hyperplastic nodules *(67)*. However, both numerical and structural aberrations are uncommon in benign hyperplastic nodules, affecting <10% of lesions *(66)*.

By contrast, follicular adenomas frequently display abnormal karyotypes. Ignoring case reports, which are subject to strong positive reporting bias, several cytogenetic investigations of follicular adenomas have found karyotypic abnormalities in an average of 30% (range 15–60%) of adenomas *(65,68–74)*. These are not uniform and have included both numerical and structural abnormalities. Trisomy of chromosome 7 has been the most frequent finding, occurring in the majority of adenomas with numerical chromosome aberrations *(65,68,72,73)*. However, the significance of this finding is debatable. Trisomy 7 is a common occurrence in a number of solid tumors, and also in benign tissues, and some have argued that it probably is of no specific significance *(75)*. In addition to trisomy 7, numerical abnormalities of every other chromosome have been reported in follicular adenomas *(65,68,70,72)*, almost invariably in the form of chromosomal gains. Structural abnormalities are also common and span a wide array of observed abnormalities. They have often included complex translocations *(68,72)* involving several chromosomes, but a number of simpler translocations, inversions, and partial deletions have also been observed *(65,67,71,72,76–79)*. These have involved chromosomes 5, 8, 9, 10, 12, 13, 14, and 19. Most of the abnormalities have only been observed in single tumors and do not often share apparently similar breakpoints.

Unlike the majority of anomalies observed in follicular adenomas, translocations involving band 19q13 have been observed repeatedly *(65,67,78,79)* and the breakpoints appear identical. In two instances the translocations have involved chromosome 5, and the breakpoints on this chromosome have also been identical. FISH analyses, using a series of cosmid probes located on 19q in a *SV40*-transformed thyroid adenoma cell line, mapped the breakpoint between the DNA polymerase delta 1 and troponin T1 genes at the boundary between chromosome bands 19q13.3 and 19q13.4. It appears likely that an oncogene (or less likely a tumor suppressor gene) of pathogenetic importance is located in this region. Potential candidate genes, which conceivably may act as oncogenes if mutated or constitutively activated, might include two zinc finger protein genes (*ZNF83* and *ZNF160*), as well as the gene coding for the gamma subunit of protein kinase C. Interestingly, translocations involving 19q13 may even occur in benign hyperplastic nodules *(67)*. This suggests that the events associated with this translocation could be among the earliest steps in follicular tumorigenesis. Furthermore, it could have diagnostic implications, as it may denote a subgroup of apparently hyperplastic nodules that in fact are destined to develop into follicular adenomas.

Another site of repeatedly observed LOH in follicular adenomas is at chromosome band 11q13, in the region of the putative MEN 1 tumor suppressor gene. Matsuo et al. *(80)* observed LOH of this region in 4 of 27 follicular adenomas, raising the possibility that the putative MEN 1 gene or other genes nearby could be involved in some follicular adenomas. It remains to be demonstrated whether tumors with genetic losses at this locus differ in progression or prognosis from other follicular adenomas.

Follicular Thyroid Carcinomas

FTCs share many cytological and histological features with follicular adenomas. On the one hand, this may lead to significant difficulties in distinguishing malignant follicular neoplasms from their benign counterparts. On the other hand, the close resemblance of benign and malignant follicular tumors argues for a possible adenoma → carcinoma pathogenetic sequence, possibly similar to that established for colon carcinoma *(81)*. Although the concept of such a progression is intuitively appealing, the present clinical and pathological paradigm is that follicular adenomas and carcinomas are distinct entities. However, this viewpoint is increasingly challenged in light of the almost continuous spectrum of cytological and histological changes observed in follicular adenomas and carcinomas; one of the major criteria for malignancy determination, capsular invasion, is occasionally observed even in adenomatous lesions. Similarly, FTC share many genetic abnormalities with follicular adenomas, again suggesting the possibility of a gradual transition from one into the other. However, multiple genomic abnormalities are observed more frequently in follicular carcinomas.

DNA aneuploidy by flow cytometry is common, occurring in 41–64% of typical FTC and in 27–80% of Hürthle cell follicular carcinomas *(64)*. In both groups, but particularly in the Hürthle cell cancers, DNA aneuploidy seems to be an independent risk factor for progression and death *(64)*. As expected from the flow cytometry data, numerical chromosome aberrations are common in follicular thyroid cancers. However, in contrast to follicular adenomas, follicular carcinomas have aberrations involving complex chromosomal rearrangements with multiple identifiable marker chromosomes *(65,69,82)*, though simple deletions and deletions/rearrangements may also be seen *(65)*. Among a plethora of structural cytogenetic abnormalities, alterations of 3p are the most commonly observed changes *(82,83)* (Fig. 1). This suggests that a tumor suppressor gene resides in this region, particularly since chromosome 3 is also the chromosome most commonly lost *(69)*. Molecular studies have corroborated the cytogenetic studies, with frequent observations of LOH of alleles mapped to 3p *(69)*. The fact that LOH at 3p has also been found in both a primary tumor and its metastasis further suggests that 3p loss is a nonrandom, inheritable property of certain follicular thyroid cancers, and hence is of possible etiological and prognostic significance *(83)*. Other neoplasms, including small cell lung cancer and renal cell carcinoma also exhibit frequent LOH of several 3p regions *(84–88)*, giving rise to the concept that several tumor suppressor genes may be located on the short arm of chromosome 3. Proof that 3p contains at least one tumor suppressor comes from the recent positional cloning of the *VHL* gene *(26)*. The *VHL* gene is also frequently mutated in patients with renal cell carcinoma, particularly clear cell carcinoma *(89,90)*. However, in several follicular thyroid cancers exhibiting 3p LOH, no mutations in the *VHL* gene were found (Linehan and Eberhardt, unpublished observations), suggesting that this gene is not involved in follicular thyroid carcinogenesis.

Interestingly, 3p LOH seems to be limited to follicular thyroid carcinomas. Matsuo et al. *(80)* were unable to detect LOH using probes from a relatively small region between 3p21.2 and 3p21.3 in

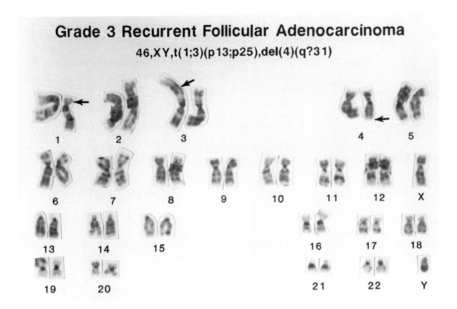

Grade 3 Recurrent Follicular Adenocarcinoma

46,XY,t(1;3)(p13;p25),del(4)(q?31)

Fig. 1. Karyotype of a recurrent grade 3 follicular carcinoma demonstrating a balanced chromosomal rearrangement of chromosome 3. Karyotype: 46,XY,t(1;3)(p13;p25),del(4)(q?31).

27 follicular adenomas. Also, Herrmann et al. *(69)*, using length RFLP probes mapping to a larger region of 3p, found no evidence for 3p LOH among six papillary and three follicular adenomas, whereas all six follicular carcinomas that were studied exhibited loss at the 3p locus. Although the number of patients examined by Herrmann et al. *(69)* was small, the general conclusions of that study have been confirmed in follow-up studies of follicular adenomas and papillary and follicular carcinomas with a larger patient cohort (Wu, Maciel, Eberhardt, and Jenkins, unpublished observations) (Fig. 2). Taken together, these studies suggest that loss of one or more 3p tumor suppressor genes could be specific for follicular thyroid carcinomas and might be viewed as a key event in the adenoma → carcinoma progression hypothesis. Further, 3p loss might help clinically to distinguish follicular adenomas from carcinomas.

Other loci exhibiting LOH have been found on chromosomes 10, 11, 16, and 17, but less frequently, raising doubt about the

Map of Chromosome 3 Deletions in FTC and FA

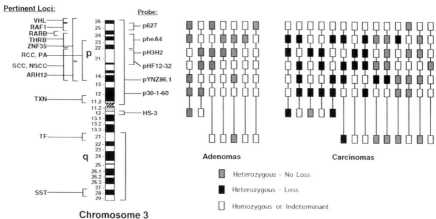

Fig. 2. Map of chromosome 3 allele loss in follicular adenomas and carcinomas of the thyroid.

importance of any of these sites *(69)*. It should be noted, that chromosomes 11 and 10 contain genes known to be involved in MEN 1 and MEN 2, respectively, and chromosome 17 contains p53, so further study of the tumors exhibiting LOH in these loci is needed. Overall the frequency of *RET* and *p53* mutations is apparently low in FTC *(91)*, arguing against a crucial role in thyroid tumor development. However, alterations of either gene may still be relevant to clinical behavior, and this aspect needs to be explored further.

Papillary Thyroid Carcinomas

PTC are quite distinct from benign and malignant follicular tumors in cytological and histological appearance, though they may include various admixtures of follicular elements *(92)*. In most countries they outnumber FTC. PTC tend to have a somewhat less aggressive course than FTC and, because there is no benign counterpart to PTC, their differential diagnosis from benign lesions is generally not a problem. There is no morphologic or clinical evidence that hyperplastic nodules or follicular adenomas ever undergo gradual change to a malignant papillary tumor. Thus, unlike FTC, a simple pathogenetic sequence of adenoma → carcinoma is less likely for PTC. Nevertheless, the cell of origin of PTC is also believed to be the normal glandular follicular epithelium. It is intriguing to speculate on how a single cell of origin can give rise to two such distinct types of malignant neoplasm, and cytogenetic and molecular genetic studies have begun to help scientists understand this problem.

DNA aneuploidy, as determined by flow cytometry, is much less common in PTC than in FTC, and may in fact be even less common than in follicular adenomas. Most studies show that no more than 20% of PTC are aneuploid *(64,65)*.

Most classical cytogenetic studies have supported the flow cytometric studies in showing a relatively lower frequency of numerical chromosome aberrations in PTC when compared to FTC *(65,68,69,82,93–95)*. Abnormal chromosome numbers are usually found in less than 20% of cases. By contrast, structural chromosome changes have been observed in >50% of PTC studied *(68,69, 82,93–95)*. Structural abnormalities involving chromosomes 1, 5, 7, 8, 9, 10, 11, 12, 16, 17, 19, 21, and 22 have been reported. Significantly, chromosome 10 has been involved in more than half of the cases with structural abnormalities, often appearing as simple inversions *(82)*.

Molecular genetic studies have revealed that the structural chromosomal changes involving chromosome 10 frequently involve an intrachromosomal inversion of the *RET* proto-oncogene. Usually the inversion involves the *H4* (D10S170) gene resulting in the formation of a chimeric fusion oncogene, *PTC1 (96,97)*. The *H4* gene contains no significant homology to known genes, but contains an open reading frame of 585 amino acids with extensive putative alpha-helical domains similar to tropomyosin, vimentin, keratin, and myosin heavy chain; a putative SH3 binding site within the carboxy terminus suggests that *H4* might be a cytoskeletal protein *(98)*. The rearranged *PTC1* gene encodes a fusion protein containing the N-terminus of *H4* translocated upstream of the *RET* tyrosine kinase domain, such that *PTC1* expression is driven by the *H4* gene promoter *(99)*. Interestingly, the *H4* gene contains a putative oligomerization domain (coiled-coil) and oligomerization of *H4* has been observed in vitro *(99)*. Since oligomerization of receptor tyrosine kinases appears to be an obligate step in their activation, oligomerization of *PTC1* may account, in part, for its oncogenic properties *(99)*. In addition, its constitutive expression by the *H4* promoter may well play an important role in its oncogenic activity *(99)*.

In addition to the predominant *PTC1* rearrangement, translocation of the *RET* locus to band 17q23 has been shown to result in formation of the so called *PTC2* oncogene by fusion with part of the gene coding for the regulatory subunit of protein kinase A *(97,100)*. Finally, another intrachromosomal rearrangement involving the *RET* and the *ele1* gene leads to formation of the *PTC3* chimeric oncogene *(97)*. FISH analysis indicates that the *ele1* gene is localized to band 10q11.2, the subband that contains RET, and karyotyping of two *PTC3* positive tumors failed to show evidence of chromosome 10 abnormalities *(101)*. Thus *PTC3* appears to be characterized by a cytogenetically undetectable paracentric inversion within 10q11.2 *(102)*.

Combined, the three *PTC* chromosomal rearrangements are observed in about 30% of PTC *(97)*. These studies suggest that *RET* activation is a very common feature of PTC. In addition, *PTC* activation has been observed in 11 of 26 occult papillary thyroid carcinomas, suggesting that *PTC* gene activation represents an early, possibly crucial, event in the process of thyroid oncogenesis *(103)*. Furthermore, *RET* activation is specific for the PTC subtype *(104)*, again suggesting that it represents an early event in the transformation of a normal thyroid epithelial cell into a cancer with papillary features. Accordingly, one hypothesis is that *RET* activation leads directly to papillary cancer formation, without intervening steps.

The mechanisms leading to the rearrangements of chromosome 10 with the resultant oncogenes have not been fully elucidated. Theoretically, any event potentially leading to an increased frequency of chromosomal breakage and subsequent rearrangement could be responsible for the *RET* gene rearrangements. This is consistent with the observation that nonspecific mutagenic stimuli such as radiation exposure result in an increased risk of PTC. This observation has been recently confirmed by the Chernobyl atomic reactor disaster where a significant increase in pediatric (5–8 yr) PTC has been observed *(105)*. Evidence that such radiation-induced lesions are a result of an increased frequency of *RET* gene rearrangements has recently been shown in vitro using X-irradiation of human undifferentiated thyroid carcinoma and fibrosarcoma cells that lack *RET* oncogene rearrangement *(106)*. In these studies rearrangements typical of in vivo thyroid cancer and atypical rearrangements not observed in vivo were seen *(106)*. Furthermore, 7 of 11 tumors from patients examined after the Chernobyl disaster displayed evidence of *RET* gene rearrangement *(107,108)*. Thus increased radiation exposure may be one mechanism for generating activated *PTC* oncogenes. In addition, it appears that the *RET* gene has not been subjected to detailed sequence analysis in nonmedullary thyroid cancers. Thus the question of whether mutational activation of the *RET* gene underlies additional thyroid cancers (other than the 30% that result from activation by rearrangement) is still an open question. So far neither *RET* oncogene activation as a whole, nor the various means of *RET* activation, has been correlated with clinical outcome, and no other consistent chromosomal changes have been observed in PTC.

In conclusion, cytogenetic changes are common in benign and malignant thyroid tumors and even occur in hyperplastic nodules. A gradual stepwise progression from hyperplastic nodules to follicular adenomas, possibly initiated by oncogene activation on chromosome 19, seems plausible. Similarly, follicular adenomas may progress to follicular carcinomas by loss of tumor suppressor function from chromosome arm 3p, and possibly from chromosome 11. FTC often exhibit gross chromosomal instability and thus a number of additional tumorigenic events may well occur subsequent to the early events, perhaps leading to more aggressive clinical behavior. Finally, PTC also arise from follicular glandular epithelium, but they do not seem to follow a gradual stepwise course of tumorigenesis. Rather, a single event, for example *RET* oncogene activation in approx 30% of tumors, seems to initiate these tumors. The underlying genetic alterations for the remaining 70% of PTC have not yet been ascertained. PTC generally display fewer cytogenetic and molecular genetic changes than follicular tumors. Thus it is possible that they are also genomically more stable, with a lesser tendency to dedifferentiate and progress clinically.

MEN

A recent excellent review of the MEN syndromes has been published *(109)*. The following briefly summarizes the current knowledge of MEN biology. By definition MEN involves occurrence of tumors in two or more endocrine glands within an individual. The disease is subdivided into two major classifications, type 1 and type 2. Both types of disease are familial and inherited in an autosomal dominant manner, although apparently sporadic development of the disease can occur. Primary hyperparathyroidism is the most common manifestation of MEN 1, affecting over 90% of patients, followed by pancreatic endocrine tumors (gastrinomas, insulinomas, glucagonomas, tumors producing vasoactive intestinal peptides [*VI*Pomas], tumors producing peptides of undetermined function, and combinations of the aforementioned) in >60% of patients, and pituitary adenomas (mostly prolactinomas and somatotrophomas) in about 30% of patients. Occasionally, other tumors, including lipomas, carcinoid tumors, and adrenal cortical tumors, are found in association with MEN 1. Patients with MEN 2 suffer mainly from MTC and pheochromocytoma. Three subcategories of the disease are recognized. MEN 2A is the dominant subtype, which includes MTC in association with pheochromocytoma and parathyroid tumors. MEN 2B usually lacks parathyroid involvement, and manifests a Marfanoid patient habitus and the occurrence of mucosal neuromas *(6,7)*. Patients with familial medullary thyroid cancer (FMTC) lack pheochromocytoma, parathyroid tumors, and the phenotypic signs of MEN 2B. The cumulative incidence of MTC approaches 100% in groups of MEN 2 patients. Pheochromocytomas, usually bilateral, occur in about 50% of MEN 2A and MEN 2B patients. Parathyroid tumors are the least common tumor in both groups, occurring in 10–30% of individuals *(6,7,110)*.

MEN 1

It was recognized early that MEN 1 was inherited in an autosomal dominant fashion, and subsequent molecular genetic linkage analysis and LOH studies have largely confirmed the putative "one disease gene" theory of the disorder. Initial studies showed extensive LOH on chromosome 11 in tumor specimens from two affected brothers *(111)*. Deletion mapping and genetic linkage studies have since mapped the responsible gene to a small region on 11q13 *(5,9,11,12,52,112)*. In the majority of tumors in MEN 1 patients, LOH of this region can be demonstrated, and linkage analysis invariably confirms that the retained allele is inherited from the affected parent *(7,8,113)*. 11q13 LOH is also observed in most parathyroid and pancreatic endocrine tumors and, with lesser frequency, in pituitary and adrenocortical lesions from MEN 1 patients *(7,114)*. MEN 1, therefore, fits the model classical familial tumor syndrome as a "one gene-double hit" disease; the paradigm being familial retinoblastoma. A germline mutation in the tumor suppressor gene is inherited, and subsequent clinical manifestations are likely to result from somatic mutation of the remaining wild type allele. The exact mechanisms of tumorigenesis will await identification and characterization of the MEN 1 gene.

There has been speculation that individuals with MEN 1 may have some generalized increase in chromosomal instability. Studies have reported somewhat increased frequencies of chromosomal breakage in normal lymphocytes from MEN 1 patients *(115,116)*—that could conceivably predispose individuals to LOH. The cause of increased chromosome breakage in MEN 1 patients remains obscure, although the mutated putative tumor suppressor gene at 11q13 might interfere with DNA repair, causing genetic instability. Clearly, these findings should be confirmed and explored in greater detail. However, the fact that cultured tumor cells from MEN 1 patients grow poorly in culture unless supplemented with serum from MEN 1 patients hints at the possibility of an autocrine or paracrine factor *(10)*. A second genetic lesion in MEN 1 tumorigenesis, at a locus distinct from 11q13, is possible, but neither molecular nor cytogenetic studies have provided evidence for additional, consistent lesions *(117)*.

On a practical level, the close linkage shown for the putative MEN 1 gene has made presymptomatic carrier detection feasible *(7,8)*. Whether detection will result in improved outcome for the identified carriers, or decreased health care costs by reducing unnecessary biochemical screening tests in noncarriers, remains to be demonstrated.

MEN 2

Initial cytogenetic studies of tumors from MEN 2 patients found evidence for deletions involving chromosome band 20p12.2 *(35,118)*, which, however, were not confirmed by other groups *(61)*. Subsequent LOH studies pointed toward loss of genetic material on chromosome 22 *(60)*, a finding which, though subsequently confirmed in some pheochromocytomas *(36)*, generally also failed to be independently confirmed. Finally, genetic linkage studies suggested linkage of the MEN 2A and 2B to chromosome 10 *(119,120)*, subsequently confirmed by high resolution mapping to the paracentromeric region of chromosome 10 *(121)*. Because LOH studies failed to show significant genomic deletions in this region *(122,123)*, oncogene activation rather than tumor suppressor loss was suspected to be the molecular mechanism of MEN 2 tumori-genesis. The region identified by linkage studies was known to harbor a candidate oncogene, the *RET* proto-oncogene, and mutations in this gene have now been identified in over 90% of individuals with MEN 2A and MEN 2B *(56)*. *RET* is a member of the receptor tyrosine kinase family and is involved in transduction of signals for cell proliferation and differentiation. *RET* mutations in MEN 2A and FMTC patients are clustered in exons 10 and 11 in an extracellular cysteine-rich domain in immediate proximity to the plasma membrane *(109)*. By far the most commonly affected site is codon CYS_{634}, which accounts for most mutations *(56,110)*, although a number of nearby cysteine residues are also affected. Mutations of more distal codons may correlate with incomplete expression in the familial MTC syndrome, and mutations that change the CYS_{634} codon to ARG are a strong predictor of associated parathyroid involvement *(110)*. In contrast, over 90% of patients with MEN 2B have a mutation in *RET* codon Met_{918}; often to a threonine.

Whether *RET* mutations are the sole cause of MEN 2, and whether these mutations account for the complete spectrum of observed variation in disease expression remains to be confirmed. As discussed in the section on adrenal tumors, some investigations have indicated a possible cofactor in the form of tumor suppressor loss on 1p. LOH from this region is observed in the majority of pheochromocytomas from patients with MEN 2 and in a much smaller number of MTCs from MEN 2 patients *(31,58)*, raising the possibility that loss from 1p is a required cofactor for the expression of pheochromocytoma in MEN 2 patients. Alternatively, the *RET* oncogene mutation may lead to a generalized increase in chromosomal instability, similar to that suggested for MEN 1. The resultant increase in chromosomal breakage may occur preferentially at predisposed sites and selectively inactivate additional tumor suppressor loci. Further studies are necessary to clarify this issue.

Regardless of potential cofactors, identification of *RET* mutations as the most likely primary cause of MEN 2 has enabled the development of highly accurate presymptomatic genetic screening, which is further facilitated by the extremely frequent involvement of a small number of codons. This allows cost-effective and highly accurate identification of presymptomatic carriers, who can be offered prophylactic thyroidectomy. Thus, the development of MTC, the major cause of mortality in this disorder, can be avoided *(124)*. Furthermore, there is reason to screen patients with sporadic MTC for *RET* mutations, because a significant percentage of patients (20%) have new germline mutations. The offspring of such patients are at risk for MEN 2A or FMTC. The improved understanding of MEN 2 represents the most significant practical achievement of molecular genetic techniques in human endocrine neoplasms thus far, and is a model for the potential clinical benefits which may be gained by application of molecular genetics.

Conclusion and Future Outlook

Cytogenetic and molecular genetic techniques have begun to unravel the process of tumorigenesis in many endocrine neoplasms. Because of the relative rarity of these tumors, few studies have led to the development of reliable diagnostic and prognostic markers. However, the MEN syndromes demonstrate the potential clinical value of cytogenetic and molecular genetic approaches to endocrine neoplasia. In addition, studies of thyroid epithelial tumors suggest viable hypotheses of thyroid tumorigenesis, and have potential for identification of diagnostic markers, that could improve preoperative diagnosis and prognostic staging.

Further advances in the understanding of the genetic basis of endocrine tumors may rely on development of new, accurate, and relatively rapid genetic screening techniques, capable of detecting most chromosomal deletions, rearrangements and amplifications. Comparative genomic hybridization is one such technique, evolved from cytogenetic methods, and particularly FISH, which should see increased application in endocrine tumors in the future. The technique is capable of detecting most large genomic deletions (>12 Mb) and nearly all genomic amplifications *(125)*. Other recent techniques, such as representational difference analysis (RDA) *(126)*, also have potential for expediting the laborious process of detailed LOH and linkage analysis *(127,128)*. RDA is also useful in detecting oncogenic viral genome sequences *(129)*, and is likely to be an important tool in molecular genetic analyses. Finally, specific pools of DNA sequences corresponding to both abnormal or normal chromosomes can be used as probes in FISH experiments to reveal sites of chromosomal rearrangements *(130)*. The coming years will show an impact of these newer techniques on the genetic analysis of endocrine tumors.

Acknowledgments

Stefan Grebe's work on this chapter was undertaken during the tenure of a Research Training Fellowship awarded by the International Agency for Research on Cancer.

References

1. Teyssier JR. The chromosomal analysis of human solid tumors. A triple challenge. Cancer Genet Cytogenet 37:103–125, 1989.
2. Arnold A. Parathyroid adenomas: clonality in benign neoplasia. In: Cossman, J. (ed.), Molecular Gentics in Cancer Diagnosis. New York: Elsevier: pp. 398–408, 1990.
3. Arnold A, Kim HG: Clonal loss of one chromosome 11 in a parathyroid adenoma. J Clin Endocrinol Metabol 69:496–499, 1989.
4. Arnold A, Kim HG, Gaz RD, Eddy RL, Fukushima Y, Byers M G, Shows TB: Molecular cloning and chromosomal mapping of DNA rearranged with the parathyroid hormone gene in a parathyroid adenoma. J Clin Invest 83:2034–2040, 1989.

5. Friedman E, De Marco L, Gejman PV, Norton JA, Bale AE, Aurbach GD, Marx SJ: Allelic loss from chromosome 11 in parathyroid tumors. Cancer Res 52:6804–6809, 1992.

6. Caruso DR, O'Dorisio TM, Mazzaferri EL: Multiple endocrine neoplasia. Curr Opin Oncol 3:103–108, 1991.

7. Larsson C, Nordenskjold M: Multiple endocrine neoplasia. Cancer Surv 9:703–723, 1990.

8. Larsson C, Nordenskjold M: Family screening in multiple endocrine neoplasia type 1 (MEN 1). Ann Medicine 26:191–198, 1994.

9. Bystrom C, Larsson C, Blomberg C, Sandelin K, Falkmer U, Skogseid B, Werner S, Nordenskjold M: Localization of the MEN1 gene to a small region within chromosome 11q13 by deletion mapping in tumors. Proc Natl Acad Sci USA 87:1968–1972, 1990.

10. Brandi ML: Parathyroid tumor biology in familial multiple endocrine neoplasia type 1: a model for cancer development. Henry Ford Hosp Med J 40:181–185, 1992.

11. Radford DM, Ashley SW, Wells SA Jr, Gerhard DS: Loss of heterozygosity of markers on chromosome 11 in tumors from patients with multiple endocrine neoplasia syndrome type 1. Cancer Res 50:6529–6533, 1990.

12. Nakamura Y, Larsson C, Julier C, Bystrom C, Skogseid B, Wells S, Carlson M, Taggart T, O'Connell P: Localization of the genetic defect in multiple endocrine neoplasia type 1 within a small region of chromosome 11. Am J Hum Genet 44:751–755, 1989.

13. Szabo J, Heath B, Hill VM, Jackson CE, Zarbo RJ, Mallette LE, Chew SL, Besser GM, Thakker RV, Huff V: Hereditary hyperparathyroidism—jaw tumor syndrome: the endocrine tumor gene HRPT2 maps to chromosome 1q21–q31. Am J Hum Genet 56:944–950, 1995.

14. Motokura T, Bloom T, Kim HG, Juppner H, Ruderman JV, Kronenberg HM, Arnold A: A novel cyclin encoded by a bcl1-linked candidate onco-gene. Nature 350:512–515, 1991.

15. Zukerberg LR, Yang WI, Gadd M, Thor AD, Koerner FC, Schmidt EV, Arnold A: Cyclin D1 (PRAD1) protein expression in breast cancer—approximately one-third of infiltrating mammary carcinomas show overex-pression of the cyclin D1 oncogene. Modern Pathol 8:560–567, 1995.

16. Henry I, Grandjouan S, Coullin P, Barnchard F, Huerre-Jeanpierre G, Glaser T, Lenoir G, Chaussain JL, Junien C: Tumor-specific loss of 11p15.5 alleles in del11p13 Wilms tumor and familial adrenocortical carcinoma. Proc Natl Acad Sci USA 86:3247–3251, 1989.

17. Byrne JA, Simms LA, Little MH, Algar EM, Smith PJ: Three non-overlap-ping regions of chromosome arm 11p allele loss identified in infantile tumors of adrenal and liver. Genes Chromosome Cancer 8:104–111, 1993.

18. Beckers A, Abs R, Willems PJ, van der Auwera B, Kovacs K, Reznik M: Aldosterone-secreting adrenal adenoma as part of multiple endocrine neo-plasia type 1 (MEN1): loss of heterozygosity for polymorphic chromosome

11 deoxyribonucleic acid markers, including the MEN1 locus. J Clin Endocrinol Metabol 75:564–570, 1992.

19. Iida A, Blake K, Tunny T, Klemm S, Stowasser M, Hayward N, Gordon R, Imai T: Allelic losses on chromosome band 11q13 in aldosterone-producing adrenal tumors. Genes Chromosome Cancer 12:73–75, 1995.

20. Malkin D: p53 and the Li-Fraumeni syndrome. Biochem Biophys Acta 1198:197–213, 1994.

21. Malkin D: p53 and the Li-Fraumeni syndrome. Cancer Genet Cytogenet 66:83–92, 1993.

22. Ohgaki H, Kleihues P, Heitz PU: p53 mutations in sporadic adrenocortical tumors. Intl J Cancer 54:408–410, 1993.

23. Chang F, Syrjanen S, Syrjanen K: Implications of the p53 tumor-suppressor gene in clinical oncology. J Clin Oncol 13:1009–1022, 1995.

24. Lane DP: p53 and human cancers. Br Med Bull 50:582–599, 1994.

25. Levine AJ, Perry ME, Chang A, Silver A, Dittmer D, Wu M, Welsh D: The 1993 Walter Hubert Lecture: the role of the p53 tumour-suppressor gene in tumorigenesis. Br J Cancer 69:409–416, 1994.

26. Latif F, Tory K, Gnarra J, Yao M, Duh F-M, Orcutt ML, Stackhous T, Kuzmin I, Modi W, Geil L, Schmidt L, Zhou F, Li H, Wei MH, Chen F, Glenn G, Choyke P, Walther MM, Weng Y, Duan DSR, Dean M, Glavac D, Richards FM, Crossey PA, Ferguson-Smith MA, Le Paslier D, Chumakov I, Cohen D, Chinault AC, Maher ER, Linehan WM, Zbar B, Lerman MI: Identification of the von Hippel-Lindau disease tumor suppressor gene. Science 260:1317–1320, 1993.

27. Kibel A, Iliopoulos O, Decaprio JA, Kaelin WG: Binding of the VonHippel-Lindau tumor suppressor protein to elongin B and C. Science 269:1444–1446, 1995.

28. Krumm A, Meulia T, Groudine M: Common mechanisms for the control of eukaryotic transcriptional elongation. Bioessays 15:659–665, 1993.

29. Frischauf AM: Positional cloning uncovers a new old oncogene. Human Mol Genet 2:847, 848, 1993.

30. Moley JF, Brother MB, Fong CT, White PS, Baylin SB, Nelkin B, Wells SA, Brodeur GM: Consistent association of 1p loss of heterozygosity with pheochromocytomas from patients with multiple endocrine neoplasia type 2 syndromes. Cancer Res 52:770–774, 1992.

31. Yang KP, Nguyen CV, Castillo SG, Samaan NA: Deletion mapping on the distal third region of chromosome 1p in multiple endocrine neoplasia type IIA. Anticancer Res 10:527–533, 1990.

32. Khosla S, Patel VM, Hay ID, Schaid DJ, Grant CS, van Heerden JA, Thibodeau SN: Loss of heterocygosity suggests mulitple genetic alterations in phaeochromocytoma and medullary thyroid carcinomas. J Clin Invest 87:1691–1699, 1991.

33. Butler MG, Rames LJ, Joseph GM: Cytogenetic studies of individuals from four kindreds with multiple endocrine neoplasia type II syndrome. Cancer Genet Cytogenet 28:253–260, 1987.

34. Zatterale A, Stabile M, Nunziata V, Di Giovanni G, Vecchione R: Multiple endocrine neoplasia type 2 (Sipple's syndrome): clinical and cytogenetic analysis of a kindred. J Med Genet 21:108–111, 1984.

35. Babu VR, van Dyke DL, Jackson CE: Chromosome 20 deletions in human endocrine neoplasia types 2A and 2B: a double blind study. Proc Natl Acad Sci USA 81:2525–2528, 1984.

36. Tanaka N, Nishisho I, Yamamoto M, Miya A, Shin E, Karakawa K, Fujita S, Kobayashi T, Rouleau GA, Mori T: Loss of heterozygosity on the long arm of chromosome 22 in pheochromocytoma. Genes Chromosome Cancer 5:399–403, 1992.

37. Van Dekken H, Bosman FT, Teijgeman R, Vissers CJ, Tersteeg TA, Vooijs GP, Verhofstad AA: Identification of numerical chromosome aberrations in archival tumours by in situ hybridization to routine paraffin sections: evaluation of 23 phaeochromocytomas. J Pathol 171:161–171, 1993.

38. Klein FA, Kay S, Ratliss JE, White FKH, Newsome HH: Flow cytometric determinations of ploidy and proliferation patterns of adrenal neoplasms: an adjunct to histological classification. J Urol 134:862–866, 1985.

39. Hosaka Y, Rainwater LM, Grant CS, Farrow GM, van Heerden JA, Lieber MM: Phaeochromocytoma: nuclear deoxyribunucleic acid patterns studied by flow cytometry. Surgery 100:1003–1008, 1986.

40. Amberson JB, Vaughan ED, Gray CF, Naus GJ: Flow cytometric determination of nuclear DNA content in benign adrenal phaeochromocytomas. Urology 30:102–104, 1987.

41. Nativ O, Grant CS, Sheps SG, O'Fallon JR, Farrow GM, van Heerden JA, Lieber MM: The clinical significance of nuclear DNA ploidy pattern in 184 patients with phaeochromocytoma. Cancer 69:2683–2687, 1992.

42. Martinez AJ: The pathology of non-functional pituitary adenomas. Pathol Res Practice 183:613–616, 1988.

43. Kovacs K, Horvath E: Pathology of pituitary tumors. Endocrinol Metabol Clin North Am 16:529–551, 1987.

44. Mark J: Two benign intracranial tumors with an abnormal chromosomal picture. Acta Neuropathol 14:174–184, 1969.

45. Anniko M, Holm LE, Tribukait B, Wersall J: Aneuploid DNA pattern in human pituitary adenomas. Arch Oto Rhino Laryngol 230:1–4, 1981.

46. Anniko M, Holm LE, Wersall J: Aggressive pitutitary tumor growth. Arch Oto Rhino Laryngol 238:53–62, 1983.

47. Rey JA, Bello MJ, de Campos JM, Kusak ME, Martinez-Castro P, Benitez J: A case of pituitary adenoma with 58 chromosomes. Cancer Genet Cytogenet 23:171–174, 1986.

48. Dietrich CU, Pandis N, Bjerre P, Schroder HD, Heim S: Simple numerical chromosome aberrations in two pituitary adenomas. Cancer Genet Cytogenet 69:118–121, 1993.

49. Capra E, Rindi G, Santi G, Spina MP, Scappaticci S: Chromosome abnormalities in a case of pituitary adenoma. Cancer Genet Cytogenet 68: 140–142, 1993.

50. Rock JP, Babu VR, Drumheller T, Chason J: Cytogenetic findings in pituitary adenoma: results of a pilot study. Surg Neurol 40:224–229, 1993.
51. Boggild MD, Jenkinson S, Pistorello M, Boscaro M, Scanarini M, Perrett CW, Thakker RV, Clayton RN: Molecular genetic studies of sporadic pituitary tumors. J Clin Endocrinol Metabol 78:387–392, 1994.
52. Yoshimoto K, Iwahana H, Kubo K, Saito S, Itakura M: Allele loss on chromosome 11 in a pituitary tumor from a patient with multiple endocrine neoplasia type 1. Jpn J Cancer Res 82:886–889, 1991.
53. Thakker RV, Pook MA, Wooding C, Boscaro M, Scanarini M, Clayton RN: Association of somatotrophinomas with loss of alleles on chromosome 11 and with gsp mutations. J Clin Invest 91:2815–2821, 1993.
54. Spada A, Vallar L, Faglia G: Cellular alterations in pituitary tumors. Eur J Endocrinol 130:43–52, 1994.
55. Narod SA, Sobol H, Nakamura Y, Calmettes C, Baulieu JL, Bigorgne JC, Couette J, de Gennes JL, Duprey J: Linkage analysis of hereditary thyroid carcinoma with and without pheochromocytoma. Hum Genet 83:353–358, 1989.
56. Ledger GA, Khosla S, Lindor NM, Thibodeau SN, Gharib H: Genetic testing in the diagnosis and management of multiple endocrine neoplasia type II. Ann Int Med 122:118–124, 1995.
57. Kubo K, Yoshimoto K, Yokogoshi Y, Tsuyuguchi M, Saito S: Loss of heterozygosity on chromosome 1p in thyroid adenoma and medullary carcinoma, but not in papillary carcinoma. Jpn J Cancer Res 82:1097–1103, 1991.
58. Mathew CG, Smith BA, Thorpe K, Wong Z, Royle NJ, Jeffreys AJ, Ponder BA: Deletion of genes on chromosome 1 in endocrine neoplasia. Nature 328:524–526, 1987.
59. Samaan NA, Yang KP, Schultz P, Hickey RC: Diagnosis, management, and pathogenetic studies in medullary thyroid carcinoma syndrome. Henry Ford Hosp Med J 37:132–137, 1989.
60. Takai S, Tateishi H, Nishisho I, Miki T, Motomura K, Miyauchi A, Ikeuchi T, Yamamoto K, Okazaki M: Loss of genes on chromosome 22 in medullary thyroid carcinoma and pheochromocytoma. Jpn J Cancer Res 78:894–898, 1987.
61. Wurster-Hill DH, Noll WW, Bircher LY, Devlin J, Schultz E: A cytogenetic study of familial medullary carcinoma of the thyroid. Cancer Res 46:2134–2138, 1986.
62. Cooley LD, Elder FFB, Knuth A, Gagel RF: Cytogenetic characterization of three human and three rat medullary thyroid carcinoma cell lines. Cancer Genet Cytogenet 80:138–149, 1995.
63. Le Coniat M, Vecchione D, Pacot A, Bernheim A, Berger R, Gardet P: Cytogenetic studies on patients with medullary carcinoma of the thyroid. Cancer Genet Cytogenet 25:303–307, 1987.
64. Hay ID: Cytometric DNA ploidy analysis in thyroid cancer. Diagn Oncol 1:181–185, 1991.

65. Teyssier JR, Liautaud-Roger F, Ferre D, Patey M, Dufer J: Chromosomal changes in thyroid tumors. Relation with DNA content, karyotypic features, and clinical data. Cancer Genet Cytogenet 50:249–263, 1990.

66. Roque L, Gomes P, Correia C, Soares P, Soares J, Castedo S: Thyroid nodular hyperplasia: chromosomal studies in 14 cases. Cancer Genet Cytogenet 69:31–34, 1993.

67. Belge G, Thode B, Bullerdiek J, Bartnitzke S: Aberrations of chromosome 19. Do they characterize a subtype of benign thyroid adenomas? Cancer Genet Cytogenet 60:23–26, 1992.

68. Bondeson L, Bengtsson A, Bondeson AG, Dahlenfors R, Grimelius L, Mark J: Chromosome studies in thyroid neoplasia. Cancer 64:680–685, 1989.

69. Herrmann MA, Hay ID, Bartelt DH, Jr., Ritland SR, Dahl RJ, Grant CS, Jenkins RB: Cytogenetic and molecular genetic studies of follicular and papillary thyroid cancers. J Clin Invest 88:1596–1604, 1991.

70. Taruscio D, Carcangiu ML, Ried T, Ward DC: Numerical chromosomal aberrations in thyroid tumors detected by double fluorescence in situ hybridization. Genes Chromosome Cancer 9:180–185, 1994.

71. Bartnitzke S, Herrmann ME, Lobeck H, Zuschneid W, Neuhaus P: Cytogenetic findings on eight follicular thyroid adenomas including one with a t(10;19). Cancer Genet Cytogenetics 39:65–68, 1989.

72. Roque L, Castedo S, Gomes P, Soares P, Clode A, Soares J: Cytogenetic findings in 18 follicular thyroid adenomas. Cancer Genet Cytogenet 67:1–6, 1993.

73. Sozzi G, Miozzo M, Cariani TC, Bongarzone I, Pilotti S, Pierotti MA: A t(2;3)(q12–13;p24–25) in follicular thyroid adenomas. Cancer Genet Cytogenet 64:38–41, 1992.

74. Herrmann MA, Hay ID, Bartelt DH Jr, Spurbeck JL, Dahl RJ, Grant CS: Cytogenetics of six follicular thyroid adenomas including a case report of an oxyphil variant with t(8;14)(q13;q24.1). Cancer Genet Cytogenet 56:231–235, 1991.

75. Johansson B, Heim S, Mandahl N, Mertens F, Mitelman F: Trisomy 7 in nonneoplastic cells. Genes Chromosome Cancer 6:199–205, 1993.

76. Belge G, Thode B, Bullerdiek J, Bartnitzke S: Deletion of part of the long arm of chromosome 13 as the only karyotypic aberration in a follicular thyroid adenoma. Cancer Genet Cytogenet 56:277–280, 1991.

77. Olah E, Balogh E, Bojan F, Juhasz F, Stenszky V, Farid NR: Cytogenetic analyses of three papillary carcinomas and a follicular adenoma of the thyroid. Cancer Genet Cytogenet 44:119–129, 1990.

78. Roque L, Castedo S, Clode A, Soares J: Translocation t(5;19): a recurrent change in thyroid follicular adenoma. Genes Chromsome Cancer 4:346, 347, 1992.

79. Dal Cin P, Sneyers W, Aly MS, Segers A, Ostijn F, Van Damme B, VanDen Berghe H: Involvement of 19q13 in follicular thyroid adenoma. Cancer Genet Cytogenet 60:99–101, 1992.

80. Matsuo K, Tang SH, Fagin JA: Allelotype of human thyroid tumors: loss of chromosome 11q13 sequences in follicular neoplasms. Mol Endocrinol 5:1873–1879, 1991.

81. Boland CR: The biology of colorectal cancer. Implications for pretreatment and follow-up management. Cancer 71:4180–4186, 1993.

82. Jenkins RB, Hay ID, Herath JF, Schultz CG, Spurbeck JL, Grant CS, Dewald GW: Frequent occurrence of cytogenetic abnormalities in sporadic nonmedullary thyroid carcinoma. Cancer 66:1213–1220, 1990.

83. Roque L, Castedo S, Clode A, Soares J: Deletion of 3p25→pter in a primary follicular thyroid carcinoma and its metastasis. Genes Chromosome Cancer 8:199–203, 1993.

84. Gazdar AF: The molecular and cellular basis of human lung cancer. Anticancer Res 14:261–267, 1994.

85. Kratzke RA, Shimizu E, Kaye FJ: Oncogenes in human lung cancer. Cancer Treat Res 63:61–85, 1992.

86. Kovacs G: Molecular differential pathology of renal cell tumours. Histopathology 22:1–8, 1993.

87. Sekido Y, Bader S, Latif F, Gnarra JR, Gazdar AF, Linehan WM, Zbar B, Lerman MI, Minna JD: Molecular analysis of the von Hippel-Lindau disease tumor suppressor gene in human lung cancer cell lines. Oncogene 9:1599–1604, 1994.

88. Minna JD: The molecular biology of lung cancer pathogenesis. Chest 103:449S–456S, 1993.

89. Foster K, Prowse A, van den Berg A, Fleming S, Hulsbeek MM, Crossey PA, Richards FM, Cairns P, Affara NA, Ferguson-Smith MA, et al.: Somatic mutations of the von Hippel-Lindau disease tumour suppressor gene in nonfamilial clear cell renal carcinoma. Human Mol Genet 3:2169–2173, 1994.

90. Gnarra JR, Lerman MI, Zbar B, Linehan WM: Genetics of renal-cell carcinoma and evidence for a critical role for von Hippel-Lindau in renal tumorigenesis. Semin Oncol 22:3–8, 1995.

91. Farid NR, Shi Y, Zou M: Molecular basis of thyroid cancer. Endocrine Rev 15:202–232, 1994.

92. Rosai J, Carcangiu ML, DeLellis RA: Atlas of Tumor Pathology. Tumors of the Thyroid Gland. Washington, DC: Armed Forces Institute of Pathology.

93. Antonini P, Venuat AM, Caillou B, Berger R, Schlumberger M, Bernheim A, Parmentier C: Cytogenetic studies on 19 papillary thyroid carcinomas. Genes Chromosome Cancer 5:206–211, 1992.

94. Herrmann ME, Talpos GB, Mohamed AN, Saxe A, Ratner S, Lalley PA, Wolwan SR: Genetic markers in thyroid tumors. Surgery 110: 941–947 1991.

95. Sozzi G, Bongarzone I, Miozzo M, Cariani CT, Mondellini P, Calderone C, Pilotti S, Pierotti MA, Della Porta G: Cytogenetic and molecular genetic characterization of papillary thyroid carcinomas. Genes Chromosome Cancer 5:212–218, 1992.

96. Pierotti MA, Santoro M, Jenkins RB, Sozzi G, Bongarzone I, Grieco M, Monzini N, Miozzo M, Herrmann MA, Fusco A, Hay ID, Della Porta G, Vecchio G: Characterization of an inversion on the long arm of chromo-

some 10 juxtaposing D10S170 and ret and creating the oncogenic sequence ret/ptc. Proc Natl Acad Sci USA 89:1616–1620, 1992.

97. Bongarzone I, Butti MG, Coronelli S, Borrello MG, Santoro M, Pilotti S, Fusco A, Della Porta G, Pierotti MA: Frequent activation of ret protoonco-gene by fusion with a new activating gene in papillary thyroid carcinomas. Cancer Res 54:2979–2985, 1994.

98. Grieco M, Cerrato A, Santoro M, Fusco A, Melillo RM, Vecchio G: Cloning and characterization of H4 (D10S170), a gene involved in RET rearrange-ments in vivo. Oncogene 9:2531–2535, 1994.

99. Tong Q, Li YS, Smanik PA, Fithian LJ, Xing SH, Mazzaferri EL, Jhiang SM: Characterization of the promoter region and oligomerization domain of H4 (D10S170), a gene frequently rearranged with the ret proto-oncogene. Oncogene 10:1781–1787, 1995.

100. Sozzi G, Bongarzone I, Miozzo M, Borrello MG, Blutti MG, Pilotti S, Pierotti MA: A t(10;17) translocation creates the RET/PTC2 chimeric trans-forming sequence in papillary thyroid carcinoma. Genes Chromosome Cancer 9:244–250, 1994.

101. Amorosi A, Cicchi P, Tonelli F, Falchetti A, Bandini S, Tanini A, Brandi ML: Multiple endocrine neoplasia type 1: a model for the analysis of tumor clonality and its biological significance. Serono Symp 83:89–98, 1991.

102. Minoletti F, Butti MG, Coronelli S, Miozzo M, Sozzi G, Pilotti S, Tunnacliffe A, Pierotti MA, Bongarzone I: The two genes generating RET/PTC3 are localized in chromosomal band 10q11.2. Genes Chromsome Cancer 11:51–57, 1994.

103. Viglietto G, Chiappetta G, Martineztello FJ, Fukunaga FH, Tallini G, Rigopoulou D, Visconti R, Mastro A, Santoro M, Fusco A: RET/PTC oncogene activation is an early event in thyroid carcinogenesis. Oncogene 11:1207–1210, 1995.

104. Santoro M, Carlomagno F, Hay ID, Herrmann MA, Grieco M, Melillo R, Pierotti MA, Bongarzone I, Della Porta G, Berger N, Peix JL, Paulin C, Fabien N, Jenkins RB, Fusco A: A *RET* oncogene activation in human thy-roid neoplasms is restricted to the papillary cancer subtype. J Clin Invest 89:1517–1522, 1992.

105. Nikiforov Y, Gnepp DR: Pediatric thyroid cancer after the Chernobyl disas-ter. Pathomorphologic study of 84 cases (1991–1992) from the Republic of Belarus. Cancer 74:748–766, 1994.

106. Ito T, Seyama T, Iwamoto KS, Hayashi T, Mizuno T, Tsuyama N, Dohi K, Nakamura N, Akiyama M: In vitro irradiation is able to cause RET onco-gene rearrangement. Cancer Res 53:2940–2943, 1993.

107. Ito T, Seyama T, Iwamoto KS, Mizuno T, Tronko ND, Komissarenko IV, Cherstovoy ED, Satow Y, Takeichi N, Dohi K, et al.: Activated RET onco-gene in thyroid cancers of children from areas contaminated by Chernobyl accident. Lancet 344:259, 1994.

108. Fugazzola L, Pilotti S, Pinchera A, Vorontsova TV, Mondellini P, Bongarzone I, Greco A, Astakhova L, Butti MG, Demidchik EP, Pacini F, Pierotti MA: Oncogenic rearrangement of the *RET* proto-oncogene in

papillary thyroid carcinomas from children exposed to the Chernobyl nuclear accident. Cancer Res 55:5617–5620, 1995.

109. DeLellis RA: Biology of disease. Multiple endocrine neoplasia syndromes revisited: clinical, morphologic and molecular features. Lab Invest 72:494–505, 1995.

110. Ponder BA: The gene causing multiple endocrine neoplasia type 2 (MEN 2). Ann Med 26:199–203, 1994.

111. Larsson C, Skogseid B, Oberg K, Nakamura Y, Nordenskjold M: Multiple endocrine neoplasia type 1 gene maps to chromosome 11 and is lost in insulinoma. Nature 332:85–87, 1988.

112. Friedman E, DeMarco L, Bale AE, Aurbach GD, Spiegel AM, Marx SJ: Allelic loss in parathyroid tumors: localizing the meni gene to a small region on 11q13. Serono Symp 83:69–76, 1991.

113. Skogseid B, Larsson C, Oberg K: Genetic and clinical characteristics of multiple endocrine neoplasia type 1. Acta Oncologica 30:485–488, 1991.

114. Thakker RV: The role of molecular genetics in screening for multiple endocrine neoplasia type 1. Endocrinol Metabol Clin North Am 23: 117–135, 1994.

115. Scappaticci S, Maraschio P, del Ciotto N, Fossati GS, Zonta AF: Chromosome abnormalities in lymphocytes and fibroblasts of subjects with multiple endocrine neoplasia type 1. Cancer Genet Cytogenet 52:85–92, 1991.

116. Hecht F, Hecht BK: Unstable chromosomes in heritable tumor syndromes. Multiple endocrine neoplasia type 1 (MEN1). Cancer Genet Cytogenet 52:131–134, 1991.

117. Scappaticci S, Brandi ML, Capra E, Cortinovis M, Maraschio PF: Cytogenetics of multiple endocrine neoplasia syndrome. II. Chromosome abnormalities in an insulinoma and a glucagonoma from two subjects with MEN1. Cancer Genet Cytogenet 63:17–21, 1992.

118. Emmertsen K, Lamm LU, Rasmussen KZ, Elbrond O, Hansen HH, Henningsen K, Jorgensen J, Petersen GB: Linkage and chromosome study of multiple endocrine neoplasia IIa. Cancer Genet Cytogenet 9:251–259, 1983.

119. Simpson NE, Kidd KK, Goodfellow PJ, McDermid H, Myers S, Kidd JRJ, Duncan AM, Farrer LA, Brasch K, et al.: Assignment of multiple endocrine neoplasia type 2A to chromosome 10 by linkage. Nature 328:528–530, 1987.

120. Mathew CG, Chin KS, Easton DF, Thorpe K, Carter C, Liou GI, Fong SL, Haak H, Kruseman AC, et al.: A linked genetic marker for multiple endocrine neoplasia type 2A on chromosome 10. Nature 328:527–528, 1987.

121. Lichter JB, Wu J, Miller D, Goodfellow PJ, Kidd KK: A high-resolution meiotic mapping panel for the pericentromeric region of chromosome 10. Genomics 13:607–612, 1992.

122. Nelkin BD, Nakamura Y, White RW, de Bustros AC, Herman J, Wells SAJ, Baylin SB: Low incidence of loss of chromosome 10 in sporadic and hereditary human medullary thyroid carcinoma. Cancer Res 49:4114–4119, 1989.

123. Okazaki M, Miya A, Tanaka N, Miki T, Yamamoto M, Motomura KM, Mori T, Takai S: Allele loss on chromosome 10 and point mutation of ras oncogenes are infrequent in tumors of MEN 2A. Henry Ford Hosp Med J 37:112–115, 1989.

124. Wells SA, Chi DD, Toshima K, Dehner LP, Coffin CM, Dowton B, Ivanovich JL, DeBenedetti MK, Dilley WG, Moley JF, Norton JA, Donis-Keller H: Predictive DNA testing and prohylactic thyroidectomy in patients at tisk for multiple endocrine neoplasia type 2A. Ann Surg 220:237–250, 1994.

125. Houldsworth J, Chaganti RS: Comparative genomic hybridization: an overview. Am J Pathol 145:1253–1260, 1994.

126. Lisitsyn N, Lisitsyn N, Wigler M: Cloning the differences between two complex genomes. Science 259:946–951, 1993.

127. Lisitsyn NA, Lisitsina NM, Dalbagni G, Barker P, Sanchez CA, Gnarra J, Linehan WM, Reid BJ, Wigler MH: Comparative genomic analysis of tumors: detection of DNA losses and amplification. Proc Natl Acad Sci USA 92:151–155, 1995.

128. Lisitsyn NA, Segre JA, Kusumi K, Lisitsyn NM, Nadeau JH, Frankel WN, Lander ES: Direct isolation of polymorphic markers linked to a trait by genetically directed representational difference analysis. Nature Genet 6:57–63, 1994.

129. Chang Y, Cesarman E, Pessin MS, Lee F, Culpepper J, Knowles DM: Identification of herpesvirus-like DNA sequences in AIDS-associated Kaposi's sarcoma. Science 266:1865–1869, 1994.

130. Telenius H, Pelmear AH, Tunnacliffe A, Carter NP, Behmel A, Nordenskjold M, Pfragner R, Ponder BA: Cytogenetic analysis by chromosome painting using DOP-PCR amplified flow-sorted chromosomes. Genes Chromosome Cancer 4:257–263, 1992.

Chapter 15

Pancreatic Exocrine Tumors

Constance A. Griffin

Introduction

The most common tumor arising from the exocrine pancreas is adenocarcinoma. Currently the fifth leading cause of cancer death in the United States *(1)*, the overall 5-yr survival rate for this cancer is <5%. Most tumors occur in the head of the pancreas and symptoms include jaundice, weight loss, and abdominal pain. Patients with localized tumors who undergo resection (pancreaticoduodenectomy) have a 5-yr survival rate approaching 20%; positive prognostic signs include the absence of metastases to lymph nodes, negative resection margins, tumor size <2 cm, absence of blood vessel invasion, and diploid DNA content *(2–6)*. The ability to diagnose accurately an intrabdominal carcinoma as pancreatic in origin by fine needle aspiration and one or several molecular diagnostic tests would be a valuable aid to the clinical managment of this aggressive neoplasm. Similarly, prognosticators that could be determined prior to surgery in patients might allow appropriate decisions to be made regarding which patients are most likely to benefit from aggressive surgery and which from experimental therapy. It is likely that elucidation of genetic changes will provide such information. The goal of this chapter is to review known genetic alterations in pancreatic cancer.

From: *Human Cytogenetic Cancer Markers*   Edited by S. R. Wolman and S. Sell
Humana Press Inc., Totowa, NJ

Pathophysiology

The pancreas consists of an exocrine portion, which secretes fluids necessary for digestion of protein, carbohydrate, and fat, and an endocrine portion, which secretes hormones required for carbohydrate metabolism. Neoplasms arise in both the exocrine and endocrine pancreas, and chromosome abnormalities have been reported in both *(7–11)*. "Carcinoma of the pancreas" refers to carcinoma arising in the exocrine portion, and this chapter will focus on these neoplasms. The exocrine pancreas is made of many small secretory glands aggregated into lobules; the lobules are separated by relatively small amounts of connective tissue stroma. The extensive ductal system in the pancreas is produced by progressive anastomosis of the secretory glands or acini. Carcinoma of the pancreas appears to arise from the ductal epithelium, rather than acini. Most are adenocarcinomas.

A stepwise progression from adenoma through dysplastic adenoma through carcinoma *in situ* to invasive cancer has long been recognized in the genesis of carcinoma of the colon *(12)*. A corresponding genetic multistep model of tumorigenesis has also been proposed based on the observations of mutations in k-ras, p53, and DCC genes *(13)*. Thus it is not surprising that several authors have suggested a similar progression for carcinoma of the pancreas. The morphologic evidence for this is circumstantial, but strongly suggestive *(14,15)*; ductal lesions have been observed that progress from nonpapillary hyperplasia, through papillary hyperplasia, through atypical papillary hyperplasia to invasive cancer *(14–16)*. An example of a normal duct is shown in Fig. 1A, and markedly atypical papillary hyperplasia (clearly separate from invasive adenocarcinoma) is shown in Fig. 1B. Additionally supporting this theory is the morphology of early pancreatic lesions appearing in hamsters treated with dihydroxy-di-n-propyl-nitrosamine (DHPN) to induce pancreatic duct carcinomas. The early lesions resemble the atypical epithelial proliferation in human pancreas *(14)*.

Cytogenetic and molecular genetic studies of adenocarcinoma of the pancreas are complicated by significant proliferation of non-neoplastic reactive stroma and lymphocytes that are interspersed with the neoplastic epithelial cells. We have found that as much as

80% of the gross tumor mass is made up of normal cells. A representative field of a pancreatic carcinoma is shown in Fig. 1C; the ductal carcinoma comprises only a minority of the cells, and the majority of the cells are nonneoplastic stromal cells.

The tumors that have been studied using cytogenetic and molecular genetic methods usually have been obtained from patients who are deemed to have a resectable tumor on clinical evaluation. Fewer than 10% of patients have tumors confined to the pancreas at diagnosis *(17)*, and 40% have locally advanced disease. Potentially curative surgery is a pancreaticoduodenectomy *(5)*, yet tumors are relatively advanced even in patients who are eligible for this procedure, as evidenced by the frequency of local lymph node involvement and perineural invasion discovered on microscopic evaluation.

Aneuploidy

A gross measurement of genetic imbalance in tumors can be obtained by the ascertainment of aneuploidy. Determination of DNA content, by either flow cytometry or absorption photocytometry, is often used to detect aneuploidy. Aneuploidy is associated with a poor prognosis in some tumors, including melanoma, colorectal cancer, and node-negative breast cancer *(18–22)*. Prognosis has also been correlated with tumor DNA content in pancreatic cancer, with a survival advantage for patients whose tumors are diploid over those that are aneuploid *(6,23,24)*. In one study, tetraploidy was also associated with a better outcome than nontetraploid tumors *(23)*.

Determination of Specific Chromosome Abnormalities

Determination of specific chromosome abnormalities can lead to the identification of genes that are directly involved in the neoplastic process. The utility of this approach in directing efforts to the 9q34 and 22q11 regions in chronic myelogenous leukemia and the subsequent identification of involvement of the *ABL* and *BCR* genes, to name merely one classic example, is well known *(25)*. Chromosome analysis may provide similar important leads in the study of pancreas cancer. Because an adequate number of metaphases

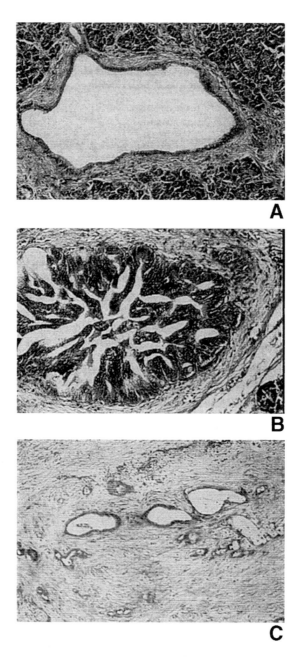

Fig. 1. (**A**) Example of a normal pancreatic duct. (**B**) Example of markedly atypical papillary hyperplasia of a duct from a specimen with invasive adenocarcinoma of the pancreas. (**C**) Representative field of carcinoma of the pancreas from one of our tumors. Carcinoma is present in the ducts: nonneoplastic stromal proliferation comprises the majority of the field.

is required for cytogenetic metaphase analysis, let us consider the culture methods that have been used to study this tumor.

Culture Methods

Despite the sizable infiltration of the tumor mass with nonneoplastic and stromal inflammatory cells, we have found clonal chromosome abnormalities in 44/62 (71%) of primary exocrine pancreatic tumors studied, using short-term culture *(9,10)*. To determine whether use of a complex medium improved the frequency of obtaining clonally abnormal karyotypes, we compared our standard tissue culture medium (RPMI with 16% fetal calf serum, 200 μm L-glutamine, 50 U/mL penicillin and streptomycin, 2.5 μg/mL fungizone) with a medium specifically formulated to support epithelial cell growth *(10)*. The latter included RPMI 1640 with 15% fetal calf serum that was rigorously screened for support of human tumor growth, 200 μm L-glutamine, 50 U/mL penicillin and streptomycin, 20 μg/mL gentamicin, 1% nonessential amino acids, 1% sodium pyruvate, 100 U/mL regular human or porcine insulin, and 1 μg/mL each of insulin-like growth factors I and II. Tumors were manually dissected, then digested with collagenase type II for 2–16 h before being centrifuged and set up in short-term culture in both media. All specimens were harvested as primary cultures at 1–12 d of culture, most within 7 d. The sole determinant of time of harvest was evidence of mitotic activity on phase microscopic monitoring, which was performed daily. Comparisons were made in 30 specimens. In 15 tumors, all cultures regardless of media used contained abnormal metaphases, but up to twice as many metaphases were obtained in the epithelial cell medium. For three tumors, only the epithelial medium cultures yielded clonal chromosome abnormalities. Whereas our comparisons were not performed in a way to allow statistical analyses, there appeared to be a trend suggesting that the use of epithelial medium enhanced the chance of detecting chromosomal abnormalities *(10)*.

The short-term culture methods employed by Johansson et al. *(7)* with 17 successfully cultured exocrine tumors also included exposure to collagenase, followed by culture in RPMI 1640 or Dulbecco's MEM/F12, both with HEPES buffer, supplemented with 5% fetal calf serum, glutamine, penicillin, streptomycin, amphotericin B, and epidermal growth factor. Clonal chromosome abnormalities were detected in nine tumors (53%). In later study reporting 17 additional exocrine tumors, the same workers added hydrocortisone, cholera toxin, dibutyl cyclic AMP, insulin, transferring, selenious acid, bovine serum albumin, and linoleic acid to their basal medium *(8)*. Abnormal karyotypes were obtained in 13 of the 17 (76%) tumors grown in this way.

Summary of Cytogenetic Analyses

Prior to the first reported cytogenetic series of 17 primary tumors in 1992 *(7)*, only a few case reports and cell lines of pancreatic cancer had been studied *(26–34)*. The majority were metastatic tumors. Although clonal karyotypic changes were found, no consistent chromosome abnormalities were identified. In the past 3 yr, a significant number of karyotypic analyses have been reported *(7–10)*, which are summarized here.

We have studied karyotypes from 62 primary adenocarcinomas of the pancreas. All tissue was obtained from patients who were surgically explored at The Johns Hopkins Hospital between September 1991 and January 1994. Patients ranged from 40–88 yr of age. Specimens were cultured and harvested as primary cultures (1–18 d in culture, most within 7 d), and slides were made and examined as described *(9,10)*. Clonal abnormalities were defined and described according to ISCN nomenclature *(35)*. Because only patients eligible for surgical resection were studied, 94% of tumors in our series originated from the head of the pancreas, and 73% were moderately differentiated. Using the staging system of Hermreck et al. *(36)*, 3 were stage I, 11 were stage II, 45 were stage III, and 3 were stage IV.

The modal number ranged from near diploid through near triploid, with occasional near tetraploid tumors. Karyotypes were generally complex (greater than three abnormalities), including both numerical and structural chromosome abnormalities. Many tumors contained at least one, and often several marker (unidentifiable) chromosomes. A representative karyotype is shown in Fig. 2. In our combined series of 44 cases with abnormal karyotypes *(9–10)*, the most frequent whole chromosomal gains were chromosomes 20 (8 tumors) and 7 (7 tumors). Losses were much more frequent: chro-

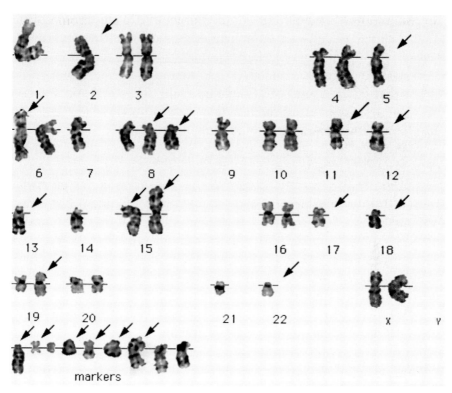

Fig. 2. Representative karyotype from a moderately differentiated adenocarcinoma of the pancreas. Clonal abnormalities (arrows) illustrated in this metaphase include –2, –5, add(6)(q24), del(8)(p13) × 2, –11, –12, –13, add(15)(p11), der(15)t(11;15)(q13;p13), –17, –18, add(19)(q11), –22, +mar1, +mar2, +mar3, +mar4, +mar5, +mar6. (case 31, ref. *10*).

mosome 18 was lost in 22 tumors, followed in frequency by chromosomes 13 (16 tumors), 12 (13 tumors), 17 (13 tumors), and 6 (12 tumors). Deletions of portions of 6q were common, seen in nine chromosomes. Structural abnormalities were frequent. Two hundred nine chromosome breakpoints were identified. Excluding Robertsonian translocations, the chromosomal arms most frequently involved were 1p(12); 6q(11); 7q and 17p (nine each); 3p, 11p, 1q, and 19q (eight each).

Analysis of other series of primary pancreatic adenocarcinomas have been reported by Johansson et al. *(7)* and Bardi et al. *(8)*. In the total of 34 cases they examined, abnormal karyotypes were obtained in 22 tumors. Abnormal but simple karyotypes were observed in 37%. The remainder were complex, with modal numbers including near-diploid, near-triploid, and near-tetraploid tumors. Numerical chromosome changes included –18 (11 tumors), –Y (7 tumors), +20 (8 tumors), +7, +11, and –12 (7 tumors each). Structural abnormalities were frequent, with structural rearrangements of 1p (9 tumors), proximal 1q (8 tumors), and proximal 6q (8 tumors).

The combined data from the 66 reported tumors with abnormal karyotypes *(7–10)* show that chromosomes 7 and 20 are the chromosomes most frequently gained. Whole chromosome losses most frequently involved chromosome 18. Regions of partial chromosome loss are delineated in the ideogram in Fig. 3A; the chromosomal arms most frequently identified with deletions include 1p, 1q, 3p, 6q, 7q, and 8p. The ideogram in Fig. 3B summarizes the location of 307 identified breakpoints involved in structural rearrangments in the same tumors. The combined data show that, excluding translocations involving the centromere region of acrocentric chromosomes, the areas most frequently involved in structural changes are 1p, pericentromeric region of 1, 6q, distal 7p, 8p, pericentromeric region of 9, 17p, and mid 19q. Genes in these regions may be particularly important in the biology of adenocarcinoma of the pancreas.

Correlations of degree of histologic differentiation and karyotype would be of interest, but are limited because of the preponderance of moderately well-differentiated tumors that come to surgery. Nonetheless, the trend is for the highest frequency of abnormal karyotypes in the least differentiated neoplasms. We obtained an abnormal karyotype from 75% of poorly differentiated tumors and 53% of moderate to well-differentiated tumors. Johansson et al. and Bardi et al. *(7,8)* obtained abnormal karyotypes from 90% of poorly differentiated tumors, 50% of moderately differentiated tumors, and 60% of well-differentiated tumors. The frequent presence of normal cells probably accounts for the normal karyotypes in the remainder.

Correlation of Cytogenetic and Molecular Analyses

The standard approach that has been fruitful in other tumors in the search for allelic loss that leads to the identification of tumor suppressor genes has been hampered in pancreas cancer by the significant

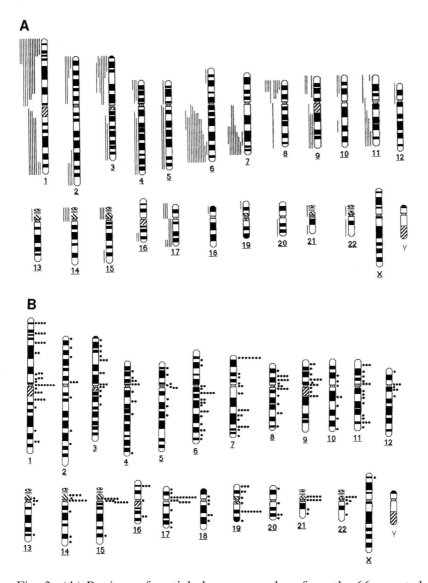

Fig. 3. (**A**) Regions of partial chromosome loss from the 66 reported tumors with abnormal karyotypes (7–10) are delineated in this ideogram. The chromosomal arms most frequently identified with deletions include 1p, 1q, 3p, 6q, 7q, and 8p. (**B**) Summary of the location of 307 identified breakpoints involved in structural rearrangements in the same tumors. The combined data show that, excluding translocations involving the centromere region of acrocentric chromosomes, the areas most frequently involved in structural changes are 1p, pericentromeric region of 1, 6q, distal 7p, 8p, pericentromeric region of 9, 17p, and mid 19q.

host desmoplastic response described earlier. The first reported allelotype utilized seven tumors enriched for tumor cells by cryostat microdissection and found loss of sequences from 18q and 17p *(37)*. A recently published polymerase chain reaction-based allelotype study of 18 pancreatic cancers used tumor xenografts to enrich for tumor cells; this study utilizing 283 polymorphic markers showed high frequency allelic loss (>60%) involving 1p, 9p, 17p, and 18q, and moderately frequent allelic loss (40–60%) involving 3p, 6p, 6q, 8p, 10q, 12q, 13q, 18p, 21q, and 22q *(38)*. Our cytogenetic data suggest that, for some of these genes, the mechanism of loss of normal alleles may be at the level of the whole chromosome. Loss of expression of the *DCC* gene, which is localized to 18q21, has been reported in adenocarcinoma of the pancreas *(39)*. Chromosome 18 loss was particularly common in both our series and Johansson's and Bardi's series, observed in 33 of the 66 tumors with abnormal karyotypes (50%). *TP53* mutations have been reported in pancreas cancer *(40–42)*. Involvement of 17p in translocations, addition of unidentified material, and loss of an entire copy of chromosome 17 were also common in the karyotypic analyses cited *(7,8)*, again providing cytogenetic evidence suggesting that loss of 17p material may be the mechanism of inactivation of one *TP53* allele. We observed loss of chromosome 13 frequently and a translocation at 13q12 in one tumor. From one tumor with monosomy 13 was found a homozygously deleted region (*DPC*, for deleted in pancreatic carcinoma) at 13q12.3; the *BRCA2* breast cancer susceptibility locus encompasses the entire *DPC* locus *(43–45)*. The specific gene involved in pancreas cancer in the *DPC* region has not yet been isolated.

In contrast, molecular analyses have demonstrated involvement of other genes for which few clues have been derived from cytogenetics. Although not found in all studies *(37)*, somatic mutations have been found in some studies that are predicted to lead to a truncated *APC* gene product in pancreatic cancer *(46,47)*. Nevertheless few instances of 5q involvement in either deletions or translocations were observed in karyotypic analyses. Similarly, the frequent somatic mutations and homozygous deletions of the p16 (*MTS1*) gene and allelic deletions of 9p21–p22 reported in 85% of pancreatic adenocarcinomas *(48)* are not correlated with a high frequency of recognized cytogenetic abnormalities of 9p. The unidentifiable marker chromosomes in many of our karyotypes may well involve at least some of these chromosome regions. Involvement of some relevant genes may also occur only at a submicroscopic level. This seems likely for genes such as *KRAS2*, where mutations have been found in up to 100% of pancreas cancers studied *(49–51)*.

Genetic instability, as measured by replication errors in microsatellite loci, has been found in 6 of 9 tumors *(52)*, and in one of 20 tumors *(38)*, but was not found in 27 other tumors *(37)*. The limited data would suggest that widespread microsatellite instability is not common in pancreas cancer. However, a recently reported cytogenetic analysis of a poorly differentiated carcinoma of the tail of the pancreas revealed 54 near-diploid, karyotypically abnormal, and unrelated clones *(53)*. All chromosomes except chromosome 15 were involved; nearly half of the most common breakpoints in this polyclonal tumor were the same as have been identified in other cases (1q21, 6q21, 7p22, 8p21, 16p13). It is tempting to speculate that the multiple abnormal clones in this case are the end product of a mutation causing genomic instability manifested at the chromosomal level.

Deletions of 6q Verified by Fish

An area of consistent genomic loss particularly indicated by cytogenetic analyses is 6q, and we have used FISH to begin to delineate the region of smallest deletion on 6q. FISH was performed using a biotin-labeled 6q24-qter probe that was made by microdissection *(54)*. The probe was hybridized to metaphases that showed apparent 6q deletions *(10)* using previously described methods *(54,55)*. We analyzed between 16 and 39 metaphases per case with fluorescence *in situ* hybridization (FISH) to determine whether sequences homologous to this probe were indeed lost from the genome or were translocated elsewhere onto marker (unidentifiable) chromosomes. In three of four cases studied, we confirmed that one copy (relative to diploid) of the region 6q24-qter was lost from the genome. A representative metaphase from each case is shown in Fig. 4. That apparent losses in complex karyotypes need to be verified is illustrated by case 24, which appeared by classical cytogenetic analysis to have a del(6)(q22). However, FISH showed that 6q24-qter sequences were retained on an unidentifiable metacentric chromosome (Fig. 4B).

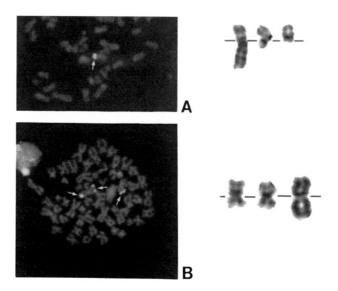

Fig. 4. Summary of analysis of four cases of adenocarcinoma of the pancreas in which the G-banded karyotype appeared to show deletion of the distal portion of 6q. To the left are representative metaphases of FISH using a probe for the region 6q24-qter probe *(9)*. To the right are the normal (if present) and derivative copies of chromosome 6. (**A**) Case 20: FISH showed one signal; karyotyping showed one normal 6, del(6)(q?13) × 2. (**B**) Case 24: FISH showed one signal on a metacentric chromosome that is probably a normal 6, and one signal on either end of a metacentric chromosome which was not identifiable by G-banding; karyotyping showed del(6)(q22) × 2 and a metacentric marker chromosome not otherwise identifiable as a 6.

The apparent deletions of 6q observed in our specimens range from 6q11-qter to 6q23-qter. Deletions encompassing wide areas of 6q, but also translocations involving 6q13, 6q15, and an intersititial deletion involving 6q13–16 were observed by Johansson et al. *(7)* and Bardi et al. *(8)*. The smallest overlapping region of deletion appears to be from 6q24 to q25. Several other lines of evidence suggest the presence of tumor suppressor genes on 6q. Karyotypic evidence of 6q deletions have been reported in ovarian carcinoma, adenocarcinoma of the salivary gland, and in melanoma *(56–58)*. Loss of heterozygosity (LOH) of DNA sequences from 6q have been reported in ovarian carcinoma and melanoma *(59–63)*. The introduction of a normal copy of chromosome 6 into melanoma cell

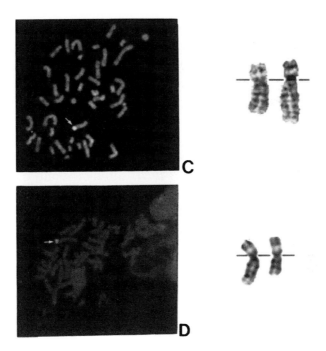

Fig. 4. (*continued*) (**C**) Case 31: FISH showed one signal; karyotyping showed one normal 6 and add(6)(q24). (**D**) Case 34: FISH showed one signal; karyotyping showed one normal 6 and del(6)(q23q25). Reprinted from ref. *10* with permission.

lines via microcell-mediated chromosome transfer resulted in loss of tumorigenicity of those cells when injected into nude mice *(64)*. More than one tumor suppressor gene may be located on 6q, however, as the apparent regions of common deletion in the tumors are large. In salivary tumors the region deleted appears to be 6q25–qter *(65,66)*; in ovarian tumors 6q24–27 *(56–58)*, and in melanoma 6q22–23 and 6q24–27 *(67–69)*.

Double Minute Chromosomes in Pancreas Cancer

Of particular interest, we have found double minute chromosomes (dmin) in 21 of 98 tumors *(9,10, and unpublished)*; they were observed in 31% of those tumors that had abnormal karyotypes. The percentage of cytogenetically abnormal metaphases in which dmin were observed ranged from 16–75/case, and the number of dmin observed ranged from one to four per metaphase. Dmin are one of two cytogenetic manifestations of gene amplification, and, to our knowledge, these tumors represent the first primary adenocarcinomas of the pancreas with such evidence of gene amplification. A representative metaphase from each of three primary specimens in which dms were seen is illustrated in Fig. 5.

Amplification of specific genes has been shown to correlate with poor prognosis in a number of solid tumors including neuroblastoma (*NMYC* amplification) *(70)*, salivary gland carcinomas (*HER2/neu ERBB2*) *(71)*, gastric carcinoma (*C-MET*) *(72)*, and gliomas (*EGFR*) *(73)*. We hypothesize that pancreas cancers also have amplified genes, and that these genes provide a growth advantage to the tumor. Identification of such genes would provide important information about the biology of this particular neoplasm. The protein products of several receptors and oncogenes, measured by immunohistochemistry and/or *in situ* hybridization, have been reported to be elevated in pancreas cancers as compared with normal pancreas acini and ducts. These include epidermal growth factor, epidermal growth factor receptor, transforming growth factor α, *ERBB2*, *ERBB3*, *C-MET*, hepatocyte growth factor and *MET/HGF* receptor *(74–80)*. However, in cases where it has been sought, DNA amplification of these genes has not been found. Whether this is a result of the inability to detect amplification by Southern blotting because of the large number of admixed normal cells in these neoplasms, or because these genes are indeed not amplified, is unknown. We are using chromosome microdissection to determine the areas of the genome that are consistently amplified. Whether the amplified DNA contains a gene or genes that are already known or includes a new gene, identification of such genes may significantly further our understanding of this tumor's biology and provide important prognostic information about this aggressive tumor.

Acknowledgments

The author thanks Patricia Long for expert production of illustrations, Ralph Hruban for materials for Fig. 1, and Elizabeth Boswell for secretarial assistance. This work was supported by RO1-CA-56130, 2P30-CA06973, and 1P50CA62924 from the NCI.

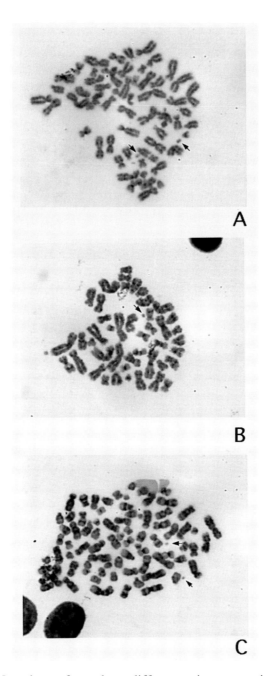

Fig. 5. Metaphases from three different primary specimens of adenocarcinoma of the pancreas in which double minute chromosomes were
seen. All examples shown are from tumors that had visible dmins in multiple metaphases. (**A**) Case 20, (**B**) case 32, and (**C**) case 36. Arrows indicate dmins. Reprinted from ref. *10* with permission.

References

1. Boring CC, Squires TS, Tong T: Cancer Statistics, 1991. Cancer 41: 19–36, 1991.
2. Cameron JL, Crist DW, Sitzmann JV, Hruban RH, Boittnot JK, Seidler AJ, Coleman J: Factors influencing survival after pancreaticoduodenectomy for pancreatic cancer. Am J Surg 161:120–125, 1991.
3. Crist DW, Sitzmann JV, Cameron JL: Improved hospital morbidity, mortality, and survival after the Whipple procedure. Ann Surg 206: 358–365, 1987.
4. Trede M: The surgical treatment of pancreatic carcinoma. Surgery 97: 28–35, 1985.
5. Yeo CJ, Cameron JL, Lillemoe KD, Sitzmann JV, Hruban RH, Goodman SN, Dooley WC, Coleman J, Pitt HA: Pancreaticoduodenectomy for cancer of the head of the pancreas: 201 consecutive cases. Ann Surg, 221:721–731, 1995.
6. Allison DC, Bose KK, Hruban RH, Piantadosi S, Dooley WC, Biotnott JK, Cameron JL. Pancreatic cancer cell DNA content correlates with long-term survival after pancreatoduodenectomy. Ann Surg 214:648–656, 1991.
7. Johansson B, Bardi G, Heim S, Mandahl N, Mertens R, Bak-Jenson E, Andren-Sanberg A, Mitelman F. Non-random chromosomal rearrangements in pancreatic carcinomas. Cancer 69:1674–1681, 1992.
8. Bardi G, Johansson B, Pandis N, Mandahl N, Bak-Jensen E, Andren-Sandberg A, Mitelman F, Heim S: Karyotypic abnormalities in tumours of the pancreas. Br J Cancer 67:1106–1112, 1993.
9. Griffin CA, Hruban RH, Long PP, Morsberger LA, Douna-Issa F, Yeo CJ: Chromosome abnormalities in pancreatic adenocarcinoma. Genes Chromosomes Cancer 9:93–100, 1994.
10. Griffin CA, Hruban RH, Morsberger LA, Ellingham T, Long PP, Jaffee EM, Hauda KM, Bohlander SK, Yeo CJ: Consistent chromosome abnormalities in adenocarcinoma of the pancreas. Cancer Res 55:2394–2399, 1995.
11. Long PP, Hruban RH, Lo R, Yeo CJ, Morsberger LA, Griffin CA: Chromosome analysis of nine endocrine neoplasms of the pancreas. Cancer Genet Cytogenet 77:55–59, 1994.
12. Morson BC: The pathogenesis of Colorectal Cancer. Philadelphia, PA: Saunders, 1978.
13. Vogelstein B, Fearon ER, Hamilton SR, Kern SE, Preisinger AC, Leppert M, Nakamura Y, White R, Smits AMM, Bos JL: Genetic alterations during colorectal-tumor development. New Engl J Med 319:525–532, 1988.
14. Kloppel G, Bommer G, Ruckert K, Seifert G: Intraductal proliferation in the pancreas and its relationship to human and experimental carcinogenesis. Virchows Arch A Path Anat Histol 387:221–233, 1980.
15. Cubilla AL, Fitzgerald PJ: Morphological patterns of primary nonendocrine human pancreas carcinoma. Cancer Res 35:2234–2248, 1975.
16. Chen J, Baithun SI: Histogenesis of pancreatic carcinomas: a study based on 248 cases. J Pathol 146:65–76, 1985.

17. Reber HA, MD, Ashley SW, MD, McFadden D, MD: Curative Treatment for Pancreatic Neoplasms. Surg Clin North Am 75:905–912, 1995.
18. Armitage NC, Robins RA, Evans DF: The influence of tumour cell DNA abnormalities on survival in colorectal cancer. Br J Surg 72:828–830, 1985.
19. Clark GM, Dressler LG, Owens MA: Prediction of relapse or survival in patients with node-negative breast cancer by DNA flow cytometry. N Engl J Med 320:627–633, 1989.
20. Heimann TM, Miller F, Martinelli G: Significance of DNA contect abnormalities in small rectal cancers. Am J Surg 159:199–203, 1990.
21. Jones DJ, Moore M, Schofield PF: Prognostic significance of DNA ploidy in colorectal cancer: a prospective flow cytometric study. Br J Surg 75:28–33, 1988.
22. Kheir SM, Bines SD, Vonroenn JH: Prognostic significance of DNA aneuploidy in stage 1 cutaneous melanoma. Ann Surg 207:455–461, 1988.
23. Bottger TC, Storkel S, Wellek S, et al.: Factors influencing survival after resection of pancreatic cancer: a DNA analysis and histomorphologic study. Cancer 73:63–73, 1994.
24. Porschen R, Remy U, Bevers G, et al.: Prognostic significance of DNA ploidy in adenocarcinoma of the pancreas. Cancer 71:3846–3851, 1993.
25. Heisterkamp N, Stam K, Groffen J: Structural organization of the bcr gene and its role in the Ph translocation. Nature 315:758–761, 1989.
26. Casalone R, Meriggi F, Forni E, Pasquali F: Cytogenetic findings in a case of anaplastic carcinoma of the pancreas. Cancer Genet Cytogenet 29:253–259, 1987.
27. Teyssier JR: Nonrandom chromosomal changes in human solid tumors: application of an improved culture method. J Natl Cancer Inst 79:1189–1198, 1987.
28. Johansson B, Mandahl N, Heim S, Mertens F, Andren-Sandberg A, Mitelman F: Chromosome abnormalities in a pancreatic adenocarcinoma. Cancer Genet Cytogenet 37:209–213, 1989.
29. Bullerdiek J, Bartnitzke S, Kahrs E, Schloot W: Further evidence for nonrandom chromosome changes in carcinoma cells: a report of 28 cases. Cancer Genet Cytogenet 16:33–43, 1985.
30. Lieber M, Mazzetta J, Nelson-Rees W, Kaplan M, Todaro G: Establishment of a continuous tumor-cell line (PANC-1) from a human carcinoma of the exocrine pancreas. Int J Cancer 15:741–747, 1975.
31. Yunis AA, Arimura GK, Russin DJ: Human pancreatic carcinoma (MIA PaCa-2) in continuous culture: sensitivity to asparaginase. Int J Cancer 19:128–135, 1977.
32. Morgan RT, Woods LK, Moore GE, Quinn LA, McGavran L, Gordon SG: Human cell line (COLO 357) of metastatic pancreatic adenocarcinoma. Int J Cancer 25:591–598, 1980.
33. Korc M, Meltzer P, Trent J: Enhanced expression of epidermal growth factor receptor correlates with alterations of chromosome 7 in human pancreatic cancer. Proc Natl Acad Sci USA 83:5141–5144, 1986.
34. Madahar C, Parsa I: Progression in a chemically induced transplantable human pancreas carcinoma. Int J Pancreat 2:183–194, 1987.

35. Mitelman F. (ed.): ISCN 1991 Guidelines for Cancer Cytogenetics. Basel, Switzerland: Karger, 1991.
36. Hermreck AS, Thomas CY, IV, Friesin SR: Importance of pathologic staging in the surgical management of adenocarcinoma of exocrine pancreas. Am J Surg 127:653–657, 1974.
37. Seymour AB, Hruban RH, Redston M, Caldas C, Powell SM, Kinzler KW, Yeo CJ, Kern SE: Allelotype of Pancreatic Adenocarcinoma. Cancer Res 54:2761–2764, 1994.
38. Hahn SA, Seymour AB, Shamsul Hoque ATM, Schutte M, da Costa LT, Redston MS, Caldas C, Weinstein CL, Fischer A, Yeo CJ, Hruban RH, Kern SE: Allelotype of Pancreatic Andenocarcinoma Using Xenograft Enrichment. Cancer Res 55:4670–4675, 1995.
39. Hoehne MW, Halatsch M-E, Kahl GF, Weinel RJ: Frequent loss of expression of the potential tumor suppressor gene DCC in ductal pancreatic adenocarcinoma. Cancer Res 52:2616–2619, 1992.
40. Barton CM, Staddon SL, Hughes CM, Hall PA, O'Sullivan C, Kloeppel G, Theis B, Russell RCG, Neoptolemos J, Williamson RCN, Lane DP, Lemoine NR: Abnormalities of the p53 tumour suppressor gene in human pancreatic cancer. Br J Cancer 64:1076–1082, 1991.
41. Ruggeri B, Zhang S-Y, Caamano J, DiRado M, Flynn SD, Klein-Szanto, AJP: Human pancreatic carcinomas and cell lines reveal frequent and multiple alterations in the p53 and Rb-1 tumor-suppressor genes. Oncogene 7:1503–1511, 1992.
42. Redston MS, Caldas C, Seymour AB, Hruban RH, da Costa L, Yeo CJ, Kern SE: p53 Mutations in pancreatic carcinoma and evidence of common involvement of homocopolymer tracts in DNA microdeletions. Cancer Res 54:3025–3033, 1994.
43. Schutte M, da Costa LT, Hahn SA, Moskaluk C, Hoque ATMS, Hruban RH, Kern SE: Identification by representational difference analysis of a homozygous deletion in pancreatic carcinoma that lies within the BRCA2 region. Proc Natl Acad Sci USA 92:5950–5954, 1995.
44. Schutte M, Rozenblum E, Moskaluk CA, Guan X, Hoque ATMS, Hahn SA, da Costa LT, de Jong PJ, Kern SE: An integrated high-resolution physical map of the DPC/BRCA2 region at chromosome 13q12[1]. Cancer Res 55:4570–4574, 1995.
45. Wooster R, Neuhausen SL, Mangion J, Quirk Y, Ford D, Collins N, Nguyen K, Seal S, Tran T, Averill D, Fields P, Marshall G, Narod S, Lenoir GM, Lynch H, Feunteun J, Devilee P, Cornelisse CJ, Menko FH, Daly PA, Ormiston W, McManus R, Pye C, Lewis CM, Cannon-Albright LA, Peto J, Ponder BAJ, Skolnick MH, Easton DF, Goldgar DE, Stratton MR: Localization of breast cancer susceptibility gene, BRCA2, to chromosome 13q12–13. Science 265:2088–2090, 1994.
46. Horii A, Nakatsuru S, Miyoshi Y, Ichii S, Nagase H, Ando H, Yanagisawa A, Tsuchiya E, Kato Y, Nakamura Y: Frequent somatic mutations of the *APC* gene in human pancreatic cancer. Cancer Res 52:6696–6698, 1992.

47. Horii A, Nakatsuru S, Miyoshi Y, Ichii S, Nagase H, Kato Y, Yanagisawa A, Nakamura Y: The *APC* gene, responsible for familial adenomatous polyposis, is mutated in human gastric cancer. Cancer Res 52:3231–3233, 1992.

48. Caldas C, Hahn SA, da Costa LT, Redston MS, Schutte M, Seymour AB, Weinstein CL, Hruban RH, Yeo CJ, Kern SE: Frequent somatic mutations and homozygous deletions of the p16 (MTS1) gene in pancreatic adenocarcinoma. Nat Genet 8:27–32, 1994.

49. Hruban RH, van Mansfeld ADM, Offerhaus GJA, van Weering DHJ, Allison DC, Goodman SN, Kensler TW, Bose KK, Cameron JL, Bos JL: K-ras oncogene activation in adenocarcinoma of the human pancreas: a study of 82 carcinomas using a combination of mutant-enriched polymerase chain reaction analysis and allele specific oligonucleotide hybridization. Am J Pathol 143:545–554.

50. Urban T, Ricci S, Grange, JD, Lacave R, Boudghene F, Breittmayer F, Languille O, Roalnd J, Bernaudin JF: Detection of c-Ki-ras mutation by PCR/RFLP analysis and diagnosis of pancreatic adenocarcinomas. J Natl Cancer Inst 85:24, 1993.

51. Bernaudin JF, Urban T, Ricci S: Re: Detection of c-Ki-ras mutation by PCR/RFLP analysis and diagnosis of pancreatic adenocarcinomas. J Natl Cancer Inst 86:17, 1994.

52. Han HJ, Yanagisawa A, Kato Y, Park JG, Nakamura Y: Genetic instability in pancreatic cancer and poorly differentiated type of gastric cancer. Cancer Res 53:5087–5089, 1993.

53. Gorunova L, Johansson B, Dawiskiba S, Andren-Sandberg A, Jin Y, Mandahl N, Heim S, Mitelman F: Massive cytogenetic heterogeneity in a pancreatic carcinoma-54 karyotypically unrelated clones. Genes Chromosomes Cancer 14:259–266, 1995.

54. Bohlander SK, Espinosa R, Le Beau MM, Rowley JD, Diaz, MO: A Method for the rapid sequence-independence amplification of microdissected chromosomal material. Genomics 13:1322–1324, 1992.

55. Hawkins, AL, Jones RJ, Zehnbauer BA, Zicha MS, Collector MJ, Sharkis SJ, Griffin CA: Fluorescent *in situ* hybridization to determine engraftment status after murine bone marrow transplant. Cancer Genet Cytogenet 64:145–148, 1992.

56. Atkin NB, Baker MC: Specific chromosome changes in ovarian cancer. Cancer Genet Cytogenet 3:275–276, 1981.

57. Trent JM, Salmon SE: Karyotypic analysis of human ovarian carcinoma cells cloned in short term agar culture. Cancer Genet Cytogenet 3:279–291, 1981.

58. Whang-Peng J, Knutsen T, Douglass EC, Chu E, Ozols, KF, Hogan MW, Young RC: Cytogenetic studies in ovarian cancer. Cancer Genet Cytogenet 11:91–106, 1984.

59. Saito S, Saito H, Koi S, Sagae S, Kudo R, Saito J, Noda K, Nakamura Y: Fine-scale deletion mapping of the distal long arm of chromosome 6 in 70 human ovarian cancers. Cancer Res 52:5815–5817, 1992.

60. Zhang JP, Robinson WR, Ehlen T, Yu MC, Dubeau L: Distinction of low grade from high grade human ovarian carcinomas on the basis of losses of

heterozygosity on chromosomes 3, 6, and 11 and HER-2/neu gene amplification. Cancer Res 51:4045–4051, 1991.

61. Lee JH, Kavanagh JJ, Wildrick DM, Wharton JT, Blick M: Frequent loss of heterozygosity on chromosomes 6q, 11, and 17 in human ovarian carcinomas. Cancer Res 50:2724–2728, 1990.

62. Ehlen T, Dubeau L: Loss of heterozygosity on chromosomal segments 3p, 6q and 11p in human ovarian carcinomas. Oncogene 5:219–223, 1990.

63. Millikin D, Meese E, Vogelstein B, Witkowski C, Trent J: Loss of heterozygosity for loci on the long arm of chromosome 6 in human malignant melanoma. Cancer Res 51:5449–5453, 1991.

64. Trent JM, Stanbridge EJ, McBride HL, Meese EU, Casey G, Araujo DE, Witowski CM, Nagle RB: The expression of tumorigenicity in human melanoma cell lines is controlled by the introduction of human chromosome 6. Science 247:568–571, 1990.

65. Stenman G, Sandros J, Dahlenfors R, Juberg-Ode M, Mark J: 6q- and loss of the Y chromosome: two common deviations in malignant human salivary gland tumors. Cancer Genet Cytogenet 22:283–293, 1986.

66. Stenman G, Sandros J, Mark J, Edstrom S: Partial 6q deletion in a human salivary gland adenocarcinoma. Cancer Genet Cytogenet 39:153–156, 1989.

67. Trent JM, Rosenfeld SB, Meyskens FL: Chromosome 6q involvement in human malignant melanoma. Cancer Genet Cytogenet 9:177–180, 1983.

68. Trent JM, Thompson FH, Meyskens FL: Identification of a recurring translocation site involving chromosome 6 in human malignant melanoma. Cancer Res 49:420–423, 1989.

69. Becher R, Gibas Z, Sandberg AA: Chromosome 6 in malignant melanoma. Cancer Genet Cytogenet 9:173–175, 1983.

70. Look AT, Hayes FA, Shuster JJ, Douglass EC, Castleberry RP, Bowman LC, Smith EI, Brodeur GM: Clinical relevance of tumor cell ploidy and N-myc gene amplication in childhood neuroblastoma: a pediatric oncology group study. J Clin Oncol 9:581–591, 1991.

71. Press MF, Pike mC, Hung G, Zhou JY, Ma Y, George J, Dietz-Bank J, James W, Slamon DJ, Batsakis JG, El-Naggar AK: Amplification and overexpression of HER-2/neu in carcinomas of the salivary gland: correlation with poor prognosis. Cancer Res 54:5675–5682, 1994.

72. Kuniyasu J, Yasui W, Kitadai Y, Yokozaki H, Ito H, Tahara E: Prequent amplification of the C-Met gene in scirrhous type stomach cancer. Biochem Biophys Res Comm 189:227–232, 1992.

73. Hurtt MR, Moossy J, Donovan-Peluso M, Locker J: Amplification of epidermal growth factor receptor gene in gliomas: histopathology and prognosis. J Neuropathol Exp Neurol 51:84–90, 1992.

74. Korc M, Chandrasekar B, Yamanaka Y, Friess H, Buchier M, Beger HG. Overexpression of the epidermal growth factor receptor in human pancreatic cancer is associated with concomitant increase in the levels of epidermal growth factor and transforming growth factor alpha. J Clin Invest 90:1352–1360, 1992.

75. Barton CM, Hall PA, Hughes CM, Gullick WJ, Lemoine NR: Transforming growth factor alpha and epidermal growth factor in human pancreatic cancer. J Pathol 163:111–116, 1991.

76. Yamanaka Y, Friess H, Kobrin MS, Buchler M, Kunz J, Beger HG, Korc M. Overexpression of HER2/neu oncogene in human pancreatic carcinoma. Human Pathol 24:1127–1134, 1993.

77. Yamanaka Y: The immunohistochemical expression of epidermal growth factors, epidermal growth factor receptors and c-erbB-2 oncoprotein in human pancreatic cancer. Nippon Ika Daigaku Zasshi-J Nippon Med Sch 59(1):51–61, 1992.

78. Lemoine NR, Lobresco M, Leung H, Barton C, Hughes CM, Prigent SA, Gullick WJ, Kloppel G: The erbB-3 gene in human pancreatic cancer. J Pathol 168:269–273, 1992.

79. Prat M, Narsimhan RP, Crepaldi T, Nicotra MR, Natali PG, Comoglio PM: The receptor encoded by the human c-MET oncogene is expressed in hepatocytes, epithelial cells and solid tumors. Int J Cancer 49:323–328, 1991.

80. Furukawa T, Duguid WP, Kobari M, Matsuno S, Tsao MS, Hepatocyte growth factor and Met receptor expression in human pancreatic carcinogenesis. Am J Pathol 147:889–895, 1995.

Chapter 16

Soft Tissue Sarcomas

Julia A. Bridge

Introduction

Pathologic Classification and Diagnostic Difficulties

Soft tissue sarcomas constitute approx 1% of all malignancies and approx 2% of all cancer deaths *(1)*. Soft tissues are embryologically derived from mesoderm and neuroectoderm and comprise >50% of total body weight. Histologically, soft tissue sarcomas resemble the cell types of the tissues of origin: fibrous tissue, adipose tissue, blood vessels, striated and smooth muscles, nerve, and other supporting tissues. Soft tissue sarcomas may arise anywhere in the body, but the majority occur in the large muscles of the extremities, chest wall, mediastinum, and retroperitoneum *(2)*.

The pathogenesis of most soft tissue sarcomas is unknown. In some instances, environmental factors play a role. For example, some sarcomas appear to be induced by radiation (post radiation sarcoma). Other influences include hereditary or genetic factors. The autosomal dominant disorder neurofibromatosis type I (von Recklinghausen disease) illustrates a hereditary disease in which affected individuals are at an increased risk of developing a neurofibrosarcoma or malignant peripheral nerve sheath tumor (MPNST).

From: *Human Cytogenetic Cancer Markers*   Edited by S. R. Wolman and S. Sell
Humana Press Inc., Totowa, NJ

Comprehensive histopathological classifications for soft tissue tumors have been submitted by the Armed Forces Institute of Pathology (AFIP) *(3)* and the World Health Organization *(4)*. These systems are primarily categorized by the line of differentiation of the tumor. Fibrous tumors, fibrohistiocytic tumors, lipomatous tumors, smooth muscle tumors, skeletal muscle tumors, synovial tumors, neural tumors, extraskeletal cartilaginous and osseous tumors, pluripotential mesenchymal tumors, and unclassified tumors comprise a portion of the histological classification provided by Enzinger and Weiss *(2)* in their authoritative book on the pathology of soft tissue tumors.

Histopathological classifications for soft tissue tumors have reduced some of the diffficulties encountered in evaluating these tumors. However, because of overlapping and/or poorly differentiated features, many sarcomas remain diagnostically challenging. The "small round cell tumors" (a term descriptive of the histologic appearance) exemplify a group of clinically and etiologically diverse neoplasms that are histologically similar. This group, Ewing's sarcoma, primitive neuroectodermal tumor (PNET), small cell osteosarcoma, rhabdomyosarcoma, neuroblastoma, and lymphoma cannot be distinguished solely by standard light microscopy (Fig. 1). An accurate diagnosis is essential for purposes of treatment and prognosis, as each neoplasm is biologically distinct. Sarcoma diagnostic dilemmas may be resolved by immunohistochemical and ultrastructural examination, but these forms of analysis are frequently not informative if the tumor shows aberrant antigen expression or has progressed to a less differentiated state *(5)*.

Cytogenetic and, more recently, molecular genetic studies of soft tissue sarcomas have revealed characteristic abnormalities that are independent of the level of differentiation of a tumor. These genetic markers have added a new dimension to the formulation of a diagnosis and the resolution of cellular origin *(6,7)*. Identification of the aberrant chromosomal bands cytogenetically has served as a foundation for molecular approaches to establishing the affected genes and to recognize the associated consequences of these gene alterations. In some instances, recognition of the cytogenetic abnormality is the first clue that a mutated gene resides at a particular locus. Chimeric genes or fusion genes resulting from chromosomal rearrangements, such as the 11;22 translocation in Ewing's sarcoma,

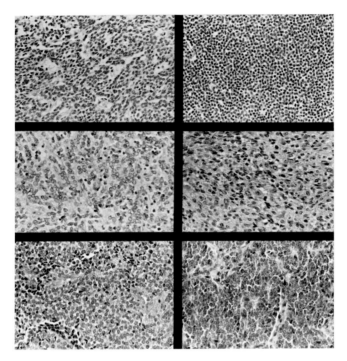

Fig. 1. Light microscopic appearance of several different "small round cell tumors" showing histomorphologic similarities. Upper left: peripheral primitive neuroectodermal tumor; upper right: small noncleaved cell lymphoma; middle left: neuroblastoma; middle right; embryonal rhabdomyosarcoma; lower left: Ewing's sarcoma; and lower right: Askin tumor (courtesy of Dr. Frederic B. Askin, Johns Hopkins Hospital, Baltimore, MD) *(6)*.

appear to have important implications not only for causation of the neoplastic state, but also in the diagnosis. Furthermore, recognition of these sarcoma-specific anomalies is imperative for development of novel therapeutic strategies based on the underlying genetic or biological events.

Cytogenetic Methodologies

Representative, aseptically collected tumor tissue should be transported to the laboratory in sterile culture media or buffer solution for cytogenetic studies as soon as possible following surgical removal. Tumor samples processed immediately yield better results in tissue culture, but successful growth of cells can also be obtained from samples processed 24–48 h after removal. Necrotic and non-neoplastic tissues should be dissected from the sample. Larger samples are preferable (1–2 cm^3), but specimens obtained by needle biopsy can also be analyzed successfully.

Tumors are prepared for culture by mechanical and enzymatic disaggregation into single cells or small clusters. In some high-grade tumors, metaphase cells can be extracted directly from disaggregated tissue if less than 1 h has passed from time of biopsy, obviating the need for culture (8). The duration of culture is individualized for each tumor, flask, and dish. Harvest or culture arrest is carried out when "peak" mitotic activity is observed (6). The length of culture should not extend beyond 2–3 wk, however, as this may result in overgrowth of normal supporting stromal cells (fibroblasts).

Fluorescence In Situ Hybridization (FISH)

Specific nucleic acid sequences can be visualized in individual metaphase and interphase cells with FISH. This technique can be performed on fresh or aged samples (such as blood smears or touch and cytospin preparations), paraffin-embedded tissue sections, and disaggregated cells retrieved from fresh, frozen, or paraffin embedded material (9,10).

FISH is a valuable technique for defining chromosomal rearrangements in soft tissue sarcomas. Bicolor FISH with whole chromosome paint probes, breakpoint spanning yeast artificial chromosomes, or cosmids from loci flanking or overlapping translocation breakpoints can be used diagnostically. A significant advantage of FISH is that it is not dependent on the acquisition of metaphase cells. The translocation or rearrangement of interest can be identified in interphase cells. With this approach, cryptic or masked translocations may be seen, a phenomenon similar to that described in chronic myelogenous leukemia (11).

In addition to translocations, supernumerary ring chromosomes are often encountered in sarcomas, particularly those of intermediate or borderline malignancy (Table 1) (6). Traditional FISH, and recently, comparative genomic hybridization (CGH) have uncovered the chromosomal composition of these rings as well as some associated gene amplifications in well-differentiated liposarcoma and dermatofibrosarcoma protuberans (12–16).

Table 1
Ring Chromosomes in Sarcomas of Borderline or
Low-Grade Malignancy

Neoplasm	Ring chromosome composition	Gene amplification
Dermatofibrosarcoma protuberans	17q23–24 22cen 22q11–12	?ZNF74
Myxoid malignant fibrous histiocytoma	?	MDM2
Well-differentiated liposarcoma	12q13–15 12q21.3–22	SAS MDM2
Parosteal osteosarcoma	?	?

For neoplasms of mixed cellular lineage, FISH can be combined with immunocytochemical studies to simultaneously determine the cytogenetic aberrations and immunophenotypic features of individual cells. For example, analysis of a dedifferentiated chondrosarcoma with a rhabdomyosarcomatous component showed that both the chondrocytic and rhabdomyoblastic cells arose from the same abnormal clone, supporting the theory of a common primitive mesenchymal progenitor with the ability to differentiate or express features of more than one line of mesenchymal differentiation *(17)*.

Reverse Transcription Polymerase Chain Reaction (RT-PCR)

The polymerase chain reaction technique uses specific synthetic oligonucleotides to amplify a section of a given gene in vitro (described in Chapter 4). With the additional step of reverse transcription, PCR can be carried out on RNA. This is particularly useful in evaluating gene rearrangements that occur as a result of chromosomal translocation in soft tissue sarcomas. Ewing's sarcoma, peripheral PNETs, alveolar rhabdomyosarcoma, desmoplastic small round cell tumor, clear cell sarcoma, myxoid liposarcoma, and possibly synovial sarcoma and myxoid chondrosarcoma, are characterized by reciprocal translocations that result in the formation of chimeric genes with the properties of transcriptional regulators and these fusion genes can be reliably identified with this approach (Table 2) *(5,18–24)*.

Table 2
Characteristic and Variant Cytogenetic Translocations
and Associated Fusion Genes in Soft Tissue Sarcomas

Neoplasm	Translocation	Fusion gene(s)
Ewing's sarcoma and peripheral primitive neuroectodermal tumors	t(11;22)(q24;q12)	EWS/FLI-1
	t(21;22)(q22;q12)	EWS/ERG
Clear cell sarcoma	t(12;22)(q13–14;q12)	EWS/ATF-1
Desmoplastic small round-cell tumor	t(11;22)(p13;q12)	EWS/WT-1
Alveolar rhabdomyosarcoma	t(2;13)(q35;q14)	PAX3/FKHR
	t(1;13)(p36;q14)	PAX7/FKHR
Myxoid liposarcoma	t(12;16)(q13–15;p11)	TLS/CHOP
Synovial sarcoma	t(X;18)(p11.2;q11.2)	SYT/SSX

Deletions and Tumor Suppressor Genes

Neuroblastoma

Neuroblastoma is the third most common childhood malignancy, with over 70% of tumors occurring in children <4 yr of age *(2)*. Neuroblastoma most commonly arises in the retroperitoneum, particularly the adrenal gland. Microscopically, neuroblastoma is composed of small round regular cells with polygonal, deep staining nuclei, and little cytoplasm. Homer Wright rosettes, a histologic configuration of tumor cells arranged around a central area filled with tangled neurites, neurosecretory granules and synaptic endings, are present in approx 25–33% of cases. Less differentiated neuroblastomas must be distinguished from nucleated erythrocytes of erythroblastosis fetalis and other small round cell tumors such as Ewing's sarcoma, rhabdomyosarcoma, and lymphoma.

Considerable efforts have been directed at defining reliable prognostic parameters for neuroblastoma. Clinical staging, age of the patient at diagnosis, site of primary tumor, catecholamine excretion pattern, serum ferritin, serum neuron specific enolase, and a number of histologic features have been described as prognostic factors *(25)*. Recently, genetic markers have been shown to be of prognostic value.

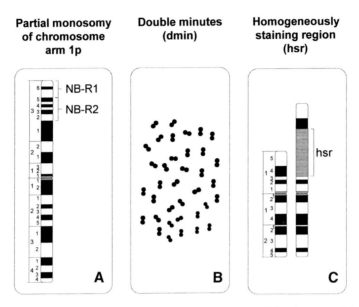

Fig. 2. The most common cytogenetic abnormalities in neuroblastoma include: partial monosomy of the short arm of chromosome 1 including two putative tumor suppressor gene regions (NB-R1 and NB-R2) (**A**), dmin (**B**), and hsr (**C**). The hsr in part C is illustrated on chromosome 11, but hsr in neuroblastomas have been identified on at least 18 of the 24 different chromosomes. The dmin and hsr are cytogenetic manifestations of N-*myc* amplification in neuroblastoma.

Neuroblastoma is characterized cytogenetically by two different types of chromosomal abnormalities each succeeded by specific biological consequences. These are either deletion of a portion or all of the short arm of chromosome 1 *(26,27)*, or the presence of double minutes (dmin) or homogeneously staining regions (hsr) (Fig. 2) *(6)*.

A deletion of the short arm of chromosome 1 was first described by Brodeur et al. *(28,29)* in 1975 as the most common cytogenetic abnormality in neuroblastoma. Partial 1p monosomy is found in 25–30% of primary tumors and 80% of cell lines *(30)*. Loss of 1p sequences not apparent cytogenetically may be detected by FISH or loss of heterozygosity (LOH) studies *(31,32)*. In some neuroblastomas, the deleted 1p material is replaced by 17q material. This translocation takes place in the S/G2 phase of the cell cycle and results in LOH 1p *(33,34)*. Nonhomologous mitotic recombination in the S/G2 phase is a novel mechanism of LOH.

Recent investigations suggest that possibly two tumor suppressor genes are located on 1p (the first an interstitial deletion encompassing a small region of 1p36 [NB-R1] and the other, a deletion within the region of 1p32–p35, [NB-R2]) and that each is associated with distinct biological behavior. Specifically, tumors of patients involving NB-R1 appear to be in the triploid range and this group rarely progresses to stage IV. Tumors of patients in the NB-R2 are more often in the diploid or tetraploid range, show N-*myc* amplification and progress to stage IV disease *(35,36)*. Interestingly, another common pediatric tumor, Wilms' tumor, is associated with two distinct regions of deletion within the same chromosomal arm (11p) *(37,38)*.

Homogeneously Staining Regions, Double Minutes, Ring Chromosomes and Gene Amplification

Neuroblastoma

Amplification of N-*myc*, a proto-oncogene located at 2p23–24, is visible cytogenetically in the form of dmin and hsr in neuroblastoma and is associated with stage III or IV (stage C/D) disease. Genomic amplification of the N-myc proto-oncogene correlates with both advanced disease stage and rapid tumor progression, independent of the other poor prognostic factors with which it is frequently associated *(39,40)*. One exception is that the presence of N-myc amplification in localized neuroblastoma does not necessarily portend an adverse outcome *(41)*.

Stage IV-S (stage D-S) is a special manifestation of neuroblastoma with remote sites of involvement, but which behaves similarily to early stage disease. Cytogenetic and molecular genetic studies of D-S have not shown associated abnormalities of 1p or N-*myc* amplification *(42)*.

Dermatofibrosarcoma Protuberans

Dermatofibrosarcoma protuberans is described as a neoplasm of intermediate or borderline malignancy. This neoplasm arises in

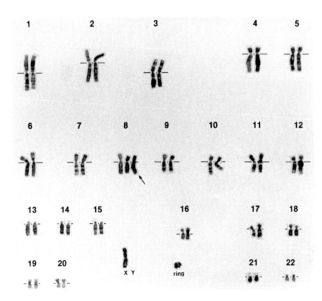

Fig. 3. Representative karyotype of a dermatofibrosarcoma protuberans from the shoulder of a 46-yr-old male showing a ring chromosome. Trisomy 8 was also a clonal finding, but loss of the Y chromosome was seen in this metaphase only *(43)*.

the dermis and is characterized by locally aggressive behavior with a tendency to recur, but rarely metastasize. Distinguishing dermatofibrosarcoma protuberans from other fibrohistiocytic neoplasms such as benign and malignant fibrous histiocytoma may be diagnostically difficult. If myxoid areas are prominent, it may be difficult to differentiate from myxoid liposarcoma. Each of these lesions is characterized by separate cytogenetic findings that can be used to assist in the diagnosis.

The observation of a ring chromosome in dermatofibrosarcoma protuberans, first described by Bridge et al. *(43)* (Fig. 3), has come to be recognized as the characteristic chromosomal anomaly of this neoplasm *(6)*. The ring chromosome is detected either as the sole anomaly or it may be accompanied by simple chromosomal trisomies. Importantly, the presence of ring chromosomes (in the absence of other complex karyotypic rearrangements) is not confined to dermatofibrosarcoma protuberans, but is also characteristic of other mesenchymal neoplasms of borderline biological behavior,

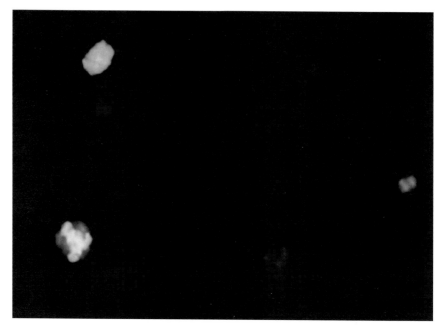

Fig. 4. Dual color FISH of a dermatofibrosarcoma protuberans metaphase cell with digoxigenin-labeled chromosome 17 paint (rhodamine detection) and biotin-labeled chromosome 22 paint (FITC detection) *(47)*. The normal chromosome 17 homolog is located in the upper left, the normal chromosome 22 homolog in the upper right, and the ring chromosome composed of three distinct regions of chromosome 17 sequences (red) separated by three regions of chromosome 22 sequences (green) in the lower left. (Courtesy of Dr. Jonathan A. Fletcher, Brigham and Women's Hospital, Boston, MA.) (*See* color insert following p. 212.)

including myxoid malignant fibrous histiocytoma, atypical lipomatous tumor or well-differentiated liposarcoma, and parosteal osteosarcoma.

Combined approaches including karyotyping, chromosome painting by FISH and CGH have revealed that the ring chromosomes in dermatofibrosarcoma protuberans are composed of a 22 centromere and sequences from chromosomes 17 and 22 (Figs. 4 and 5) *(16,44–47)*. Amplification of chromosome 17 and 22 sequences have also been demonstrated by CGH in cytogenetically normal cases. The amplified sequences include 22q11–12 and 17q23–24.

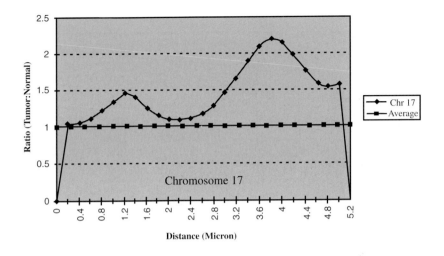

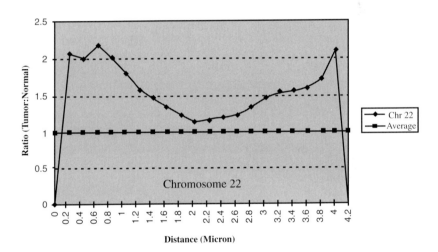

Fig. 5. CGH profiles, with pter at left and qter at right, for chromosomes 17 and 22 in a case of dermatofibrosarcoma protuberans *(47)*. Peaked line shows ratio of dermatofibrosarcoma protuberans DNA (FITC) to control DNA (rhodamine) signal intensity across the designated chromosomes, whereas the baseline was established from average FITC:rhodamine signal intensity readings in nonamplified chromosomes from the same metaphase. Amplification of chromosome 17 and 22 sequences is most pronounced in regions corresponding to 17q21→qter and 22q12→qter, respectively. Spurious amplification is also seen in the chromosome 22 pericentromeric region owing to incomplete competition of repetitive satellite sequences. (Courtesy of Dr. Jonathan A. Fletcher, Brigham and Women's Hospital, Boston, MA.)

Three cases of dermatofibrosarcoma protuberans and one case of giant cell fibroblastoma (a juvenile form of dermatofibrosarcoma protuberans) have shown a translocation between chromosomes 17 and 22 [t(17;22)(q22;q13)], suggesting that these regions are critical *(45,48,49)*. A 2;17 translocation [t(2;17)(q33;q25)] has also been reported in a case of dermatofibrosarcoma protuberans not showing a ring chromosome *(50)*. One group of investigators observed contiguous chromosome 17 and 22 sequences in one ring chromosome case (within resolution limits of dual color chromosome painting) and hypothesized that the rings in dermatofibrosarcoma protuberans are complex chromosome structures that evolved from a fusion between 17q22–23 and 22q12–13 *(49)*. Dermatofibrosarcoma protuberans would, therefore, share a common key event in their pathogenesis; a molecular juxtaposition of 17q22–23 and 22q12–13, achieved by visible chromosome rearrangements (rings and translocations); and/or molecularly recognizable hybrid transcripts. Notably, in addition to the potential significance of a 17;22 fused transcript, there is over-representation of 17 and 22 sequences even in cases showing translocations *(49)*. The relevance of this low-level amplification with respect to dermatofibrosarcoma protuberans pathogenesis is unclear.

Myxoid Malignant Fibrous Histiocytoma (MFH)

MFH is the most common soft tissue sarcoma of late adult life *(2)*. Five histologic variants of MFH have been described;

1. Storiform/pleomorphic (most common);
2. Giant cell;
3. Inflammatory;
4. Angiomatoid; and
5. Myxoid.

Reported prognostic factors include tumor size, location (particularly depth), presence of neutrophils, mitotic activity, vascular invasion, cellularity, histologic subtype and grade (extent of necrosis), DNA ploidy, and cytogenetic findings *(6)*.

Ring chromosomes in the absence of other complex chromosomal abnormalities is the characteristic cytogenetic finding in myxoid MFH, distinguishing it from other MFH subtypes and from other types of sarcomas, such as myxoid liposarcoma, with which it may be confused *(51)*. Multiple complex chromosomal abnormalities including telomeric associations and dicentric chromosomes are common findings in the other histologic variants of MFH. Notably, myxoid MFH also differs by its better prognosis. Thus, the cytogenetic findings also serve as prognostic markers for this neoplasm. The particular chromosomal sequences constituting these rings have not yet been identified, although *MDM2* amplification reportedly correlates with the presence of ring chromosomes in MFH *(15)*. *MDM2*, the human homolog of the murine dmin type 2 gene, has been cloned and mapped to 12q13–14 *(52)*.

Well-Differentiated Liposarcoma

The biological behavior of liposarcomas closely parallels the histologic subtype; therefore, any diagnostic inaccuracy can significantly affect a patient's clinical management. Well-differentiated liposarcoma is a low-grade malignant neoplasm. Atypical lipoma and atypical intramuscular lipoma are terms that are synonymous with subcutaneous and muscular forms of well-differentiated liposarcoma. The presence of large unidentifiable "giant rod-shaped marker" chromosomes and/or ring chromosomes typifies this neoplasm (Fig. 6) *(53,54)*. Other chromosomal abnormalities may accompany these marker and ring chromosomes, but often they are observed as isolated anomalies.

With the use of CGH and FISH with a chromosome 12 painting probe, investigators have shown that chromosome 12 sequences are present in the supernumerary ring chromosomes and giant rod-shaped marker chromosomes *(12,13,55)*. Specifically, the 12q13–15 and 12q21.3–22 regions have been identified in such markers *(55)*. In addition to the constant chromosome 12 contribution, sequences have been added variably from chromosomes 1, 4, and 16. Analyses of *SAS, MDM2,* and *GADD153/CHOP* known to be in the region of 12q13–14 have revealed constant coamplification of *SAS* and *MDM2* *(14)*. *GADD153/CHOP*, which is critically rearranged in myxoid liposarcoma, is generally not amplified, although 1 of 19 liposarcomas evaluated in a separate study has shown amplification of *GADD153/CHOP* along with *MDM2 (56)*.

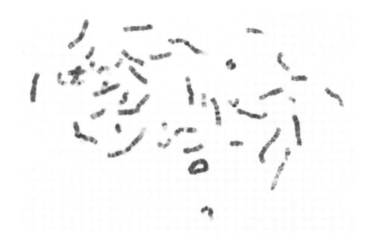

Fig. 6. Metaphase spread demonstrating ring chromosomes in a well-differentiated liposarcoma.

Translocations and Gene Rearrangements

Ewing's Sarcoma and Primitive Neuroectodermal Tumors

Ewing's sarcoma and peripheral primitive neuroectodermal tumors (pPNETs) and a class of biphenotypic childhood sarcomas with myogenic and neural differentiation are characterized cytogenetically by a highly recurrent reciprocal translocation between chromosomes 11 and 22 [t(11;22)(q24;q12)] (Fig. 7) *(57–61)*. This translocation is observed in >85% of these tumors and results in the fusion of the 3′ portion (the DNA-binding domain) of the *FLI-1* gene on chromosome 11 with the 5′ portion (the amino terminus) of the *EWS* gene on chromosome 22 *(62)*. Consequently, a hybrid EWS/FLI-1 protein is formed that behaves as an aberrant transcription factor.

FLI-1 is a member of the *ETS* family of transcription factors, a family defined by the presence of an 85 amino acid domain, called the *ets* domain, that mediates sequence-specific DNA binding *(63,64)*. The function of the *EWS* gene is unknown. It is structurally related to *TLS*, the amino terminus of which is fused to the *CHOP* DNA-binding protein in the 12;16 translocation characteristic of

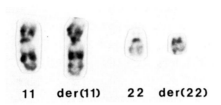

11   der(11)   22   der(22)

Fig. 7. Characteristic cytogenetic translocation in Ewing's sarcoma and pPNET, t(11;22)(q24;q12). The normal homologs are on the left of each pair.

myxoid liposarcoma *(65,66)*. Sequence analyses of *EWS* and *TLS* have revealed no well-characterized functional motifs or predicted structures, although when the amino termini of *EWS* and *TLS* are fused to *FLI-1*, they appear to perform similar functions in transformation *(67)*. *EWS/FLI-1* contributes to the transformed phenotype of Ewing's sarcoma cells by inducing the deregulated activation of genes, or the unscheduled activation of genes, or both, that are normally responsive to *FLI-1* or to other close members of the *ETS* family. Ewing's sarcoma and related tumors are characterized by an elevated level of c-*myc* expression. *EWS/FLI-*1 is a transactivator of the c-*myc* promoter, suggesting that upregulation of c-*myc* expression is under control of *EWS/FLI-1 (68)*.

Considerable heterogeneity exists with respect to specific *EWS/FLI-1* breakpoints. However, all *EWS/FLI-1* fusions have shown an intact *FLI-1* DNA-binding domain, suggesting that this function is necessary for biologic activity *(19,69,70)*. In contrast to normal *FLI-1*, the *EWS/FLI-1* fusion transforms NIH3T3 cells and this activity requires both *EWS* and *FLI-1* sequences.

In addition to the *EWS/FLI-1* fusion that occurs with the classic 11;22 translocation, the *EWS* gene can be fused to *ERG*, a closely related transcription factor, located at the chromosomal breakpoint 21q22. *ERG* is also a member of the *ETS* gene family. Thus, investigations have shown that fusion of *EWS* to different members of the *ETS* family may result in the expression of similar disease phenotypes and that oncogenic conversion is achieved by the linking of the two domains with no marked constraint on the connecting peptide.

Correlations between the different molecular breakpoints or fusion gene partners and clinical behavior are few. In one study, fusion of exon 7 of *EWS* with exon 6 of *FLI-1* predominated over fusion of exon 7 of *EWS* with exon 5 of *FLI-1* in localized non-metastatic Ewing's sarcoma by a ratio of 14:1, and was more abundant in tumors affecting the long bones (ratio of 9:0) *(71)*. In central axis tumors and metastatic disease there was little difference between the two types of fusions. So far, no relationship between the different chimeric transcripts (*EWS/FLI-1* and *EWS/ERG*) and any other clinical parameters have been identified *(72)*.

MIC2p antigen, a membrane protein of unknown function, is often used as a marker of Ewing's sarcoma and pPNETs. Unfortunately, it is occasionally present in other types of neoplasms, and, therefore, immunoreactivity cannot eliminate other possible diagnoses. The RT-PCR method is highly advantageous in confirming or establishing the diagnosis of Ewing's sarcoma or pPNET because of its ability to detect either fusion gene combination (Fig. 8) *(20,73)*. PCR is a rapid and sensitive method that is not limited by the quantity of available tissue and, therefore, can also be applied to fine needle biopsy specimens. Recently, a multiplex RT-PCR assay has been developed that allows identification of either the *EWS/FLI-1* or the *PAX3/FKHR* (associated with alveolar rhabdomyosarcoma) chimeric transcripts in a single reaction *(74)*.

FISH is also a valuable technical adjunct for defining the rearrangements. Bicolor FISH with cosmids from loci flanking or overlapping the 7-kb region called EWSR1 on chromosome 22 and the 40- to 50-kb region called EWSR2 on chromosome 11 allows localization of the two breakpoints of the t(11;22)(q24;q12) within a 10-kb resolution *(75)*. With either the PCR or the FISH approach, cryptic or masked translocations may be seen, a phenomenon similar to that described in chronic myelogenous leukemia.

Clear Cell Sarcoma of Tendons
and Aponeuroses (Malignant Melanoma of Soft Parts)

Clear cell sarcoma is a rare malignant neoplasm that most commonly arises in proximity to tendons and aponeuroses in the extremities (particularly the foot and ankle) of young adults. It derives its

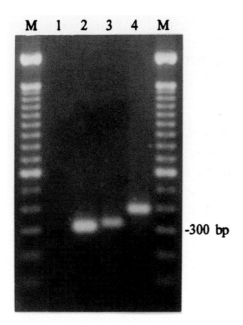

Fig. 8. RT-PCR analysis of *EWS/FLI-1* chimeric transcript expression in a Ewing's sarcoma patient sample. PCR analysis was performed on oligo-dT reverse-transcribed total RNA samples with primers 22.3 and 11.3. Amplified PCR products were separated by electrophoresis on a 2% agarose gel and visualized with ethidium bromide staining. M, 100bp marker; lane 1, negative control (Ewing's sarcoma patient sample RNA without primers); lane 2, Ewing's sarcoma patient sample RNA quality control with β-actin primers (314 bp); lane 3, Ewing's sarcoma patient sample showing a type I fusion (328 bp); and lane 4, positive control, Ewing's sarcoma cell line (SK-ES-1) with a type II fusion (394 bp).

name from the clear histologic appearance of the tumor cell cytoplasm secondary to abundant intracellular glycogen. The demonstration of melanin, melanosomes, and premelanosomes in clear cell sarcoma has led to a hypothesized neural crest origin for this neoplasm *(76–78)* and a proposal that it be renamed "malignant melanoma of soft parts" *(76)*.

Clear cell sarcoma is characterized cytogenetically by a 12;22 translocation [t(12;22)(q13;q12–13)](Fig. 9) *(79)*. In the absence of a 12;22 translocation, other structural rearrangements or extra copies of chromosome 22 have been seen in all but one reported

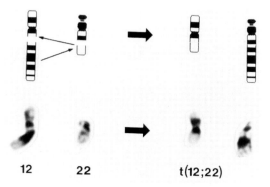

Fig. 9. Schematic and partial karyotype of the typical 12;22 translocation in clear cell sarcoma *(6)*.

case (Fig. 10) *(6)*. Diagnostically important, recognition of the
12;22 translocation (which is not seen in malignant melanoma) is
useful in distinguishing clear cell sarcoma from metastatic cutaneous malignant melanoma and also from other soft tissue sarcomas
with which diagnostic confusion may occur (fibrosarcoma, synovial
sarcoma, epithelioid malignant schwannoma, hemangiopericytoma,
alveolar soft-part sarcoma, and hemangioendothelioma).

In addition to the observation of t(12;22) or other structural or
numerical anomalies of chromosome 22, extra copies of chromosome 8 have been detected in over half of the reported cases, indicating that this polysomy may also be an important nonrandom
event in this tumor *(80)*. Overrepresentation of chromosome 8 is
seen frequently in hematologic disorders, both as a primary and a
secondary event *(81)*. In some forms of leukemia, trisomy 8 is associated with an intermediate to poor prognosis. Trisomy 8 has also
been described as a nonrandom secondary change in Ewing's sarcoma *(82)* and myxoid liposarcoma *(83)*. The clinical significance
of trisomy 8 in these mesenchymal neoplasms is not yet known.

The 12;22 translocation in clear cell sarcoma also results in the
formation of a chimeric protein detectable by RT-PCR. With this
translocation, the N-terminal domain of *EWS* is linked to the bZIP
domain of *ATF-1*, a transcription factor normally regulated by
cAMP *(22)*. *ATF-1* has been localized to 12q13.1–13.2 *(84)*. The
bZIP domain mediates protein dimerization and DNA binding. The

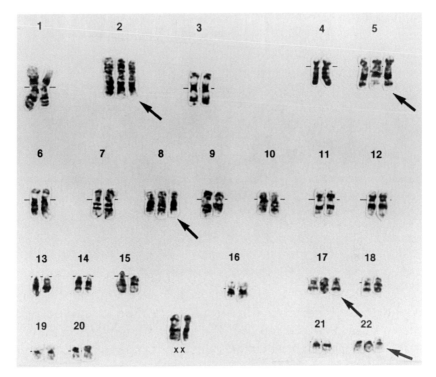

Fig. 10. In the absence of the 12;22 translocation in clear cell sarcoma, other structural or numerical anomalies of chromosome 22 are seen, such as in this case with trisomy 22. Also note the extra copy of chromosome 8, a finding which has been observed in over half of reported cases of clear cell sarcoma *(6,80)*.

structural and functional consequences of this fusion gene closely resemble those of Ewing's sarcoma, *EWS/FLI-1* or *EWS/ERG*. In both tumors, the chimeric gene generated on the der(22) chromosome codes for a protein in which the same portion of the N-terminal domain of *EWS* is linked to a DNA-binding domain of a transcription factor. Thus, Ewing's sarcoma and clear cell sarcoma appear to share a common mechanism of oncogenesis.

Desmoplastic Small Round Cell Tumor

The *EWS* gene has also been shown to be involved in another tumor, desmoplastic small round cell tumor. Desmoplastic small round cell tumor (DSRCT) is a rare primitive sarcoma primarily occurring in young males that shows widespread abdominal serosal involvement not related to a particular organ system, prominent desmoplasia, and aggressive clinical behavior *(85)*.

Cytogenetically, DSRCT is characterized by an 11;22 translocation *(6)*. In contrast to Ewing's sarcoma and pPNET, however, the breakpoint on chromosome 11 is on the short arm, t(11;22)(p13;q12). With this translocation a tumor suppressor gene, *WT1* (localized to 11p13) is juxtaposed to *EWS (21)*. *WT1* is involved in a subset of Wilm's tumors and codes for a transcription factor similar to other translocation partners of *EWS*. DSRCT represents the third primitive sarcoma in which the *EWS* gene is involved and the first instance of recurrent rearrangement of a tumor suppressor gene.

Alveolar Rhabdomyosarcoma

Alveolar rhabdomyosarcoma, a highly malignant pediatric neoplasm, is characterized cytogenetically by a (2;13)(q35;q14) translocation (Figs. 11 and 12). The solid variant pattern of alveolar rhabomyosarcoma that shares the cytologic features of typical alveolar lesions, but lacks discrete fibrous septa and clinically behaves more aggressively, has also been shown to exhibit the 2;13 translocation *(86)*. This translocation results in the fusion of the *PAX3* gene, a locus on chromosome 2 encoding a member of the paired box or *PAX* transcription factor family, with *FKHR* (or *ALV*), a chromosome 13 locus encoding a member of the fork-head transcription-factor family (Fig. 13) *(87)*. The chimeric product, the PAX3/FKHR fusion protein, is a much more potent transcriptional activator than PAX3 and may function as an oncogenic transcription factor by enhanced activation of normal *PAX3* target genes *(88)*.

In a minority of alveolar rhabdomyosarcoma cases, a variant translocation has been observed, t(1;13)(p36;q14). This variant translocation results in a rearrangement of *PAX7*, a chromosome 1 locus encoding another member of the PAX family, and generates a *PAX7/FKHR* chimeric transcript that is analogous to the 5'PAX3-3'FKHR product of the t(2;13) *(89)*.

Detection of the derivative 13 in both interphase and metaphase cells has been achieved with bicolor FISH by labeling the 3'FKHR

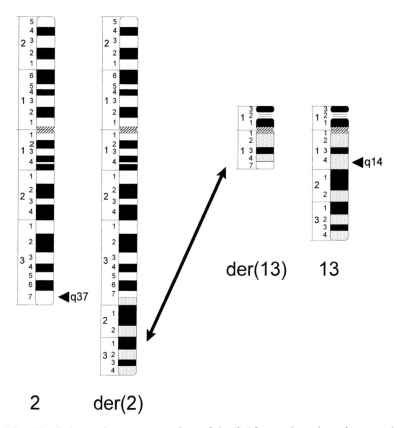

Fig. 11. Schematic representation of the 2;13 translocation characteristic of alveolar rhabdomyosarcoma.

and the 5′PAX3 cosmid probes with digoxigenin and biotin, respectively *(90)*. FISH analyses of both alveolar rhabdomyosarcoma and embryonal rhabdomyosarcoma has revealed the rearrangement only in alveolar rhabdomyosarcoma. This assay is a sensitive and rapid means of identifying the t(2;13) in alveolar rhabdomyosarcoma.

Myxoid Liposarcoma

Myxoid liposarcoma is characterized cytogenetically by a recurrent translocation involving chromosomes 12 and 16[t(12;16) (q13;p11)] demonstrable also by FISH (Fig. 14). The q13–15 breakpoint region on chromosome 12 also commonly rearranged in

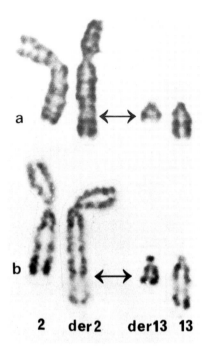

2   der2   der13   13

Fig. 12. Partial karyotype of t(2;13)(q37;q14) in alveolar rhabdomyosarcoma. Reprinted with permission from ref. *85a*.

lipomas is different than that in myxoid liposarcoma as demonstrated by high resolution chromosome banding and molecular studies *(91–93)*. Similar to other translocation-featured sarcomas, the
12;16 translocation results in the fusion or juxtaposition of two
genes, *CHOP* on chromosome 12 and *TLS* on chromosome 16 *(66)*.
CHOP is a growth-arrest and DNA-damage inducible member of
the C/EBP family of transcription factors *(94)*. *TLS*, also called
FUS, encodes a glycine-rich nuclear RNA-binding protein and
shares extensive sequence homology with *EWS*. Identification of
this translocation or rearrangement is useful diagnostically in distinguishing myxoid liposarcoma from other histologically similar
myxoid neoplasms.

Synovial Sarcoma

Synovial sarcoma, a rare neoplasm of young adults, occurs
primarily in juxta-articular locations, particularly the knee *(6)*.

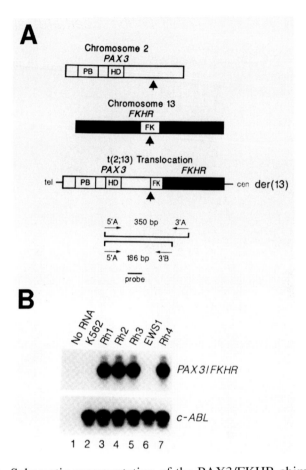

Fig. 13. Schematic representation of the PAX3/FKHR chimeric product resulting from the t(2;13) translocation. (**A**) PAX3 contains two discrete DNA-binding domains, a paired box (PB) and the paired-type homeodomain (HD), whereas FKHR contains a central forkhead DNA-binding domain (FK). The arrows indicate the position of t(2;13) breakpoints. The der(13)-encoded PAX3/FKHR polypeptide consists of the amino-terminal portion of PAX3 including the PB and HD domains, fused to a bisected FK domain of FKHR. The position of oligonucleotide primers for RT-PCR analysis, the probe for Southern blot detection, and the size of the PCR product generated are indicated. (**B**) Representative blot of RT-PCR analysis. PCR products generated with the 5′A and 3′A primers, or with primers for the ubiquitously expressed c-ABL message, were separated by gel electrophoresis, transferred to nylon membranes, and hybridized with ^{32}P-labeled probes specific for either the PAX3/FKHR transcript or c-ABL. The samples analyzed included the rhabdomyosarcoma cell line, SJ-RH1-4, the Ewing's sarcoma cell line SJ-EWS1, and the leukemic cell line K562. Reprinted with permission from ref. *74.*

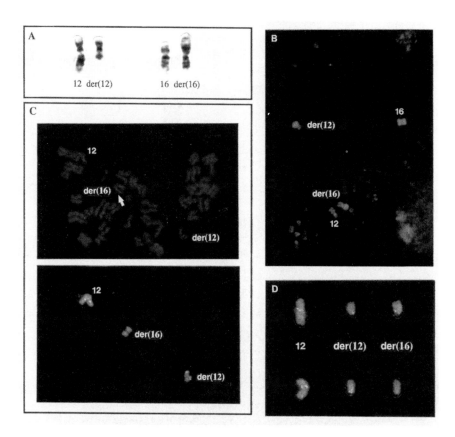

Fig. 14. FISH analysis of t(12;16) from a myxoid liposarcoma using the 100C4 YAC. (**A**) Representative GTG-banded chromosomes showing the normal homologs of chromosomes 12 and 16 and the reciprocal transloca-tion (12;16)(q13.3;p11.2). (**B**) Partial metaphase hybridized with whole chromosome probes for chromosome 12 (yellow-green) and chromosome 16 (red-orange) showing the normal and translocated derivatives of these chromosomes. (**C**) Partial metaphase with endoreduplication visualized by DAPI staining (top) and bicolor FISH (bottom) using a whole chromosome probe for chromosome 12 (red-orange) and the 100C4 YAC (yellow-green). The YAC hybridization signal is apparent on the normal 12, der(12), and der(16) chromosomes. (**D**) Examples of the normal 12, der(12), and der(16) from two additional cells showing hybridization of 100C4 to both sides of the (12;16)(q13.3;p11.2) translocation breakpoint. Reprinted with permission from ref. *90a*. (*See* color insert following p. 212.)

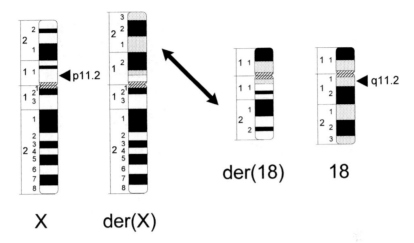

Fig. 15. Schematic of the X;18 translocation characteristic of synovial sarcoma.

Microscopically, synovial sarcoma may present as a biphasic pattern composed of epithelium-like cells and spindle-shaped cells or as a monophasic pattern composed solely of epithelium-like cells or spindle-shaped cells.

The term "synovial sarcoma" appears to be a misnomer as most immunohistochemical, electron microscopic and cytogenetic studies have shown that there is little evidence that this sarcoma arises from pre-existing synovial tissue. Moreover, synovial sarcoma occasionally occurs in areas with no apparent relationship to synovial structures, such as the head and neck region. These occurrences have also raised doubt as to the synovial origin of the neoplasm *(95,96)*.

Limon et al. *(97)* and Turc-Carel et al. *(98)* were the first to show that synovial sarcoma is characterized by a nonrandom translocation t(X;18)(p11.2;q11.2) (Fig. 15). This translocation is seen in both biphasic and monophasic synovial sarcomas. FISH studies and molecular analyses of this translocation have revealed two alternative breakpoint regions involved on Xp11.2, one residing in the ornithine aminotransferase-like 1 *(OATL1)* region and the other one in the related but distinct *OATL2* region *(99)*. Reports are contradictory as to whether a relationship exists between the different breakpoints and the resulting histopathologic appearance *(100,101)*.

Screening of a synovial sarcoma complementary DNA library with a yeast artificial chromosome spanning the X chromosome breakpoint has revealed a hybrid transcript that contains 5′ sequences (designated *SYT*), mapping to chromosome 18, and 3′ sequences, (designated *SSX*) mapping to chromosome X (SYT-SSX fusion protein) *(102)*. Neither *SYT* or *SSX* have exhibited significant homology to known gene sequences.

Conclusions

Cytogenetic and molecular genetic analyses play a direct, potentially decisive role in the examination of soft tissue sarcomas. The histological classification of mesenchymal neoplasms, especially high-grade lesions, often presents a challenge to the surgical pathologist. Electron microscopy can be helpful, but sampling errors can occur with the technique. Also many lesions defy histological classification, even with the aid of immunohistochemistry. This is partly related to the fact that many soft tissue sarcomas have a common origin from primitive mesenchymal cells. An accurate diagnosis is essential for determination of appropriate therapy. Chromosomal and molecular genetic analysis may be used not only to supplement conventional pathological examination in the differentiation of soft tissue sarcomas, but also as a vital diagnostic tool when other investigations have failed.

The multistep process of malignant transformation is complex. The development of new cytogenetic and molecular genetic techniques has led to a greater understanding of the genetic changes that occur in soft tissue sarcomas. Although soft tissue sarcomas are clinically and pathologically heterogeneous, a common form of oncogenesis has been observed in a subset of these tumors. Specifically, Ewing's sarcoma and related pPNETs, clear cell sarcoma, desmoplastic small round cell tumor, alveolar rhabdomyosarcoma, myxoid liposarcoma, and possibly synovial sarcoma are characterized by reciprocal translocations that result in the formation of chimeric genes with the properties of transcriptional regulators. The promiscuous pairing of the *EWS* gene with other genes appears to determine the phenotype of several primitive sarcomas *(21)*. The fusion protein products of these translocations promote oncogenesis by acting as aberrant transcription factors.

Less common variant translocations and related fusion genes have been detected in Ewing's sarcoma and alveolar rhabdomyosarcoma, expanding the repertoire of possible gene rearrangements involved in the pathogenesis of these neoplasms. The distinctiveness of the fusion proteins permits the use of RT-PCR and FISH for defining the cytogenetic phenotype as well as providing new diagnostic and perhaps prognostic approaches.

Amplification of genes, a well recognized mechanism of oncogenesis, has also been identified in soft tissue sarcomas. In addition to N-*myc* amplification in neuroblastoma, amplifications of genes and chromosomal sequences have been identified in the supernumerary ring chromosomes and/or giant rod marker chromosomes of well-differentiated liposarcoma, myxoid malignant fibrous histiocytoma, and dermatofibrosarcoma protuberans, sarcomas of intermediate or borderline malignancy.

Genetic studies of soft tissue sarcomas are rapidly providing a cumulatively more powerful data base that has proven to be diagnostically and, in some instances, prognostically informative. Characterization of a tumor's genetic profile with an understanding of the biologic functions of the genetic events (i.e., gene amplification and hybrid transcripts) should permit specific gene therapies. For example, the abnormal fusion transcript that occurs as the result of a translocation could be targeted and scrambled by specific oligonucleotides. The potential utilization of such biology-specific therapy could lead to improved eradication of disease in individuals with these sarcomas *(103)*.

References

1. Storm HH: Cancers of the soft tissues. Cancer Survey: Trends Cancer Incidence Mortal 19/20:197–217, 1994.
2. Enzinger FM, Weiss SW: Soft Tissue Tumors, 3rd ed. St. Louis: Mosby, 1995.
3. Lattes R: Tumors of the soft tissue. In: Atlas of Tumor Pathology. Second series. Fascicle 1/Revised. Washington, DC: Armed Forces Institute of Pathology, 1983.

4. Weiss SW, Sobin L: WHO Classification of Soft Tissue Tumors. Berlin; Germany: Springer Verlag, 1994.

5. Barr FG, Chatten J, D'Cruz DM, Willson AE, Nauta LE, Nycum LM, Biegel J, Womer RB: Molecular assays for chromosomal translocations in the diagnosis of pediatric soft tissue sarcomas. JAMA 273:553–557, 1995.

6. Sandberg AA, Bridge JA: The Cytogenetics of Bone and Soft Tissue Tumors. Austin, TX: Landes, CRC, 1994.

7. Bridge JA: Cytogenetics and experimental models of sarcomas. In: Abeloff M (ed.), Current Opinion in Oncology. Philadelphia, PA: Current Science, pp. 333–339, 1995.

8. Fletcher JA, Kozakewich HP, Hoffer FA, Lage JM, Weidner N, Tepper R, Pinkus GS, Morton CC, Corson JM: Diagnostic relevance of clonal cytogenetic aberrations in malignant soft tissue tumors. N Engl J Med 324:436–443, 1991.

9. Bridge JA: Cytogenetic and molecular cytogenetic techniques in orthopaedic surgery. Current concepts review. J Bone Joint Surg 75A:606–614, 1993.

10. Gray JW, Pinkel D, Brown JM: Fluorescence in situ hybridization in cancer and radiation biology. Radiat Res 137:275–289, 1994.

11. Giovannini M, Biegel JA, Serra M, Wang JY, Wei YH, Nycum L, Emanuel BS, Evans GA: EWS-erg and EWS-Fli1 transcripts in Ewing's sarcoma and primitive neuroectodermal tumors with variant translocations. J Clin Invest 94:489–496, 1994.

12. Pedeutour F, Suijkerbuijk RF, Van Gaal S, Van de Klundert W, Van Haelst A, Collin F, Huffermann K, Turc-Carel C: Chromosome 12 origin in rings and giant markers in well-differentiated liposarcoma. Cancer Genet Cytogenet 66:133,134, 1993.

13. Dal Cin P, Kools P, Sciot R, De Wever T, Van Damme B, Van de Ven W, Van den Berghe H: Cytogenetic and fluorescent in situ hybridization investigation of ring chromosomes characterizing a specific pathologic subgroup of adipose tissue tumors. Cancer Genet Cytogenet 68:85–90, 1993.

14. Pedeutour F, Suijkerbuijk RF, Forus A, Van Gaal J, Van de Klundert W, Coindre JM, Nicolo G, Collin F. Van Haelst U, Huffermann K, Turc-Carel C: Complex composition and co-amplification of SAS and MDM2 in ring and giant marker chromosomes in well-differentiated liposarcoma. Genes Chromosome Cancer 10:85–94, 1994.

15. Nilbert M, Rydholm A, Willén H, Mitelman F, Mandahl N: MDM2 gene amplification correlates with ring chromosomes in soft tissue tumors. Genes Chromosome Cancer 9:261–265, 1994.

16. Pedeutour F, Coindre JM, Sozi G, Nicolo G, Leroux A, Toma S, Miozzo M, Bouchot C, Hecht F, Ayraud N, Turc-Carel C: Supernumerary ring chromosomes containing chromosome 17 sequences: a specific feature of dermatofibrosarcoma protuberans? Cancer Genet Cytogenet 76:1–9, 1994.

17. Bridge JA, DeBoer J, Travis J, Johansson SL, Elmberger G, Noel SM, Neff JR: Simultaneous interphase cytogenetic analysis and fluorescence immunophenotyping of dedifferentiated chondrosarcoma: implications for histopathogenesis. Am J Pathol 144:215–220, 1994.

18. Rabbitts TH, Forster A, Larson R, Nathan P: Fusion of the dominant negative transcription regulator CHOP with a novel gene FUS by translocation t(12;16) in malignant liposarcoma. Nat Genet 4:175–180, 1993.

19. Zucman J, Melot T, Desmaze C, Ghysdael J, Plougastel B, Peter M, Zucker JM, Triche TJ, Sheer D, Turc-Carel C, Ambros P, Combaret V, Lenoir G, Aurias A, Thomas G, Delattre O: Combinatorial generation of variable fusion proteins in the Ewing family of tumours. EMBO J 12:4481–4487, 1993.

20. Delattre O, Zucman J, Melot T, Garau XS, Zucker JM, Lenoir GM, Ambros PF, Sheer D, Turc-Carel C, Triche TJ, Aurias A, Thomas G: The Ewing family of tumors: a subgroup of small-round-cell tumors defined by specific chimeric transcripts. N Engl J Med 331:294–299, 1994.

21. Ladanyi M, Gerald W: Fusion of the EWS and WT1 genes in the desmoplastic small round cell tumor. Cancer Res 54:2837–2840, 1994.

22. Zucman J, Delattre O, Desmaze C, Epstein A, Stenman G, Speleman F, Fletchers CDM, Aurias A, Thomas G: EWS and ATF-1 gene fusion induced by t(12;22) translocation in malignant melanoma of soft parts. Nat Genet 4:341–345, 1993.

23. Gill S, McManus AP, Crew AJ, Benjamin H, Sheer D, Busterson BA, Pinkerton CR, Patel K, Cooper CS, Shipley JM: Fusion of the EWS gene to a DNA segment from 9q22–31 in a human myxoid chondrosarcoma. Genes Chromosomes Cancer 12:307–310, 1995.

24. Clark J, Rocques PJ, Crew AJ, Gill S, Shipley J, Chan AM, Gusterson BA, Cooper CS: Identification of novel genes, SYT and SSX, involved in the t(X;18)(p11.2;q11.2) translocation found in human synovial sarcoma. Nat Genet 7:502–508, 1994.

25. Michon J, Delattre O, Zucker JM, Peter M, Delonlay P, Luciani S, Mosseri V, Vielh P, Neuenschwander S, Thomas G: Prospective evaluation of Nmyc amplification and deletion of the short arm of chromosome 1 in neuroblastoma tumors: A single institution study. Adv Neuroblastoma Res 4:11–17, 1994.

26. Stock C, Ambros IM, Mann G, Gadner H, Amann G, Ambros PF: Detection of 1p36 deletions in paraffin sections of neuroblastoma tissues. Genes Chromosomes Cancer 6: 1–9, 1993.

27. Weith A, Martinsson T, Cziepluch C, Bruderlein S, Amier LC, Berthold F, Schwab M: Neuroblastoma consensus deletion maps to 1p36.1–2. Genes Chromosomes Cancer 1:159–166, 1989.

28. Brodeur GM, Sekhon GS, Goldstein MN: Specific chromosomal aberration in human neuroblastoma. Am J Hum Genet 27:20A, 1975.

29. Brodeur GM, Sekhon GS, Goldstein MN: Chromosomal aberrations in human neuroblastomas. Cancer 40:2256–2263, 1977.

30. Brodeur GM, Fong CT: Molecular biology and genetics of human neuroblastoma. Cancer Genet Cytogenet 41:153–174, 1989.

31. Fong CT, Dracopoli MC, White PS, Merrill PT, Griffith RC, Housman DE, Brodeur GM: Loss of heterozygosity for chromosome 1p in human neuroblastomas: correlation with N-myc amplification. Proc Natl Acad Sci USA 86:3753–3757, 1989.

32. Van Roy N, Laureys G, Verscharaegen-Spae MR, Benoit Y, Chan A, Versteeg R. Speleman F: High resolution mapping of DNA markers on chromosome 1 and the neuroblastoma consensus deletion region using fluorescence *in situ* hybridization (FISH). Cancer Genet Cytogenet 63:168, 1992.

33. Savelyeva L, Corvi R. Schwab M, Translocation involving 1p and 17q is a recurrent genetic alteration of human neuroblastoma cells. Am J Hum Genet 55:334–340, 1994.

34. Caron H, van Sluis P, van Roy N, de Kraker J, Speleman F, Voute PA, Westerveld A, Slater R, Versteeg R: Recurrent 1;17 translocations in human neuroblastoma reveal nonhomologous mitotic recombination during the S/G2 phase as a novel mechanism for loss of heterozygosity. Am J Hum Genet 55:341–347, 1994.

35. Takeda O, Homma C, Maseki N, Sakurai M, Kanda N, Schwab M, Nakamura Y, Kaneko Y: There may be two tumor suppressor genes on chromosome arm 1p closely associated with biologically distinct subtypes of neuroblastoma. Genes Chromosomes Cancer 10:30–39, 1994.

36. Schleiermacher G, Peter M, Michon J, Hugot JP, Vielh P, Zucker JM, Magdelenat H, Thomas G, Delattre O: Two distinct deleted regions on the short arm of chromosome 1 in neuroblastoma. Genes Chromosomes Cancer 10:275–281, 1994.

37. Haber DA, Housman DE: The genetics of Wilms' tumor. Adv Cancer Res 59:41–68, 1991.

38. Slater RM, Mannens MMAM: Cytogenetics and molecular genetics of Wilms' tumor of childhood. Cancer Genet Cytogenet 61:111–121, 1992.

39. Brodeur GM, Seeger RC, Schwab M, Varmus HE, Bishop JM: Amplification of N-myc in untreated human neuroblastomas correlates with advanced disease stage. Science 224:1121–1124, 1984.

40. Seeger RC, Brodeur GM, Sather H, Dalton A, Siegel SE, Wong KY, Hammond D: Association of multiple copies of the N-myc oncogene with rapid progression of neuroblastoma. N Engl J Med 313:1111–1116, 1985.

41. Cohn SL, Look AT, Joshi W, Holbrook T, Salwen H, Chagnovich D, Chesler L, Rowe ST, Valentine MB, Komuro H, Castelberry RP, Bowman LC, Rao PV, Seeger RC, Brodeur GM: Lack of correlation of N-myc gene amplification with prognosis in localized neuroblastoma: a pediatric oncology group study. Cancer Res 55:721–726, 1995.

42. Lo R. Perlman E, Hawkins AL, Hayashi R, Wechsler DS, Look AT, Griffin CA: Cytogenetic abnormalities in two cases of neuroblastoma. Cancer Genet Cytogenet 74:30–34, 1994.

43. Bridge JA, Neff JR, Sandberg M: Cytogenetic analysis of dermatofibrosarcoma protuberans. Cancer Genet Cytogenet 49:199–202, 1990.

44. Stenman G, Andersson H, Meis-Kindblom JM, Roijer E, Kindblom L: FISH analysis of supernumerary ring chromosome in dermatofibrosarcoma protuberants. Int J Oncol 6:81–86, 1995.

45. Minoletti F, Miozo M, Pedeutour F, Sard L, Pilotti S, Azzarelli A, Turc-Carel C, Pierotti MA, Sozi G: Involvement of chromosomes 17 and 22 in

dermatofibrosarcoma protuberans. FISH study of three new cases. Genes Chromosomes Cancer 13:62–65, 1995.

46. Pedeutour F, Simon MP, Minoletti F, Sozzi G, Pierotti MA, Hecht F, Turc-Carel C: Ring chromosome 22 in dermatofibrosarcoma protuberans are low-level amplifiers of chromosome 17 and 22 sequences. Cancer Res 55:2400–2403, 1995.

47. Naeem R, Lux M, Huang S-F, Naber SP, Corson JM, Fletcher JA: Ring chromosomes in dermatofibrosarcoma protuberans are composed of interspersed sequences from chromosomes 17 and 22. Am J Pathol 147:1553–1558, 1995.

48. Craver RD, Correa H, Kao YS, Van Brunt T, Golladay ES: Aggressive giant cell fibroblastoma with a balanced 17;22 translocation. Cancer Genet Cytogenetic 80:20–22, 1995.

49. Pedeutour F, Lacour JP, Perrin C, Huffermann K, Simon MP, Ayraud N, Turc-Carel C: Another case of t(17;22)(q22;q13) in an infantile dermatofibrosarcoma protuberans. Cancer Genet Cytogenet 89:175–176, 1996.

50. Sinovic J, Bridge JA: Translocation (2;17) in recurrent dermatofibrosarcoma protuberans. Cancer Genet Cytogenet 75:156–157, 1994.

51. Örndal C, Mandahl N, Rydholm A, Willén H, Brosjö O, Heim S, Mitelman F: Supernumerary ring chromosomes; in five bone and soft tissue tumors of low or borderline malignancy. Cancer Genet Cytogenet 60:170–175, 1992.

52. Oliner JD, Kinzler KW, Meltzer PS, George DL, Vogelstein B: Amplification of a gene encoding a p53-associated protein in human sarcomas. Nature 358:80–83, 1992.

53. Sreekantaiah C, Leong SPL, Karakousis CP, McGee DL, Rappaport WD, Villar HV, Neal D, Fleming S, Wankel A, Herrington PN, Carmona R, Sandberg AA: Cytogenetic profile of 109 lipomas. Cancer Res 51:422–433, 1991.

54. Mandahl N, Höglund M, Mertens F, Rydholm A, Willén H, Brosjö O, Mitelman F: Cytogenetic aberrations in 188 benign and borderline adipose tissue tumors. Genes Chromosome Cancer 9:207–212, 1994.

55. Suijkerbuijk RF, Olde Weghuis DEM, Van Den Berg M, Pedeutour F, Forus A, Myklebost O, Glier C, Turc-Carel C, Geurts van Kessel A: Comparative genomic hybridization as a tool to define two distinct chromosome 12-derived amplification units in well-differentiated liposarcomas. Genes Chromosomes Cancer 9:292–295, 1994.

56. Forus A, Florenes VA, Moelandsmo GM, Fodstad O, Myklebost O: The protooncogene CHOP/GADD153 involved in growth arrest and DNA damage response is amplified in a subset of human sarcomas. Cancer Genet Cytogenet 78:165–171, 1994.

57. Aurias A, Rimbaut C, Buffe D, Dubousset J, Mazabraud A: Chromosomal translocations in Ewing's sarcoma. N Engl J Med 309:496–497, 1983.

58. Turc-Carel C, Philip I, Berger MP, Philip T, Lenoir GM: Translocation (11;22)(q24;q12) in Ewing sarcoma cell lines. N Engl J Med 309:497–498, 1983.

59. Whang Peng J, Triche TJ, Knutsen T, Miser J, Dopublass EC, Israel MA: Chromosome translocations in peripheral neuroepithelioma. N Engl J Med 311:584–585, 1984.

60. Stephenson CF, Bridge JA, Sandberg AA: Cytogenetic and pathologic aspects of Ewing's sarcoma and neuroectodermal tumors. Hum Pathol 23:1270–1277, 1992.

61. Sorenson PHB, Shimada H, Liu XF, Lim JF, Thomas G, Triche TJ: Biphenotypic sarcomas with myogenic and neural differentiation express the Ewing's sarcoma EWS/FLI1 fusion gene. Cancer Res 55:1385–1392, 1995.

62. Turc-Carel C, Aurias A, Mugneret F: Chromosomes in Ewing's sarcoma. I. An evaluation of 85 cases and remarkable consistency of t(11;22)(q24;q12). Cancer Genet Cytogenet 32:229–238, 1988.

63. Ben-David Y, Giddens EB, Letwin K, Bernstein A: Genes Dev 5: 908–918, 1991.

64. Nye JA, Petersen JM, Gunther CV, Jonsen MD, Graves BJ: Interaction of murine ETS-1 with GGA-binding sites establishes the ETS domain as a new DNA-binding motif. Genes Dev 67:975–990, 1992.

65. Crozat A, Aman P, Mandahl N, Ron D: Fusion of CHOP to a novel RNA-binding protein in human myxoid liposarcoma. Nat 363:640–644, 1993.

66. Rabbitts TH, Forster A, Larson R. Nathan P: Fusion of the dominant negative transcription regulator CHOP with a novel gene FUS by translocation t(12;16) in malignant liposarcoma. Nat Genet 4:175–180, 1993.

67. Lessnick SL, Braun BS, Denny CT, Mays WA: Multiple domains mediate transformation by the Ewing's sarcoma EWS/FLI-1 fusion gene. Oncogene 10:423–431, 1995.

68. Bailly RA, Bosselux R, Zucman J, Cormier F, Delattre O, Roussel M, Thomas G, Ghysdael J: DNA-binding and transciptional activation properties of the EWS-FLI-1 fusion protein resulting from the t(11;22) translocation in Ewing sarcoma. Mol Cell Biol 14:3230–3241, 1994.

69. Delattre O, Zucman J, Plougastel B, Desmaze C, Melot T, Peter M, Kovar H, Houbert I, de Jong P, Roulear G, Aurias A, Thomas G: Gene fusion with an ETS-binding domain caused by chromosome translocation in human tumours. Nature 359:162–165, 1992.

70. May WA, Gishizky ML, Lessnick SL, Lunsford LB, Lewis BC, Delattre O, Zucman J, Thomas G, Denny CT: Ewing sarcoma 11;22 translocation produces a chimaeric transcription factor that requires the DNA-binding domain encoded by FLI-1 for transformation. Proc Natl Acad Sci USA 90:5752–5756, 1993.

71. Zoubek A, Pfleiderer C, Salzer-Kuntschik M, Amann G, Windhager R, Fink FM, Koscielniak E, Delattre O, Strehl S, Ambros PF, Gadner H, Kovar H: Variability of EWS chimaeric transcripts in Ewing tumours: a comparison of clinical and molecular data. Br J Cancer 70:908–913, 1994.

72. Kretschmar CS: Ewing's sarcoma and the "peanut" tumors. N Engl J Med 331:325–327, 1994.

73. Pellin A, Boix J, Blesa JR, Noguera R, Carda C, Llombart-Bosch A: EWS/FLI-1 rearrangement in small round cell sarcomas of bone and soft

tissue detected by reverse transcriptase polymerase chain reaction amplification. Eur J Cancer 30:827–831, 1994.

74. Downing JR, Khandekar A, Shurtleff SA, Head DR, Parham DM, Webber BL, Pappo AS, Hulshof MG, Conn WP, Shapiro DN: Multiplex RT-PCR assay for the differential diagnosis of alveolar rhabdomyosarcoma and Ewing's sarcoma. Am J Pathol 146:626–634, 1995.

75. Desmaze C, Zucman J, Delattre O, Melot T, Thomas G, Aurias A: Interphase molecular cytogenetics of Ewing's sarcoma and peripheral neuroepithelioma t(11;22) with flanking and overlapping cosmid probes. Cancer Genet Cytogenet 74:13–18, 1994.

76. Chung EB, Enzinger FM: Malignant melanoma of soft parts. A reassessment of clear cell sarcoma. Am J Surg Pathol 7:405–413, 1983.

77. Amr S, Farah GR, Muhtaseb HH, Al-Hajj HA, Leven A: Clear cell sarcoma; Report of two cases with ultrastructural observation. Clin Oncol 10:59–65, 1984.

78. Kindblom LG, Lodding P, Angervall A: Clear cell sarcoma of tendons and aponeuroses. An immunohistochemical and electron microscopic analysis indicating neural crest origin. Virchows Arch Pathol Anat 409:109–128, 1983.

79. Bridge JA, Borek DA, Neff JR, Huntrakoon M: Chromosomal abnormalities in clear cell sarcoma. Implications for histogenesis. Am J Clin Pathol 93:26–31, 1990.

80. Travis JA, Bridge JA: Significance of both numerical and structural chromosomal abnormalities in clear cell sarcoma. Cancer Genet Cytogenet 64:104–106, 1992.

81. Sandberg AA. The Chromosomes in Human Cancer and Leukemia, 2nd ed. New York: Elsevier Science, 1990.

82. Mugneret F, Lizard S, Aurias A, Turc-Carel C: Chromosomes in Ewing's sarcoma. II. Nonrandom additional changes, trisomy 8 and der(16)t(1;16). Cancer Genet Cytogenet 32:239–245, 1988.

83. Sreekantaiah C, Karakousis CP, Leong SPL, Sandberg AA: Trisomy 8 as a nonrandom secondary change in myxoid liposarcoma. Cancer Genet Cytogenet 51:195–205, 1991.

84. Desmaze C, Zucman J, Delattre O, Melot T, Thomas G, Aurias A: Precise localization on chromosome 12 of the ATF-1 gene by fluorescence *in situ* hybridization. Hum Genet 93:207–208, 1994.

85. Gerald WL, Miller HK, Battifora H, Miettinen M, Silva EG, Rosai J: Intra-abdominal desmoplastic small round-cell tumor. Report of 19 cases of a distinctive type of high-grade polyphenotypic malignancy affecting young individuals. Am J Surg Pathol 15:499–513, 1991.

85a. Turc-Carel C, Lizard-Nacol S, Justrabo E, Favrot M, Philip T, Tabone E: Consistent chromosomal translocation in alveolar rhabdomyosarcoma. Cancer Genet Cytogenet 19:361–362, 1986.

86. Parham DM, Shapiro DN, Downing JR, Webber BL, Douglass EC: Solid alveolar rhabdomyosarcoma with the t(2;13): Report of two cases with diagnostic implications. Am J Surg Pathol 18:474–478, 1994.

87. Galili N, Davis RJ, Fredericks WJ, Mukhopadhyay S, Rauscher FJ, Emanuel BS, Rovera G, Barr FG: Fusion of a fork head domain gene to PAX3 in the solid tumour alveolar rhabdomyosarcoma. Nat Genet 5:230–235, 1993.

88. Fredericks WJ, Galili N, Mukhopadhyay S, Rovera G, Bennicelli J, Barr FG, Rauscher FJ: The PAX3-FKHR fusion protein created by the t(2;13) translocation in alveolar rhabdomyosarcomas is a more potent transcriptional activator than PAX3. Mol Cell Biol 15:1522–1535, 1995.

89. Davis RJ, D'Cruz DM, Lovell MA, Biegel JA, Barr FG: Fusion of PAX7 to FKHR by the variant t(1;13)(p36;q14) translocation in alveolar rhabdomyosarcoma. Cancer Res 54:2869–2872, 1994.

90. Biegel JA, Nyeum LM, Valentine V, Barr FG, Shapiro DN: Detection of the t(2;13)(q35;q14) and PAX3-FKHR fusion in alveolar rhabdomyosarcoma by fluorescence *in situ* hybridization. Genes Chromosome Cancer 12:186–192, 1995.

90a. Gemmill RM, Mendez MJ, Dougherty CM, Paulien S, Liao M, Mitchell D, Jankowski SA, Trent JM, Berger C, Sandberg AA, Meltzer PS: Isolation of a yeast artificial chromosome clone that spans the (12;16) translocation breakpoint characteristic of myxoid liposarcoma. Cancer Genet Cytogenet 62:166–179, 1992.

91. Eneroth M, Mandahl N, Heim S, Willén H, Rydholm A, Alberts KA, Mitelman F: Localization of the chromosomal breakpoints of the t(12;16) in liposarcoma to subbands 12q13.3 and 16p11.2. Cancer Genet Cytogenet 48:101–107, 1990.

92. Mrózek K, Karakousis CP, Bloomfield CD: Chromosome 12 breakpoints are cytogenetically different in benign and malignant lipogenic tumors: localization of breakpoints in lipoma to 12q15 and in myxoid liposarcoma to 12q13.3. Cancer Res 53:1670–1675, 1993.

93. Schoenmakers EFPM, Kools PFJ, Mols R, Kazmierczak B, Bartnitzke S, Bullerdiek J, Dal Cin P, De Jong PJ, Van den Berghe H, Van de Ven WJM: Physical mapping of chromosome 12q breakpoints in lipoma, pleomorphic salivary gland adenoma, uterine leiomyoma, myxoid liposarcoma. Genomics 20:210–222, 1994.

94. Ron D, Habener JF: CHOP, a novel developmentally regulated nuclear protein that dimerizes with transcription factors C/EBP and LAP and functions as a dominant negative inhibitor of gene transcription. Genes Dev 6:439–453, 1992.

95. Bridge JA, Bridge RS, Borek DA, Shaffer B, Norris CW: Translocation t(X;18) in orofacial synovial sarcoma. Cancer 62:935–937, 1988.

96. Roberts C, Seemayer TA, Bridge JA: Cancer Genet Cytogenet, in press.

97. Limon J, Dal Cin P, Sandberg AA: Translocations involving the X chromosome in solid tumors. Presentation of two sarcomas with t(X;18)(q13;p11). Cancer Genet Cytogenet 23:87–91, 1986.

98. Turc-Carel C, Dal Cin P, Limon J, Li F, Sandberg AA: Translocation X;18 in synovial sarcoma. Cancer Genet Cytogenet 23:93, 1986.

99. Shipley JM, Clark J, Crew AJ, Birdsall S, Rocques PJ, Bw S, Chelly J, Monaco AP, Abe S, Gusterson BA, Cooper CS: The t(X;18)(p11.2;q11.2) translocation found in human synovial sarcomas involves two distinct loci on the X chromosome. Oncogene 9:1447–1453, 1994.

100. de Leeuw B, Suijkerbuijk RF, Olde Weghuis DO, Meloni AM, Stenman G, Kindblom LG, Balernans M, van den Berg E, Molenaar WM, Sandberg AA, Geurts van Kessel A: Distinct Xp11.2 breakpoint regions in synovial sarcoma revealed by metaphase and interphase FISH: relationship to histologic subtypes. Cancer Genet Cytogenet 75:89–94, 1994.

101. Fligman I, Lonardo F, Jhanwar SC, Gerald WL, Woodruff J, Ladanyi M: Molecular diagnosis of synovial sarcoma and characterization of a variant SYT-SSXZ fusion transcript. Am J Pathol 147:1592–1599, 1995.

102. Clark J, Rocques PJ, Crew AJ, Gill S, Shipley J, Chan AMI, Gusterson BA, Cooper CS: Identification of novel genes, SYT and SSX, involved in the t(X;18)(p11.2;q11.2) translocation found in human synovial sarcoma. Nat Genet 7:502–508, 1994.

101. Kretschmar CS: Ewing's sarcoma and the "peanut" tumors. N Engl J Med 331:325–327, 1994.

Chapter 17

Special Techniques in Cytogenetics

Linda A. Cannizzaro

Introduction

Our perception of chromosomes has changed dramatically over the past few years. High resolution cytogenetic analyses, coupled with chromosomal *in situ* hybridization, have helped to unravel the mysteries of prokaryotic and eukaryotic chromosome structure. Molecular cytogenetic technology has proved to be a valuable resource to decipher the genetic composition of chromosomal regions involved in disease manifestation. *In situ* hybridization of DNA probes to chromosomes has resulted in mapping many genes and anonymous DNA sequences directly to definitive chromosomal regions. Information is also now available regarding the position and relationship of genes along the chromosome's length. The advent of computerized digital analysis systems has made it possible to map multiple genes or DNA sequences simultaneously.

Molecular cytogenetics has also become a powerful tool for identifying genes involved in cancer-associated chromosome alterations, and has defined how genes are repositioned as genetic material shifts during transformation of the cell. Such genetic shifts are a result of some molecular alterations that take place within the DNA itself, as the malignancy progresses to a more advanced stage.

From: *Human Cytogenetic Cancer Markers* Edited by S. R. Wolman and S. Sell
Humana Press Inc., Totowa, NJ

Despite tremendous advances in molecular cloning technology, however, some chromosomal regions, because of their specialized composition, have been difficult to study. For instance, chromosomal regions comprised primarily of multiple repeats, or complex sequences, such as CTG islands, have been difficult to separate from the rest of the genome for further study and characterization. As a result, very few DNA probes have been isolated from such regions, leaving them virtually unexplored. Unfortunately, many such regions contain genes that are altered in some form, in either a genetic or a malignant disease.

Chromosome microdissection provides a viable alternative and circumvents this problem. The technique involves dissecting DNA directly from any chromosomal region, irrespective of its structural composition. It is performed under a dissecting microscope equipped with an automated micromanipulator. Microdissection is proving to be an extremely versatile tool that can be used to dissect out even the smallest subband region, which in humans is estimated to contain 2–4 Mb of DNA. Microdissection can be performed on chromosomes from any organism, eukaryotic or prokaryotic, mammalian or nonmammalian.

Chromosome Microdissection: The Technique

Chromosome microdissection is now performed routinely in many cytogenetic laboratories. Chromosome preparations are generated using a modified fixation procedure to diminish depurination of the DNA. The preparations are banded using routine cytogenetic procedures, and the cell suspension is usually placed on coverslips. The dissections are carried out on a dissecting microscope equipped with an automated micromanipulator. The dissecting needles are easily prepared using a pipet puller and are pulled to a diameter of approx 2 μ. About 20 pieces of DNA are dissected out from one specific band or chromosome region. The DNA fragments are pooled in a tube that contains all the reagents required for polymerase chain reaction (PCR) amplification. This tube also contains a set of universal primers that facilitate amplification of chromosomal regions where the DNA sequence is not known. After amplification, the products are digested with a restriction endonuclease to generate a series of DNA microclones ranging in size from 200 bp to about 2.5 kb in length. These microclones are then analyzed on a Southern blot probed with total human genomic DNA to determine their unique or repetitive nature. Microclones that contain primarily non-repetitive sequences are selected out and propagated for sequencing and further molecular characterization analyses. Thousands of recombinant clones can be rapidly generated by this procedure.

Microdissection is becoming a standardized technique, but there is still opportunity for further exploration and development. The primary uses of chromosome microdissection at the present time include:

1. Rapid isolation of new DNA markers;
2. Isolation of DNA sequences to fill in gaps for long range physical genome mapping efforts, especially of disease-associated chromosomal regions; and
3. For use as template DNA to screen different types of DNA libraries, including cDNAs, YACs, bacteriophage P1 (alternative to yeast artificial chromosomes [YACs] with an average insert size of 95 Kb), and cosmids.

In addition to filling in gaps for physical mapping in humans, microdissection has been used to dissect chromosome regions from different organisms and species. Species-specific DNA libraries are being used for comparative mapping efforts and may be useful for mapping disease-associated loci in humans. This chapter focuses primarily on the use of microdissection in analysis of the human genome and to study chromosome regions consistently altered in malignant development and progression.

History of Chromosome Microdissection

Chromosome microdissection was initiated about 10 yr ago and was first used to dissect out either mouse or Drosophila chromosomes. The chromosome preparations were unstained and dissections were performed based on recognizable morphologic differences of particular chromosomes in the cell *(1–4)*. Such chromosome dissections were monitored under phase contrast microscopy, but the targeted DNA segments were either involved in chromosome translocations or were part of specialized structures, such as homogeneously staining regions (hsr) or double minutes (dmin), that could easily be distinguished from the other chromosomes in the metaphase. Because there were no demarcations that allowed precise identification of the selected region within the chromosome, numerous fragments needed to be dissected in order to ensure isolation of the targeted region. On the average, a minimum of 100 pieces were scraped, pooled, digested with a restriction endonuclease, then cloned into a lambda vector for further propagation and characterizations. The yield from these dissections ranged from several hundred to several thousand recombinant DNA clones with an average insert size of about 250 bp (the size of the inserts ranged from <100 bp to >400 bp) (2,5). The fixation of chromosome preparations in the standard 3:1 Carnoy's fixative caused a significant amount of depurination and is believed to have resulted in the selective recovery of only the smaller sized DNA fragments (5).

Further refinements in the procedure were made as the technique became established in an increasing number of laboratories. Depurination of DNA was minimized by modifying the fixation of the chromosome preparations by increasing the proportion of methanol to acetic acid from 3:1 to 9:1. It was also discovered that banding the chromosomes with trypsin-Giemsa (GTG) stain did not alter the viability of the DNA. This was a landmark observation that significantly improved the precision of the microdissection technique by increasing the frequency with which libraries were obtained from precisely defined chromosome regions.

Thus, these minor modifications in fixation and staining of the chromosome preparations greatly facilitated selection of an increased number of clones that originated from targeted regions in humans (6) and in Drosophila (7). The DNA isolated by microdissection of GTG-banded chromosome preparations was found to represent at least 95% of the targeted region, whereas dissections from unstained preparations (7) represented only 3–4% of the targeted region. Dissections performed from fewer metaphases could yield as much as 1 µg of DNA (7). As a result, only about 20 fragments needed to be microdissected. The fact that fewer metaphases are required to generate substantial numbers of the desired DNA markers makes the chromosome microdissection technology more cost effective and less time consuming. In addition, the use of nongene-specific DNA primers, such as Alu and other types of universal primers, has enabled generation of DNA probes from regions of the genome that have been unexplored and whose sequence composition was relatively unknown *(8,9)*. Thousands of region-specific probes could be isolated very rapidly by this strategy. This resulted in a marked increase in the number of chromosome-specific and chromosome band-specific libraries, which could be used for diagnosis of diseases localized within a specific targeted region. Based on the fact that a band-specific library can be generated from only 20–40 DNA fragments, it has been estimated that it would be possible to dissect the entire human genome within 1 yr, if two band-specific libraries were generated in parallel *(7,8,10)*.

Differential Diagnosis of Disease With Microdissected DNA

Multiple DNA markers can now be isolated easily from any chromosome region involved in a genetic or malignant disorder. In many cases, even when disease-associated chromosomal regions were known, few markers were available for diagnostic purposes that were able to detect mutations in patients affected by that specific disease. Within recent years, however, microdissection technology has generated numerous informative markers from multiple disease-associated regions. These regions include 1p36 for neuroblastoma *(11)*; 2q33-qter for Waardenburg syndrome, type II *(12)*; 3p14 for tumor suppressor loci *(13)*; 5q21 and 5q22 for adenomatosis polyposis coli (APC) *(14)*; 6q16–21 for malignant melanoma *(15,16)*; 7q22–32 for cystic fibrosis *(17)*; 8q23–q24.1 for Langer Giedion syndrome *(6,18)*; and 11p15.5 for Beckwith Wiedemann syndrome *(19)*; 11p13 for Wilm's tumor-aniridia *(20)*; 11q23 for ataxia telangiectasia (AT) *(21)*; 15q11–12 for Prader Willi/Angelman syndromes *(22)*; 22q12–13.1 for neurofibromatosis-2 *(23)*; and Xq27 for fragile X syndrome *(6,18,24)*.

It is clear that microdissected clones have become valuable diagnostic tools that are now used for a variety of clinical and research investigations. These include: refined definition of translocation breakpoints associated with a variety of malignant types and stages;

more precise definition of critical regions involved in deletions, amplifications, and other alterations in affected patients; improved identification of mutations in patients and in tumor tissues; and more precise definition of regions that show loss of heterozygosity (LOH).

Isolating New Markers for Inherited
Disorders by Chromosome Microdissection

Laboratories involved in physical mapping of specific chromosome regions, either to generate long-range physical maps or to identify a disease gene, have used microdissection to great advantage. For example, about 1500 clones have been isolated from the aniridia-Wilms' tumor locus in 11p13 by microdissection (20) in an attempt to complete a physical map of 7.5 Mb through this region. Several of these microdissected clones mapped within the aniridia region, some clones mapped within the Wilms' tumor region, and two clones were localized within both the aniridia and Wilms' tumor regions. These clones will be useful for screening a cDNA library to isolate a potential gene expressed by sequences from within this region, and are presently capable of detecting mutations within affected patients.

A similar strategy was used to isolate additional markers from the 15q11 region which is deleted in Prader Willi syndrome (PWS) (22). Approximately 5000 clones have been isolated by microdissection. About 39% of the microclones were comprised of unique sequences. Clones consisting primarily of unique sequences can then be used to screen cDNAs in order to isolate a candidate gene for this syndrome. Several of these clones are able to detect deletions in patients affected with PWS and, thus, may have diagnostic utility.

An important strategy was developed that permitted direct amplification of a target sequence dissected from one single G-banded chromosomal segment (25). In this study (25), primers were first constructed from a rat sodium channel gene. PCR was then performed using human genomic DNA as a template. A fragment that mapped to the human chromosomal region, 2q22–q23, was obtained. This fragment contained significant sequence homology to types I, II, and III of the rat brain alpha subunit sodium channel gene. This ability to generate a gene sequence from one single fragment exemplifies the possibilities for rapid isolation of genes from regions involved in human disease.

Dissected DNAs have also been amplified by primer-linker-adapter methods *(8)*. LOH analysis of select microclones from chromosome region 8q was performed on patients with tricho-rhino-phalangeal syndrome (TRPS) types I and II. These clones were able to detect deletions in patients affected by this disorder.

Additional markers have been isolated by microdissection for the region associated with Beckwith Wiedemann syndrome (BWS) in 11p15, a region that is often amplified in affected patients *(19)*. Patients with this syndrome have 75% increased risk over the general population of developing childhood tumors such as Wilms, rhabdomyosarcoma, or hepatoblastoma. These newly developed markers could be used to determine the parental origin of the amplified 11p15 region, facilitate construction of the physical map of the BWS critical region, and lead to the development of sequence tagged site *(STS)* markers for BWS.

Microdissection is also being used to generate markers from homologous chromosome regions in animal models, used to study human diseases such as diabetes. Microclones have been isolated from the mouse chromosome region, designated as the diabetes (db) locus. This was achieved by using a mouse cell line with a 4;15 translocation *(26)*. The db locus is located within the mid chromosome 4 region. After microdissection, 47 additional restriction fragment length polymorphisms (RFLPs) were isolated from the db microclone library. Select microclones from the middle of mouse chromosome 4 were also used to type the progeny of three different backcrosses, to position 7 known genes, 41 microclones, and three anonymous markers to a 21 cM region of mid mouse chromosome 4. This, ultimately, will facilitate cloning the mouse db gene.

Additional markers have also been generated from mouse chromosome 1, a region that corresponds to human chromosome region 2q *(27)*. This region is designated as the Bcg locus and confers resistance to intracellular parasites. This strategy could help in discovering markers for diagnosing related human infectious disorders.

Isolating New Markers for Malignant Disorders by Chromosome Microdissection

A number of chromosomal regions are involved in alterations manifested in association with different specific malignancies and with specific stages of malignant progression. The region 3p14 is one such chromosomal region. Microdissection libraries have been generated from this region *(13)*, and are being used to screen YACs to identify potential tumor suppressor loci. Four DNA microclones were isolated from 3p14 that have been used to detect two new breakpoints that were previously indistinguishable in renal cell carcinoma patients carrying a 3;8 translocation *(13)*. One other microclone has been isolated that maps to the homozygously deleted region of 3p14 in small cell lung carcinoma cell line U2020. In addition, microclones used to screen YAC libraries each generated 1–7 YACs for the 3p14 region, ranging between 250 and 600 kb in size. Interestingly, a low frequency of single copy microclones was obtained from this locus, which is involved in many different chromosome alterations in hematopoietic and solid tumor malignancies. The nature of these clones may provide some clues regarding the sequence composition of the 3p14 region, and lead to an understanding of why this genome region is so susceptible to mutational events.

The span of 11q13.4–q25 is another chromosomal region frequently altered in malignant disorders. At least 50 STSs have been identified from a microdissection library generated from this region *(28)*. An additional 59 single copy clones have now been sequenced from 11q14–q23 and 11q23–q25. These clones were mapped by PCR using somatic cell hybrid panels containing various deletions of 11q *(28)*. Such clones will ultimately be used to construct long-range physical maps of the region and will help to define the critical chromosome alterations in the 11q region.

Microdissection and LOH Analysis

Clones obtained from microdissection of chromosome regions consistently altered in specific malignancies have been used successfully to identify deletions in affected patients. Two microdissection libraries have been constructed from the chromosome regions associated with APC, 5q21.2–21.3 and 5q22 *(14)*. After deletion mapping with 17 single copy microclones on a somatic cell hybrid panel, 7 of these clones were localized to the critical interstitial deletion of 6–8 Mb in APC affected individuals.

LOH analysis has been successful using microdissected markers obtained from patients with constitutional disorders as well. For example, the critical region for neurofibromatosis-type 2 *(NF2)* lies within 22q12–13.1. Four clones isolated from a microdissection library were mapped to the NF2 region and all of these microclones detected polymorphisms. Forty-one patients with acoustic neurinoma were evaluated for LOH with each of these polymorphic markers *(23)*. The majority of acoustic neurinomas occur as solitary unilateral tumors. However, about 4% of patients develop bilateral tumors that are the hallmark of NF2. LOH was detected in 55% of the 41 patients evaluated with the four polymorphic markers.

Deletions have been detected in patients with severe growth and mental retardation in association with multiple anomalies. A microdissection library constructed from region 2p23–p25 yielded several microclones that were used to detect deletions in these patients *(29)*.

Using Microclones to Define Translocation Breakpoint Regions

Precise definition of translocation breakpoint regions can oftentimes be difficult or impossible in patients with malignant disorders. High resolution chromosome preparations are problematic because of the limited amounts of patient material available for study. Many samples obtained from patients undergoing radiation and chemotherapy are difficult to analyze, because of the treatments' negative effect on chromosome morphology. Presently, molecular cytogenetic analysis of cancer-associated chromosome alterations is limited by the availability of region-specific DNA probes. Microdissection has become a new resource to identify critical areas of a chromosome altered in a malignancy. Once the critically altered region is defined, the next step, the identification of a potential tumor suppressor and/or candidate gene locus, is more likely.

Microclones have helped to define the precise breakpoint region in several consistent chromosome translocations associated with malignancy. A strategy that permits direct PCR of dissected chromosome fragments, without the need to extract DNA, has been successful in differentiating molecular breakpoint regions. The technique requires only 1–4 dissected pieces *(30)* from the region under investigation. This strategy, applied to patients with AML, can be used to discriminate translocation breakpoints within the 11q23 region that appear similar cytogenetically. Two patients were diagnosed with

AML-M4, one of whom had t(6;11)(p22;q23), and the other patient t(4;11)(q21;q23); a third patient, with AML-M1, carried a t(9;11)(p22;q23). Using PCR-amplified DNA from the breakpoint region dissected out of only a few metaphases, it was determined that the t(6;11) break was proximal to the t(9;11) and the t(4;11) breaks in 11q23. There are significant advantages to using this technology in conjunction with routine cytogenetic analysis of such patient samples. First, fewer numbers of metaphases are needed for analysis; and, second, it is not necessary to establish cell lines from each patient sample. Chromosome microdissection can extract a significant amount of information from limited quantities of a patient sample. On the other hand, performing microdissection routinely on patient samples is time consuming and is not an appropriate way to handle those patient samples that require rapid turnaround time.

Specialized Uses of Microdissection that can be Applied to Diagnosis

One problem that is often encountered during routine cytogenetic workup of patient samples is the appearance of unusual looking marker chromosomes. Usually these markers are small, and because the amount of chromosome material is limited, it is often impossible to decipher the chromosomal origin of the marker with a series of chromosome-specific DNA probes. In addition, in cases where the sample is from a patient diagnosed with an advanced leukemia, lymphoma, or solid tumor, the complexity of the chromosome abnormalities increases significantly. In such cases, a structurally abnormal chromosome may be derived from pieces of three or more different chromosomes. Microdissection makes it possible to dissect out such chromosome recombinations. The fragments must first be amplified with a universal primer, then labeled with a fluorochrome during the PCR reaction. The probe, which contains DNA from the marker chromosome, is hybridized back to normal chromosome preparations to identify the origin of the unidentifiable segments *(31,15,16)*. The probes derived from amplification of microdissected DNA have been designated as "micro-FISH" probes and can be generated within 24 h *(16)*. This is a valuable tool that enhances routine cytogenetic diagnosis of unusual or highly complicated cases. Some examples of successful applications of this approach are: differentiating the X and Y specific segments of an X;Y translocation chromosome; identifying the origin of a minute marker chromosome in a mentally retarded patient *(31)*; identifying the origins of unusual markers in different types of malignancies *(15,16)*.

Microdissection can also determine the origin of sequences contained in specialized structures, such as dmins or hsrs. Dmin chromosomes are minute sized structures visible in many malignant cell types, and are manifested primarily in advanced stages of tumor progression. The origin of these structures is still unresolved, but they are believed to arise as a result of breakage and deletion of specific sequences along a chromosome *(32)*. It is not clear whether dmins arise from one or multiple sites, or whether they are reintegrated preferentially into any one specific chromosomal site. In an effort to answer some of these questions, a genomic library was constructed from approx 20 dmin dissected from HL60 leukemic cells. After PCR amplification, and FISH hybridizations to normal chromosomes, it was determined that these structures originated from a discrete area of chromosome 8, distal to the c-*myc* locus, or the 8q24.3 region. These studies found that dmin DNA in HL60 cells becomes reintegrated into five different chromosome sites; the pericentromeric regions of chromosomes 1 and 16, 8q24, 18p11, and 18q22–23. In addition, the microdissected DNA, when used as a probe in northern blots, detected multiple expressed transcripts that were distinct from those expressed by c-*myc* *(32)*.

Chromosome microdissection has also been used to determine the genetic origin of dmins in multidrug resistant hamster cells. In one case, PCR amplification was performed using primers specific for the hamster multidrug resistance (MDR) gene *(33)*. After the dmin DNA was hybridized to the hamster cells, signal was found over an abnormally banded region (ABR) in the MDR cell line, providing evidence that dmins and ABRs are related structures. Microdissection, in conjunction with gene-specific amplification and FISH analyses, can provide valuable information about the origin of the amplified sequences detected in different tumor types at specific stages of malignant progression.

The DNA that comprise dmins or hsrs appears to represent amplified domains of tumor-associated genes, usually oncogenes. Several studies using microdissected DNA obtained from either hsrs or dmins, again followed by FISH to chromosomes, have elucidated specific chromosomal sites that, in some cases, contain known oncogenes, and, in others, do not. Microdissection of 16 putative hsrs from 9 different breast cancer cell lines was performed to determine the chromosomal origin of these structures *(34,35)*. Since hsrs are large ambiguously staining segments, only one to five copies of the target region were needed for PCR amplification. After hybridization of the hsr DNA library to normal chromosomes, several chromosome regions were consistently identified as sites of gene amplification. Interestingly, the *ERBB2* oncogene was the most commonly amplified chromosome region in the breast cancer cell lines. Also, regions 13q31 and 20q12–q13.2 were frequently amplified in these cases. In 81% of the breast cancer lines studied, the hsrs consisted of sequences from two or more chromosome regions. Comparative genomic hybridization analysis (CGH) of both primary breast tumors and cell lines detected more frequent amplification distal to ERBB2, within the 17q22–q24 region *(36)*. Such differences may be attributed to technical variations, and demonstrate the need to perform complementary analyses, especially at more advanced stages of malignant progression. The ability to microdissect unusual marker chromosomes such as hsrs may shed light on how such anomalies are formed. These studies also identified additional chromosome sites of potential tumor suppressor loci or amplification, which had not yet been revealed by other means.

A similar study of dmins and hsrs was undertaken in seven ovarian carcinomas. Amplification of several specific chromosome sites, 11q13.2–14, 12p11.2–13, 16p11–p13.2, 19p, and 19q13.1–q13.2, was found. These sites may contain genes that are involved in the development or progression of ovarian carcinoma *(37)*. The two most common sites of DNA amplification included 19q13.1–q13.2 and 12p12.1, which harbor the *AKT2* and *KRAS* genes, respectively. Each of these oncogenes is amplified in ovarian cancer *(37)*. In contrast to breast cancer, where the hsrs are derived from two or more different chromosomes, hsrs manifested in ovarian cancer originate from only one or two chromosomes. This difference in sequence complexity suggests that hsrs evolve differently in ovarian and breast cancers or, perhaps, these structures formed at a different stage of progression of the malignancy.

Another recently developed strategy that complements chromosome microdissection is CGH. The chromosome location of an amplified domain in tumor DNA is first determined by CGH. Afterwards, a probe is generated from the amplified domain by microdissection *(38)*. The probes are hybridized back to normal chromosomes to confirm the location of the isolated clones. Subsequently, the amplified-domain-specific probe may be used as a marker to determine the aggressiveness of the tumor, and provide information about patient prognosis.

Isolating Pure Populations of Specific Cell Types by Chromosome Microdissection

In addition to its value in generating new markers for a variety of uses, microdissection continues to evolve in other areas. In some malignant disorders, such as Hodgkin's disease (HD), the transformed cells, Reed Sternberg cells, are only a small fraction of the diseased tissue. These cells and their variants make up only 1–5% of the cells present in the diseased lymph node. The majority of background cells are nonneoplastic lymphocytes, plasma cells, eosinophils, macrophages, and fibroblasts, in various combinations. Relatively little information is available regarding the cytogenetic and molecular alterations manifested in this tumor. Alterations are difficult to detect by Southern analysis because of the limited number of transformed cells available. Our laboratory is using microdissection to isolate pure populations of the Reed Sternberg cells in order to obtain additional molecular information regarding gene rearrangements specific to the transformed phenotype. Similar analyses are now being performed on pure populations of tumor cells in other laboratories *(39)*. Molecular analyses, such as LOH or mutation detection, can then be evaluated in the tumor cell population, without background contamination from other surrounding cell types.

Future of Chromosome Microdissection

Chromosome microdissection is a relatively new and powerful tool that can be used effectively to complement cytogenetic, molecular cytogenetic, and molecular genetic studies of hematopoietic and solid tumor malignancies. The advantages of using microdissection technology include:

1. The generation of new DNA markers from any region of the mammalian genome irrespective of its DNA composition;
2. The isolation of DNA libraries from specialized structures such as dmins or hsrs;
3. Facilitation of identification of chromosomal markers of unknown origin in patient samples or cell lines; and
4. Filling in gaps in long-range physical maps, including those constructed from chromosome regions altered in genetic disease and malignancy.

One of the drawbacks of chromosome microdissection is the amount of time required to sort through the enormous number of microclones that can be generated from the chromosome region of interest. The small size and great number of these clones requires intense effort to screen for those recombinants that primarily contain unique sequences. However, this problem can be circumvented with the use of rare-cutting restriction endonucleases. It is now possible to generate much larger fragments from the microdissected DNA pool, and then amplify these larger fragments (up to 35kb) by a modified PCR amplification technique *(40)*. This modified technique will ultimately improve the cumbersome microclone screening process. At this time, chromosome microdissection continues to be relatively unexplored territory.

Acknowledgments

The author wrote this chapter while funded by grant VM89 from the American Cancer Society.

References

1. Rohme D, Fox H, Herrmann B, Frischauf AM, Edstrom JE, Mains P, Silver LM, Lehrach H: Molecular clones of the mouse t complex derived from microdissected metaphase chromosomes. Cell 36:783–788, 1984.
2. Fisher EMC, Cavana JS, Brown SDM: Microdissection and microcloning of the mouse X chromosome. Proc Natl Acad Sci USA 82:5846–5849, 1985.
3. Wesley CS, Ben M, Kreitman M, Hagag N, Eanes WF: Cloning regions of the Drosophila genome by microdissection of polytene chromosome DNA and PCR with nonspecific primer. Nucleic Acids Res 18:599–603, 1989.

4. Weith A, Winking H, Brackmann B, Boldyreff B, Trout W: Microclones from a mouse germ line HSR detect amplification and complex rearrangements of DNA sequences. EMBO J 6:1295–1300, 1987.

5. Edstrom J, Kaiser R, Rohme D: Microcloning of mammalian metaphase chromosomes. Methods Enzymol 151:503–516, 1987.

6. Ludecke H-H, Senger G, Claussen U, Horsthemke B: Cloning defined regions of the human genome by microdissection of banded chromosomes and enzymatic amplification. Nature 338:348–350, 1989.

7. Saunders RDC, Glover DM, Ashburner M, Siden-Kiamos I, Louis C, Monastiriati M, Savakis C, Kafatos F: PCR amplification of DNA microdissected from a single polytene chromosome band: a comparison with conventional microcloning. Nucleic Acids Res 17:9027–9037, 1989.

8. Johnson DH: Molecular cloning of DNA from specific chromosomal regions by microdissection and sequence-independent amplification of DNA. Genomics 6:243–251, 1990.

9. Kao F-T, Yu J-W: Chromosome microdissection and cloning in human genome and genetic disease analysis. Proc Natl Acad Sci USA 88:1844–1848, 1991.

10. Senger G, Ludecke H-J, Horsthemke B, Claussen U: Microdissection of banded human chromosomes. Hum Genet 84:507–511, 1990.

11. Martinsson T, Weith A, Cziepluch C, Schwab M: Chromosome 1 deletions in human neuroblastomas: generation and fine mapping of microclones from the distal 1p region. Genes Chromosomes Cancer 1:67–78, 1989.

12. Hirota T, Tsukamoto K, Deng H-X, Yoshiura K-i, Ohta T, Tohma T, Kibe T, Harada N, Jinno Y, Niikawa N: Microdissection of human chromosomal regions 8q23.3–q24.11 and 2q33-qter: construction of DNA libraries and isolation of their clones. Genomics 13:349–354, 1992.

13. Bordenheuer W, Szymanski S, Lux A, Ludecke HJ, Horsthemke B, Claussen U, Senger G, Smith DI, Wang N-D, LePaslier D, Cohen D, Heppell-Parton A, Rabbitts P, Schutte J, Opalka B: Characterization of a microdissection library from human chromosome region 3p14. Genomics 19:291–297, 1994.

14. Hampton G, Leuteritz G, Ludecke H-J, Senger G, Trautman U, Thomas H, Solomon E, Bodmer WF, Horsthemke B, Claussen U, Ballhausen WG: Characterization and mapping of microdissected genomic clones from the adenomatous polyposis coli (APC) region. Genomics 11:247–251, 1991.

15. Guan X-Y, Meltzer PS, Cao J, Trent JM: Rapid generation of region-specific genomic clones by chromosome microdissection. Isolation of DNA from a region frequently deleted in malignant melanoma. Genomics 14:680–684, 1992.

16. Meltzer PS, Guan X-Y, Burgess A, Trent JM: Rapid generation of region specific probes by chromosome microdissection and their application. Nature Genet 1:24–28, 1992.

17. Weber J, Weith A, Kaiser R, Grzeschik K-H, Olek K: Microdissection and microcloning of human chromosome 7q22–32 region. Somatic Cell Mol Genet 16:123–128, 1990.

18. Ludecke H-J, Senger G, Claussen U, Horsthemke B: Construction and characterization of band-specific DNA libraries. Hum Genet 84:512–516, 1990.
19. Puech A, Ahnine L, Ludecke HJ, Senger G, Ivens A, Jeanpierre C, Little P, Horsthemke B, Claussen U, Jones C, Junien C, Henry I: 11p15.5-specific libraries for identification of potential gene sequences involved in Beckwith-Wiedemann syndrome and tumorigenesis. Genomics 13:1274–1280, 1992.
20. Davis LM, Senger G, Ludecke H-J, Claussen U, Horsthemke B, Zhang SS, Metzroth B, Hohenfellner K, Zabel B, Shows TB: Somatic cell hybrid and long-range physical mapping of 11p13 microdissected genomic clones. Proc Natl Acad Sci USA 87:7005–7009, 1990.
21. Seki N, Yamauchi M, Saito T, Katakura R, Ohta T, Yoshiura K-I, Jinno Y, Niikawa N, Hori T-A: Microdissection and microcloning of genomic DNA markers from human chromosomal region 11q23. Genomics 16:169–172, 1993.
22. Buiting K, Neumann M, Ludecke H-J, Senger G, Claussen U, Antich J, Passarge E, Horsthemke B: Microdissection of the Prader-Willi syndrome chromosome region and identification of potential gene sequences. Genomics 6:521–527, 1990.
23. Fiedler W, Claussen U, Ludecke H-J, Senger G, Horsthemke B, Van Kessel AG, Goertzen W, Fahsold R: New markers for the neurofibromatosis-2 region generated by microdissection of chromosome 22. Genomics 10:786–791, 1991.
24. Djabali M, Nguyen C, Buinno I, Oostra BA, Mattei MG, Ikeda JE, Jordon BR: Laser microdissection of the fragile X region: Identification of cosmid clones and of conserved sequences in this region. Genomics 10:1053–1060, 1991.
25. Han J, Lu C-M, Brown GB, Rado TA: Direct amplification of a single dissected chromosomal segment by polymerase chain reaction: a human brain sodium channel gene is on chromosome 2q22–q23. Proc Natl Acad Sci USA 88:335–339, 1991.
26. Bahara N, McGraw DE, Khilling R, Friedman JM: Microdissection and microcloning of mid-chromosome 4: genetic mapping of 41 microdissection clones. Genomics 16:113–122, 1993.
27. Vidal SM, Epstein DJ, Malo D, Weith A, Vekemans M, Gros P: Identification and mapping of six microdissected genomic DNA probes to the proximal region of mouse chromosome 1. Genomics 14:32–37, 1992.
28. Saejima H, Yoshiura K, Tamura T, Tokino T, Nakamura Y, Niikawa N, Jinno Y: Fifty novel sequence-tagged sites (STSs) on human chromosome 11q13.4–q25 identified from microclones generated by microdissection. Cytogenet Cell Genet 70:108–111, 1995.
29. Yu J, Qi J, Tong S, Kao F-T: A region-specific microdissection library for human chromosome 2p23–p25 and the analysis of an interstitial deletion of 2p23.3–p25.1. Hum Genet 93:557–562, 1994.
30. Cotter FE, Lillington D, Hampton G, Riddle P, Nasipuri S, Gibbons B, Young BD: Gene mapping by microdissection and enzymatic amplification: Heterogeneity in leukemia associated breakpoints on chromosome 11. Genes Chromosomes Cancer 3:8–15, 1991.
31. Deng H-X, Yoshiura K-i, Dirks RW, Harada N, Hirota T, Tsukomoto K, Jinno Y, Niikawa N: Chromosome band-specific painting: chromosome in

situ suppressor hybridization using PCR products from a microdissected chromosome band as a probe pool. Hum Genet 89:13–17, 1992.

32. Sen S, Sen P, Mulac-Jericevic B, Zhou H, Pirrotta V, Stass SA: Microdissected double minute DNA detects variable patterns of chromosomal localization and multiple abundantly expressed transcripts in normal and leukemic cells. Genomics 19:542–551, 1994.

33. Sognier MA, McCombs J, Brown DB, Lynch G, Tucker M, Eberle R, Belli JA: Use of chromosome microdissection, the polymerase chain reaction and dot blot hybridization to analyze double minute chromosomes. GATA 11:69–76, 1994.

34. Guan X-Y, Meltzer PS, Trent JM: Rapid generation of whole chromosome painting probes (WCPs) by chromosome microdissection. Genomics 22:101–107, 1994.

35. Guan X-Y, Meltzer PS, Dalton WS, Trent JM: Identification of cryptic sites of DNA sequence amplification in human breast cancer by chromosome microdissection. Nature Genet 8:155–161, 1994.

36. Kallioniemi A, Kallioniemi O-P, Piper J, Tanner M, Stokke T, Chen L, Smith HS, Pinkel D, Gray JW, Waldman FM: Detection and mapping of amplified DNA sequences in breast cancer by comparative genomic hybridization. Proc Natl Acad Sci USA 91:2156–2160, 1994.

37. Guan X-Y, Cargile CB, Anzick SL, Thompson FH, Meltzer PS, Bittner ML, Taetle R, McGill JR, Trent JM: Chromosome microdissection identifies cryptic sites of DNA sequence amplification in human ovarian carcinoma. Cancer Res 55:3380–3385, 1995.

38. Liang BC, Meltzer PS, Guan X-Y, Trent JM: Gene amplification elucidated by combined chromosomal microdissection and comparative genomic hybridization. Cancer Genet Cytogenet 80:55–59, 1995.

39. Hedrum A, Ponten F, Ren Z, Lundeberg J, Ponten J, Uhlen M: Sequence-based analysis of the human p53 gene based on microdissection of tumor biopsy samples. BioTechniques 17:118–129, 1994.

40. Barnes WM: PCR amplification of up to 35-kb DNA with high fidelity and high yield from λ bacteriophage templates. Proc Natl Acad Sci USA 91:2216–2220, 1994.

Index